Language Disorders Across the Lifespan

Language Disorders Across the Lifespan

Second Edition

Betsy Partin Vinson

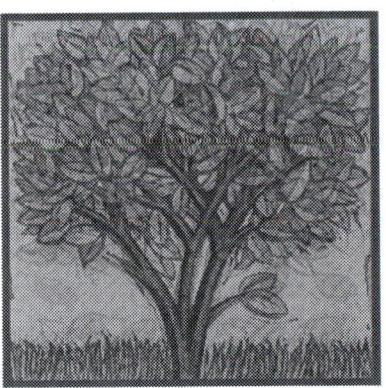

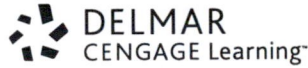

DELMAR
CENGAGE Learning™

Australia • Brazil • Japan • Korea • Mexico • Singapore • Spain • United Kingdom • United States

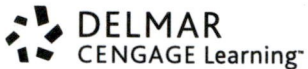
DELMAR
CENGAGE Learning

Language Disorders Across the Lifepan, Second Edition
Betsy Partin Vinson

Vice President, Health Care Business Unit: William Brottmiller

Director of Learning Solutions: Matthew Kane

Product Manager: Molly Belmont

Editorial Assistant: Angela Doolin

Marketing Director: Jennifer McAvey

Marketing Coordinator: Chris Manion

Content Project Manager: Jessica McNavich

For product information and technology assistance, contact us at
Cengage Learning Customer & Sales Support, 1-800-354-9706

For permission to use material from this text or product, submit all requests online **www.cengage.com/permissions**
Further permissions questions can be emailed to
permissionrequest@cengage.com

Library of Congress Control Number: 2006018327

ISBN-13: 978-1-4180-0954-0

ISBN-10: 1-4180-0954-7

Delmar
Executive Woods
5 Maxwell Drive
Clifton Park, NY 12065
USA

Cengage Learning is a leading provider of customized learning solutions with office locations around the globe, including Singapore, the United Kingdom, Australia, Mexico, Brazil, and Japan. Locate your local office at **www.cengage.com/global**

Cengage Learning products are represented in Canada by Nelson Education, Ltd.

To learn more about Delmar, visit **www.cengage.com/delmar**

Purchase any of our products at your local college store or at our preferred online store **www.ichapters.com**

Notice to the Reader
Publisher does not warrant or guarantee any of the products described herein or perform any independent analysis in connection with any of the product information contained herein. Publisher does not assume, and expressly disclaims, any obligation to obtain and include information other than that provided to it by the manufacturer. The reader is expressly warned to consider and adopt all safety precautions that might be indicated by the activities described herein and to avoid all potential hazards. By following the instructions contained herein, the reader willingly assumes all risks in connection with such instructions. The publisher makes no representations or warranties of any kind, including but not limited to, the warranties of fitness for particular purpose or merchantability, nor are any such representations implied with respect to the material set forth herein, and the publisher takes no responsibility with respect to such material. The publisher shall not be liable for any special, consequential, or exemplary damages resulting, in whole or part, from the readers' use of, or reliance upon, this material.

Printed in the United States of America
3 4 5 6 7   14 13 12 11 10

ED204

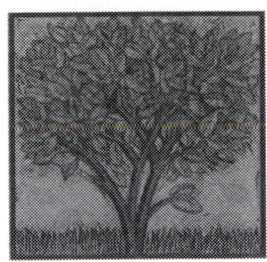

Contents

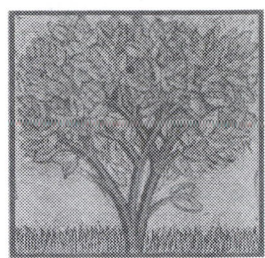

Preface

Language Disorders Across the Lifespan, 2nd edition, is an introductory undergraduate textbook designed to create a basic understanding of language disorders in children and adults. It is hoped that this understanding will serve as the foundation of a continuing curiosity about communication disorders. A wide variety of pediatric and adult communication differences, delays, and disorders from the perspectives of causes and defining characteristics are presented in a format that will facilitate the student's understanding of these aspects of communication disorders. Differences related to multicultural aspects of language and communication are incorporated into the text, as well as delays and disorders related to developmental language deficits, language-learning disabilities, reading disorders, attention deficit disorders, aphasia, dementias, and traumatic brain injury. I envisioned this book when I began teaching Introduction to Language Disorders at the University of Florida and found that there was not a book that addressed language deficits across the entire lifespan. Typically, students would have to buy two or three books to cover the lifespan; this was expensive, so I taught the course without a textbook for several years by relying on teaching packets I developed.

The primary objective of this book is to provide the undergraduate student with an overview of pediatric and adult language differences and disorders. Basic knowledge of language development and neuroanatomy is assumed, as topics related to these areas of communication sciences are addressed throughout the book. High school students who are considering entering the profession of speech-language pathology may also find that this book provides an overview of the types of language deficits with which our profession works. A second objective is to provide the student with knowledge associated with professional requirements of persons assessing and treating language-based communication disorders. Finally, it is hoped that studying this book will create in the student the desire to explore and integrate continuing study of language disorders from three perspectives: the researcher's, the clinician's, and the academician's.

Organization of the Text

Chapters 1 through 4 address language disorders in preschool children. Chapter 1 provides a review of language-learning theories, including the widely accepted work of Bloom and Lahey in defining language disorders based on form, content, and use. Chapter 2 provides a discussion of speech and language disorders associated with different syndromes. I have expanded the information on the syndromes discussed in the first edition and added several more of the most commonly seen syndromes that have language delays and disorders as part of their characteristics. Chapter 3 focuses on general assessment information as well as specific assessment and diagnostic considerations in preschool children. Chapter 4 provides information on different behavioral techniques employed in therapy at all age levels, as well as some specific suggestions for working with preschoolers. New to this edition is Chapter 5 that addresses the persistence and impact of preschool language delays and disorders on school and work performances across the lifespan.

Chapters 6 through 11 are dedicated to the school-aged child and adolescent. Because so many school districts rely on labeling disorders to determine a child's eligibility for services, these chapters are based on an etiological perspective. Chapter 6 provides definitions of language-based learning disabilities and addresses curricular issues that may be impacted by the presence of a language-based learning disability. Chapter 7 encompasses the effects of language deficits on reading and spelling. This is a "hot topic" in our profession and warranted more attention than it received in the first edition. Chapter 8 looks at the impact of attention deficit disorder with and without hyperactivity on language skills and academic performance. Although ADD/H is not a language disorder, the impact it can have on language and learning is an area of increasing study in our field. Therefore, I decided to include a separate chapter addressing this issue. Chapter 9 addresses traumatic brain injury, an area that affects all ages. I included this chapter in the school-aged section of the book because the highest incidence of brain injury is in the adolescent population. That said, the information in this chapter can be equally applied to adults who sustain a traumatic brain injury. Chapters 10 and 11 address assessment and treatment considerations in the school-aged population.

Chapters 12 and 13 address the most common language deficits in adults: dementias and aphasias. In Chapter 12, various types of dementia are discussed, as well as assessment and treatment considerations. Chapter 13 looks at the different aphasia syndromes, again including assessment and treatment factors in this population of adults with language disorders.

Features of the Book

The *marginal notes* used in the first edition have been retained based on feedback from students that they were helpful in the learning process. More *case studies* have been added to the text. *Learning objectives* are presented at the beginning of each chapter, and *study questions* are at the end of each chapter. More *illustrations* and *tables* have been added to further clarify information in the text. I have expanded the discussion of syndromes and, as mentioned above, I have added a chapter on reading and spelling disorders, and a chapter that traces the life-long persistence of language disorders identified in the preschool population.

Concluding Remarks

This book does not pretend to be a scientific approach to the study of language delays, disorders, and differences. It is clinically based on my experiences and research and literature reviews over the last 29 years as a speech-language pathologist. I am indebted to those who have taught me so much about language deficits throughout my educational and professional career. This includes my professors at Emory University, my colleagues over the years, the students I have taught, and the many patients I have had the opportunity to serve. I am also grateful to those who have taught me life skills, including patience and perseverance. These people include my parents, Clyde and Betty Partin, my husband, Tim, and my three children, Elizabeth, Jennifer, and Will. I would also like to acknowledge Laurie Traver, Molly Belmont, Kalen Conerly, Maura Brown, Jessica McNavich, and all those I do not know whom they have enlisted for support for their guidance in this project. I would also like to thank Linda Lombardino, Ph.D., a colleague here at the University of Florida, for her guidance in the chapter on reading and spelling disabilities and the contribution of the case study in Chapter 7. Thanks are also extended to the anonymous reviewers who had many helpful hints along the way. All these individuals had a vision and I hope that I have been able to fulfill that vision and that you, the undergraduate student, will benefit from this book.

Betsy Partin Vinson

I

LANGUAGE DELAYS AND DISORDERS IN PRESCHOOL CHILDREN

The American Speech-Language-Hearing Association (ASHA) defines language as

> A complex and dynamic system of conventional symbols that is used in various modes for thought and communication. Contemporary views of human language hold that: (a) language evolves within specific historical, social, and cultural contexts; (b) language, as rule governed behavior, is described by at least five parameters—phonologic, morphologic, syntactic, semantic, and pragmatic; (c) language learning and use are determined by the interaction of biological, cognitive, psychosocial, and environmental factors; and (d) effective use of language for communication requires a broad understanding of human interaction including such associated factors as nonverbal cues, motivation, and sociocultural rules. (ASHA Committee on Language, 1983, p. 44)

One of the biggest dangers in the assessment of language disorders in preschoolers is the random application of labels. Therefore, Chapter 1 addresses language disorders on the basis of the five parameters listed in the ASHA definition of language. Models of language disorders based on the features of language are presented to help the student envision and understand the roles of these features in language delays and disorders.

In Chapter 2, language disorders with definitive etiologic bases are described. The causes include Down syndrome, fragile X syndrome, Apert syndrome, Pierre-Robin sequence, cerebral palsy, hearing impairment, "failure to thrive," fetal alcohol syndrome, cytomegalovirus infection, specific language impairment, cognitive disabilities, and autism spectrum disorders.

Chapter 3 is dedicated to assessment considerations and protocols related to the preschool population. The use of standardized and nonstandardized assessment tools is discussed, as is diagnostic report writing.

Chapter 4 explores issues related to treatment of language delays and disorders in preschool children. Presymbolic and symbolic play is explained. The roles of the family and the child's general environments are addressed extensively throughout the chapter.

Finally Chapter 5 reviews the various preschool deficits explored in Chapters 1 and 2 and discusses the impact of these deficits throughout the lifespan.

It is critical for clinicians to understand the differences between language delays, language disorders, and language differences before moving on to Chapters 6–13.

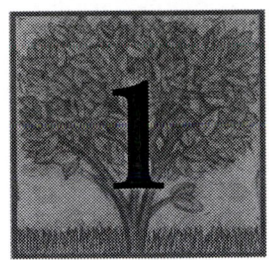

Classification of Language Abnormalities Based on Normal Development and Features of Language

▨ LEARNING OBJECTIVES

After completion of this chapter, the reader will be able to

1. Explain the differences between a language delay, a language disorder, and a language difference.

2. Differentiate between linguistic competence and linguistic performance.

3. Discuss the role of cognition in the development and organization of language.

4. Describe the role of the listener in the development and interpretation of a child's language.

5. Explain the theoretical basis for the Bloom and Lahey model of language disorders.

6. Discuss the impact of cultural influences on storytelling.

▨ INTRODUCTION

Language delay. The acquisition of normal language competencies at a slower rate than would be expected given child's chronological age and the level of functioning.

Language disorder. A disruption in the learning of language skills and behaviors. It typically includes language behaviors that would not be considered part of normally developing linguistic skills.

When discussing disturbances of language functioning in preschool children, it is necessary to distinguish among a language delay, a language disorder, and a language difference. Briefly, a **language delay** can be defined as the acquisition of normal language competencies at a slower rate than would be expected given the child's chronological age and level of functioning. A **language disorder**, in contrast to a language delay, consists of language skills and behaviors that would not be considered part of normally developing linguistic skills. When delays extend into the early elementary school-age years, they may appear as a language disorder. This is further discussed in Chapter 5. However, a language disorder may be diagnosed during any point in life, depending on a variety of etiological factors.

As discussed by Bloom and Lahey (1978), this aberration of development differs from normal development in terms of the actual behaviors demonstrated by the child, the sequence in which aspects of language are learned, and the rate at which they are learned. The American Speech-Language-Hearing Association (ASHA) defines a language disorder as "impaired comprehension and/or use of spoken, written and/or other symbol systems. This disorder may involve (1) the form of language (phonology, morphology, syntax), (2) the content of language (semantics), and/or (3) the function of language in communication (pragmatics) in any combination" (The American Speech-Language-Hearing Association, 1993, p. 40). The breakdown of the definition of language disorders into the components of language is a major topic in this first chapter.

Finally, **language difference** is the term applied to language behaviors and skills that are not in concert with those of a person's primary speech community or native language. Language differences exist owing to unfamiliarity with a language or to cultural variations of the person's native language. Individuals who speak English as a second language may experience instances in which lack of familiarity with English impairs a communicative exchange. In such instances the language is considered different, but not disordered or delayed.

Another semantic dichotomy that a clinician must understand is the difference between linguistic competence and linguistic performance as it relates to delays, disorders, and differences (Bloom & Lahey, 1978). Both of these aspects of language must be considered in terms of the person's native language as well as in any cultural setting he or she may be. **Linguistic competence** refers to the language user's underlying knowledge about the system of rules of the language he or she is using to communicate in any given setting. It is the understanding a person has of the operating principles needed to use language in a functional manner, whether it be the person's native language or not. **Linguistic performance**, on the other hand, refers to the utilization of the child's or adult's linguistic knowledge in daily communication. Whether an individual (of any age) is described as having a language delay, a language disorder, or a language difference, the assessment of language skills must address his or her linguistic competence and linguistic performance.

Language difference. Language behaviors and skills that are not in concert with those of the person's primary speech community or native language.

Linguistic competence. The language user's underlying knowledge about the system of rules of the language he or she is using.

Linguistic performance. The utilization of the person's linguistic knowledge in daily communication.

■ WHO IS AT RISK?

There are numerous factors that can place a child at risk for developing a language delay or a disorder. For example, a pregnant mother who has a dependence on nicotine, alcohol, and/or other drugs places her unborn child at undue risk for developmental problems. Also, children born with certain syndromes or sequences may be at risk. Other risk factors include prematurity, low birth weight, physical problems, emotional deficits, ear infections, sensory deficits, and illnesses. The impact of these factors is discussed at length in Chapter 2.

Another sign that a child may be at risk is the late development of speech and language. Reviewing the research literature, Plante and Beeson (2004) define late talkers as "young children (between approximately 16 and 30 months) whose language skills fall below 90 percent of their age peers. These children are slow to acquire their first fifty words and slow to combine words into phrases" (p. 177). Frequently, late talkers have none of the risk factors cited in the previous paragraph, yet they often experience language deficits as they mature. Some, but not all, children do eventually reach the language and speech levels of their age-peers. While it is difficult to predict who will continue to have problems, some factors under consideration as

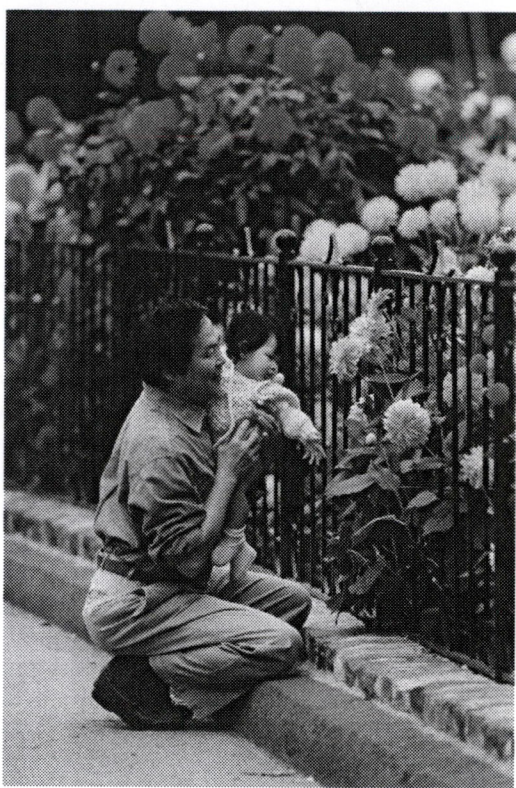

FIGURE 1–1. A variety of opportunities are needed to facilitate language development. A trip to a garden provides opportunities to stimulate the senses as well as to expand a child's language by exposing him or her to a variety of colors, smells, and textures.

having predictive power are limited vocabulary, limited use of gestures to augment communication, and poor comprehension skills (Thal et al., 1997; Thal & Tobias, 1992). That is why it is so important that parents and other caregivers to take advantage of opportunities in everyday life to develop and expand a child's language. An example of this is depicted in Figure 1–1.

■ LANGUAGE DEVELOPMENT

Robert Owens (1984) delineated five principles that must be considered when describing the development of language and communication in infants:

1. Development is predictable.

2. Developmental milestones are attained at about the same age in most children.

3. Developmental opportunity is needed.

4. Children go through developmental changes or periods.

5. Individuals differ greatly. (Rossetti, 1986, p. 18)

While it is not the intent of this book to provide a treatise on language development, a brief review of philosophies dedicated to explaining the growth of language in a child is offered. The reader is referred to the reference list at the end of this chapter for in-depth resources addressing the broad scope of language development and to further study the components of each of the theories mentioned in this section.

McLaughlin (1998) describes two approaches to the study of language development. One is to describe the sequence of language acquisition based on normative development. The other approach addresses the question of how language develops, looking at the underlying processes and mechanisms. McLaughlin refers to various "-isms" when exploring the question of how language develops. One of these "-isms" is **nativism**. Those who are proponents of this school of thought believe that when a child is born, he or she has all the language aspects, and that the knowledge of language comes to fruition as the child matures biologically. This viewpoint closely ties in with the "nature" side of the nature versus nurture philosophy of child development. McLaughlin cites Parker and Riley (1994) in saying that language development is inherent in a child's genetic makeup or nature. The concept of nativism is often associated with **mentalism**, which also holds that "knowledge primarily derives from inborn mental processes" (McLaughlin, 1998, p. 129). Those who ascribe to the nativism theory believe that the structure of language is independent of the use of language (Hulit & Howard, 2002).

Nativism. The capacity to develop language is innate, with language knowledge coming to fruition as the child matures biologically.

Mentalism. Often associated with nativism, the mentalism philosophy posits that one's knowledge is derived from innate mental processes.

Nativism is on the opposite side of theories of language development from the empirical perspective which holds that children are genetically equipped to learn, but the individual is not born with the knowledge he or she gains over the life span. **Empiricism** and **behaviorism** embrace the nurture side of the argument with regard to what constitutes the process of developing language (McLaughlin, 1998). Behaviorists and empiricists tend to believe that children are relatively passive in their language acquisition, and that "their emerging language is determined not by self-discovery or creative experimentation but by the selective reinforcements received from their speech and language models" (Hulit and Howard, 2002). Arguments can be made for the role of nature and the role of nurture in a child's development of language. McLaughlin (1998) points out that most of today's researchers favor a compromise between nature and nurturing. This compromise is referred to as **interactionism**. Proponents of interactionism ask, "What is the nature of the interaction between childrens' genetic makeup and their experiences that results in language learning?" (McLaughlin, 1998, p. 129).

Empiricism. The belief that a child's language is not innate but develops as a result of experiences.

Behaviorism. Like empiricism, the belief that a child's language is not innate but develops when verbalizations are positively reinforced.

Piaget put forth a model based on the interaction between cognition and language. He paid particular attention to the ages of birth to 2 years, a period of tremendous development of cognition and, coincidentally, speech and language. Hulit and Howard (2002) summarize this relationship as follows:

> It should be noted that all theorists accept that a relationship exists between cognitive development and language development. What separates cognitive theorists from others is their belief that language does not hold an absolutely unique position in overall development. They believe that language itself is not innate, even though the cognitive precursors for language are innate. (p. 33)

Cognitive theorists also believe that language is a result of cognitive development and organization. It is not genetically preordained, nor is it structured around learning principles. Rather, these theorists believe that language is rooted in environmental opportunities and cognitive processes, and that language is one ability, among others, that is developed for the manipulation and representation of concepts the child has learned (Hulit & Howard, 2002).

Transformational generative grammar (TGG). A grammar system in which there is a deep structure and a surface structure and a set of rules that govern the combining of words.

Linguistic universals. A belief that there are some commonalities and similarities in the form and content of all languages.

Language acquisition device (LAD). The LAD is not a specific structure, but rather a conglomeration of innate capacity of language that governs the input and output of language form.

Other researchers and practitioners look at language development in terms of the features of language (form, content, and use). Chomsky studied the "structure of language and the structure of the mind" (McLaughlin, 1998, p. 146), and his theory became known as **transformational generative grammar (TGG)** based on linguistic universals and the language acquisition device. **Linguistic universals** are the "shared principles" that underlie the variety of languages and form the foundation for a relatively universal structure of language. For example, all languages have a basic subject/predicate structure of language, and a method for negation. In keeping with the belief that there are certain universals in language, Chomsky's theory holds that language structure is an innate capacity specific to human beings (McLaughlin, 1998). Chomsky also proposed the concept of a **language acquisition device (LAD)** that serves as the neurological foundation for language development. The LAD is not a specific structure in the brain; rather it is a means of looking at the neurological network responsible for language development in children, even in the absence of input from adults in the child's world. Chomsky (1965) further maintains that the LAD is unique among humans.

While Chomsky studied language and its development in terms of its structure, Fillmore (1968), Chafe (1970), and others sought to explain language development in terms of the content, or semantics, of language. One notion espoused by Fillmore is that of case grammar. Fillmore believed that the semantic deep structure of a sentence is formed prior to the syntactic representation of the sentence. He looked at language in terms of the basic relationships in a sentence. In Fillmore's model of case grammar, there is an effort to study the influence that semantics has on the structure of language.

According to Fillmore, the relationship between nouns and verbs is determined by universal semantic concepts at a level beneath the deep structure (Hulit & Howard, 2002).

Fillmore further believed that there are two components to sentences. The first component is **modality** which has to do with sentence characteristics such as negation, interrogation, and verb tense. The second component is **proposition** which examines the relationship between nouns and verbs within a sentence. Fillmore maintained that "the relationship between the noun and verb in a given sentence determines the meaning underlying that sentence" (Hulit & Howard, 2002, p. 30). When contrasting Chomsky's and Fillmore's theories, it is important to note the role of cognition. In Chomsky's transformational generative grammar, cognition and interaction with the environment had no role in the development of language; rather, language required linguistic input only. In Fillmore's case grammar, language is based largely on the child's understanding of his experiences, with the revelation of cognition relying on language. This belief (**cognitive determinism**) is a driving force behind the model of language development proposed by Bloom which is explained in further detail later in this chapter. Cognitive determinism is a term to denote the belief that a child's knowledge of the world is expressed through his language, and that meaning precedes form (McLaughlin, 1998; Bloom & Lahey, 1978).

Finally, a model of language development based on pragmatics, or use, of language is presented by Searle, and referred to as **sociolinguistics**. The concept of sociolinguistics is addressed in more detail in the section "Language Differences" in this chapter. In the theory of **speech acts**, the "social, emotional, and legal ramifications" (McLaughlin, 1998) of words are studied. As explained by the speech acts theory, the speaker's intent, or use, is focused on more than the speaker's word choices. Searle goes on to delineate three types of intent: ordering, requesting, and asserting (Plante & Beeson, 2004). Speech acts are analyzed in terms of forces and components. The forces are **propositional force**, which is the "literal meaning" of a sentence, and the **illocutionary force**, which is the intention of the speech act. The three primary components of speech acts are words and propositions (otherwise known as the locutionary component of language), the intent (illocutionary component), and the perlocutionary component which is the listener's interpretation of the speech act (McLaughlin, 1998). The pragmatic theorists were the first to acknowledge the role that the listener plays in the development and interpretation of language.

■ LANGUAGE DELAYS

Some children develop language as described above, but later than one would consider to be within normal limits. Language abnormalities related to delays can be characterized in five different ways. A wide range of normal

Modality. According to Fillmore, one of two components of sentences that looks at the influence of semantics on grammar, particularly as applied to verb tense, the question form, and negation.

Proposition. According to Fillmore, the second component of a sentence that regulates the relationship between nouns and verbs.

Cognitive determinism. The belief that cognition relies on language for a child to understand his experiences; the child's knowledge of the world is expressed through his language, with meaning preceding form.

Sociolinguistics. The study of social and cultural influences on language structures.

Propositional force. The literal meaning of a sentence.

Illocutionary force. The intention of a speech act.

development of language is exhibited across a wide demographic spectrum, and the speech-language pathologist needs to analyze this knowledge through application of the principles outlined by Owens. Without this knowledge as the foundation for studying language abnormalities, he or she cannot possibly understand the complexities inherent in the diagnosis and treatment of language delays, disorders, and differences. The first three categories of language delays represent degrees of difference in delays. The last two categories of language delays represent deviations from normal schedules and sequences that are rarely seen.

The first and most prevalent characterization of children's abnormal language is language delay (Shames, Wiig, & Secord, 1994). As stated in the introduction, a child is considered to be language delayed if he or she exhibits normal language behaviors, but the language skills fall below those expected based on his or her chronological age and level of cognitive or intellectual functioning. In other words, everything he or she does typically would be observed in a normally developing child, and the behaviors are typically in the normal sequence of acquisition. However, the child with a language delay acquires these skills at a slower rate than would be expected given his or her age and other abilities. This delay can refer to the onset of usage of the language skill, the rate of progression through the acquisition process, the sequence in which the language skills are learned, or all of these (Bloom & Lahey, 1978).

A second type of delay occurs when a child exhibits a language delay with a plateau (Shames et al., 1994). Children in this category follow a normal sequence of acquisition of language skills but never acquire all of the skills expected for a child of his or her age. That is to say, the child progresses up to a point but then levels off. If the acquisition of the language skills of such a child were charted, the child's learning curve would "flatten out" or plateau. For example, a child who develops language normally until 24 months of age but then fails to progress would be characterized as having "plateaued" at 24 months. He or she may have small bursts of improvement followed by another plateau or may remain at the 24-month level. It is also possible that, once the child starts to improve, improvement may continue until he or she has caught up with age-level peers. This kind of plateau could be the result of a physical illness, trauma, or a psychological insult of some kind. However, not all plateaus are due to a developmental deficit or insult. Sometimes a plateau is indicative of progress in another area of development. For example, a child who is delayed in both speech and language skills and motor development may plateau in his or her speech and language development during periods of growth in motor skills. These types of plateaus occur because the immature central nervous system is unable to handle the simultaneous growth in two systems.

A third category of language abnormalities based on normal sequence and schedules describes children who exhibit significant language delay

(Shames et al., 1994). Again, the child acquires linguistic features in the normal sequence, but tremendous discrepancies occur between the ages the features are acquired and the age at which they are integrated. Linguistic features that frequently coincide with increasing **mean length of utterance** may be delayed in acquisition. For example, a child whose language is categorized in this manner may acquire his or her first words around 28 months of age but may not combine words until he or she is 4 to 5 years of age.

Mean length of utterance (MLU). The average length of a sample of utterances spoken by an individual.

Less frequently seen language abnormalities based on developmental schedules and sequences are the use of normal error patterns with unusual frequency or the use of unique language or phonological features that have never been documented as a normal part of acquisition (Shames et al., 1994). Both of these types of language patterns are seen relatively infrequently. An example of normal error patterns with unusual frequency would be the reversal of the position of two sounds in a word, a linguistic behavior known as **metathesis**. It is not uncommon for a child to mispronounce the word "animal" as "aminal," but with a good model he or she typically will correct the pronunciation in a relatively short period of time. If the child continued to do this reversal consistently for all similar combinations, with unusual frequency, or in many different combinations, it could indicate a language disorder. In the case described previously, the child would not make the correction and would continue to call animals "aminals."

Metathesis. The reversal of the position of two sounds in a word (e.g., *aks* for *ask*).

An example of the use of a unique language or phonological feature that has never been documented as a normal part of acquisition is documented in an unpublished thesis at the University of Florida (Schaffer, Dyson, & Vinson, 1989). The child, Edward, was born approximately 3 weeks early after a high-risk pregnancy. Developmental milestones were at the low end of the normal limits, but his speech attempts were essentially unintelligible. Edward had a speech pattern of using the phoneme /h/ for all consonants. As he learned a new phoneme or phonological process, he would then use the newly acquired sound or process in the position of all consonants. Gradually, Edward would learn where to use the new phonemes appropriately, then the /h/ would reappear in all other consonant positions. This continued until he had acquired approximately 80% of the consonant sounds. Clearly, this is not a normal pattern of acquisition with regard to sequence or schedule.

■ LANGUAGE DISORDERS

When analyzing linguistic competence, the clinician must look at the child's knowledge of language in terms of content, form, and use. The content domain includes **semantics**, meaning the knowledge and ideas children have about the objects and events in their world. The form domain consists of specific

Semantics. The knowledge and ideas a person has about the objects and events in the world that make up the content of language.

structures of language, including phonology, morphology, and syntax. Pragmatics, the broadest of the language domains, reflects the different uses, or functions, of language that the child communicates through language.

The following discussion of language deficits attributed to the features of language is based primarily on the work of Bloom and Lahey (1978). These two researchers define a language disorder as "a broad term to describe certain behaviors, or the lack of certain other behaviors, in a child that are different from the behaviors that might be expected considering the child's chronological age" (Bloom & Lahey, 1978), and their study of language disorders is based on the following premises:

1. Objects have distinctive properties, including causality, action, time, location, possession, and object permanence.

2. It is necessary to have an understanding of object categories, object knowledge, object relations, and event relations.

3. There are two aspects of language use: language functions (interaction, regulation, control) and linguistic selection (we choose words to fulfill a function based on our intent and perceptions of the listener, information sharing, and the situation).

In the Bloom and Lahey model of language development, all features of language are intertwined, so a deficit in one may be accompanied by, or result in, a deficit in another. These investigators also have developed models that represent the different types of language disorders related to the features of language. These models form the basis of the subsequent discussion in this section.

Children may have difficulty formulating ideas or conceptualizing information about the world (content), they may have difficulty learning a code to represent their knowledge (form), or they may learn a code that does not conform with that of their speech community or learn the conventional code but be unable to use it (use). In Figure 1–2, normal language is section-D. If the description of a child's language fell in area D, but later than expected, the child would exhibit a delay. Disordered language consists of a disruption within one or more of the three components or in the interaction among and between the components.

The Semantic Domain: Deficits in Content

Description of the Semantic Domain

Early semantic rules appear to be universal. Regardless of the native language, children learn that basic rules exist governing meaning and relationships between meaning units, and other rules exist that dictate the relationship of

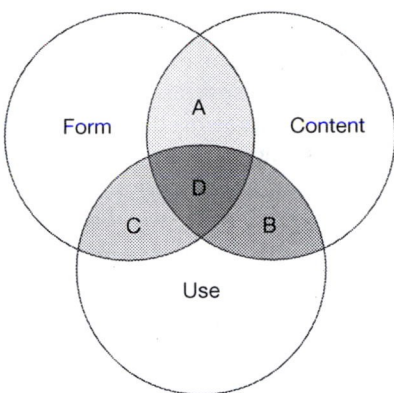

FIGURE 1–2. Bloom and Lahey's model of normal language. Complete development of the components and the interactions are denoted by the solid lines. (From *Language Disorders and Language Development* by M. Lahey. © 1988, Allyn and Bacon.)

language form to objects and events, and with words and word combinations. We also know that children combine words cross-culturally in similar ways to express basic meaning. For example, children typically use agent + action, action + state, and attribute + object to govern their early word combinations, regardless of their native language.

According to Bloom and Lahey (1978), word meaning is made up of semantic features that characterize and define the word and selection restrictions that prohibit certain word combinations (redundancy). Using this definition of word meaning, synonyms are words with identical semantic features and antonyms are words with opposite semantic features. When faced with a word that has multiple meanings, the listener must rely on selection restrictions, linguistic context, and nonlinguistic context. For example, if I saw a football player showing off, I might say, "He is a real hot dog!" Using your knowledge of semantic features and selection restrictions, you would be able to understand that this is a metaphor, and that the football player is not actually a hot dog. However, if a child has semantic deficits, he or she may envision an actual hot dog without understanding that I meant the player was being pompously demonstrative.

Language is a fundamental way of representing experience. Therefore, experiences are needed for language development and enhancement. Conceptual development occurs when a child has the ability to organize cognitively many different experiences and to reorganize these concepts as more information is learned. When children are developing their semantic repertoires, it is not uncommon for them to identify several objects by one descriptor or name based on other experiences with objects or events that have the same semantic features. A child who has been exposed primarily to dogs most likely will go through a stage in which he or she identifies all animals with four legs as dogs. However, as the child learns more about the animals and develops the restrictions that guide word selection in any given experience, he or she will begin to label animals by their correct names using conventional semantic categories. A child who was shown a Christmas tree in an office referred to it as a "hot flower." The mother explained that the child identified all trees and plants as flowers and used the word "hot" for all lights; hence, the "hot flower" in the lobby.

Another consideration in describing the concept of semantics is that a word may have two types of meaning. The first type is denotative meaning, which is the literal definition of a word as found in a dictionary. In contrast, connotative meaning is the meaning of a word based on emotional and/or associative factors. Nicolosi, Harryman, and Kresheck (1996) provide an example of connotative meaning in the use of the word "pig." "Pig" can be literally, or denotatively, defined as a large, domesticated farm animal from which pork is derived. The connotative meaning of "pig" may refer to a sloppy individual or an unsavory character. Thus, the connotative meaning depends on an interpretation by the communication partners.

Children who have weakness in conceptual development (i.e., the development of ideas about the world, which make up the content of language), fall into the category of those with semantic deficits. A pure semantic deficit is rare because conceptual knowledge is necessary to develop form and use. Some research indicates that children who are blind may, early in their language development, have language disorders that are restricted to the semantic category (Bloom & Lahey, 1978). However, they usually outgrow their deficits when they learn to compensate for the sensory deficit. Children who have hydrocephalus also demonstrate semantic deficits in many cases. Children whose language could be illustrated using the drawing in Figure 1–3 would have more advanced form and use interactions than content interactions.

They may speak in grammatically correct sentences but have little to say. The term "cocktail party speech," which is common in individuals with hydrocephaly, is an apt descriptor of content-specific disorders. Most interactions at cocktail parties consist of forms and uses that are appropriate for social interaction but are weak on content. Typically, a child with a semantic deficit may give commands and ask many questions. He or she may be extremely social and may even be described as verbally aggressive. Some children in this category may be echolalic, which means the child repeats, or echoes, what he or she hears spoken by others (Bloom & Lahey, 1978).

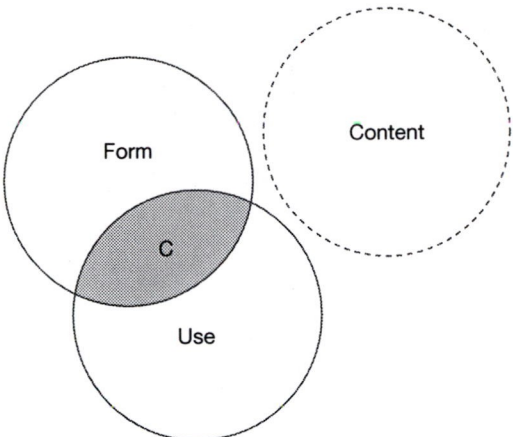

FIGURE 1–3. Bloom and Lahey's model of content disorders. Complete development of the components and the interactions are denoted by the solid lines; dashed lines represent incomplete development of the component or the interactions, or both. (From *Language Disorders and Language Development*, by M. Lahey. © 1988, Allyn and Bacon.)

Disorders of Content

Clinically, children who have semantic deficits are slow in acquiring their first words and in subsequent vocabulary development. These children have difficulty in acquiring temporal and spatial relationships. Another clinical red flag that can be indicative of a semantic deficit or disorder would be difficulty in grasping synonyms and antonyms (Lahey, 1988).

The Form Domain: Phonology, Syntax, and Morphology

Defining the Form Domain

Children who have form deficits may use gestures or primitive forms of communication because they have difficulty learning and using the conventional codes. Figure 1–4 shows a partial overlay of content and use, with the separation of form. This is a graphic representation of how knowledge and ideas about the world's objects and events and the abilities to communicate these ideas, may be intact, while the child's knowledge of the linguistic system for representing and communicating these ideas is impaired. Children who have difficulties acquiring word endings (such as -ed, -ing, -er, and -est) fall into this category, which Bloom and Lahey have designated as a disruption between form and content.

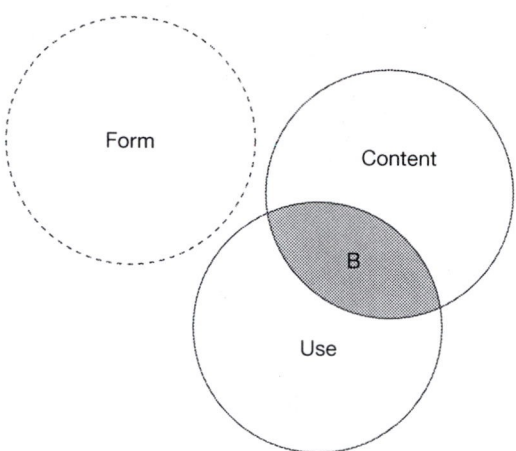

FIGURE 1–4. Bloom and Lahey's model of form disorders. (Reprinted with permission from *Language Disorders and Language Development*, by M. Lahey. © 1988, Allyn and Bacon.)

Phonology Deficits. The form of the structures puts the knowledge children have about their world into words, phrases, and sentences. Form connects sounds with the conventional system of symbols. The first form component we will discuss is **phonology**. Phonological rules govern the distribution and sequencing or organization of phonemes (sounds) within a language. Children who have phonological deficits will have difficulty establishing correct correspondences between the adult's and the child's linguistic forms. This may be evidenced in consistent misuse of specific phonemes despite being able to correctly articulate the sound. For example, the child may be able to say /s/, but when shown a saw will identify it as a "taw." Some children with phonological deficits may have more pervasive speech-motor difficulties, and the role the speech-motor deficits play in the phonological deficit needs to be clarified before a phonological approach is used as the basis for remediation.

Phonology. The distribution and sequencing or organization of phonemes within a language.

Syntax Deficits. **Syntax** refers to the appropriate, rule-based ordering of words in connected discourse. Rules exist that govern word order, sentence organization, and the definition of relationships between words, word types (questions, passive, etc.), and word classes (nouns and verbs). The psycholinguistic theory, which explains the relationship between language form and cognitive processing, helps us to understand the syntactic component of language. Noam Chomsky, the leading proponent of the psycholinguistic theory, described language from an innate, rule-governed psychological perspective and argued that universal linguistic rules of grammar underlie language acquisition. Children's knowledge of linguistic rules allows them to understand and generate language.

Syntax. Appropriate, rule-based ordering of words in connected discourse.

Clinically, syntactic deficits may be manifested as depressed utterance length, the use of telegraphic speech, frequent word reversals, and problems with the auxiliary verb system.

Morphology Deficits. Morphemes are the smallest units of meaning that make up the grammar, or **morphology**, of language. They are the rules that modify meaning at the word level. Morphological deficits are demonstrated clinically as problems with prefixes, suffixes, verb tense, plurality, and word usage. Morphemes can be free or bound. Free morphemes can stand alone and have meaning (single words), while bound morphemes must be attached to words in order to have meaning. An example of a bound morpheme is the prefix "-un." By itself, that prefix has no meaning; however, it gains meaning when attached to a word as in "undone." Thus, bound morphemes change the meaning of a word. Bound morphemes also may change the syntactic category of a word as when "-ly" is added to an adjective and changes the word into an adverb (e.g., "glad" is an adjective that becomes an adverb when "–ly" is added) (Plante and Beeson, 2004).

Morphology. Units of meaning that make up the grammar of language by modifying meaning at the word level.

The Pragmatic Domain: Deficits in the Functional Use of Language

Defining Pragmatics

Pragmatics refers to the social use of language. The person must have pragmatic competence in order to analyze and understand contexts in which language is used and the functions for which it is used. Language is used in a variety of ways for a variety of purposes, but a child with a pragmatic deficit will not be able to use language in context appropriately (Table 1–1).

Pragmatics. The social use and functions of language for communication.

At a very early age, the child develops the ability to choose alternative structures to influence the listener and create change. Prior to the development of language, the child's communicative signals are expressed through

TABLE 1–1. Uses of language.

Social	Greeting
Learning	Giving information
	Requesting information
Control	Turn-taking
	Initiating
	Maintaining
	Giving feedback

Jargon. Utterances made up of correctly articulated nonsense words with appropriate prosody.

Metalinguistics. Skills that form the basis for effective pragmatic skills by allowing the interpretation of language.

cooing, crying, **jargon**, and echolalia as he or she attempts to establish and maintain contact with other people in his or her environment. As children mature, they learn why people speak and begin to use conventional language forms and content to effectively communicate their intentions.

In the early school years, children begin to develop **metalinguistic** skills, which form the foundation for effective pragmatic skills. Embedded in metalinguistic skills are the knowledge and interpretation of rules of language. For example, the child learns that a word is a word, it is made up of sounds, it can be defined, and it can be spoken and written.

Children who have pragmatic deficits will learn the system to code ideas but will have difficulty putting it into use.

Disorders of Use

The child often will talk about something that is out of context with the conversation or topic at hand. Some authors have described the interaction pattern as intrapersonal communication because the child will ramble repetitively or tangentially with little regard for the listener (Figure 1–5) (Bloom & Lahey, 1978).

Pragmatic deficits may appear as difficulty in maintaining a topic, or lack of communication despite relatively normal use of speech sounds, morphology,

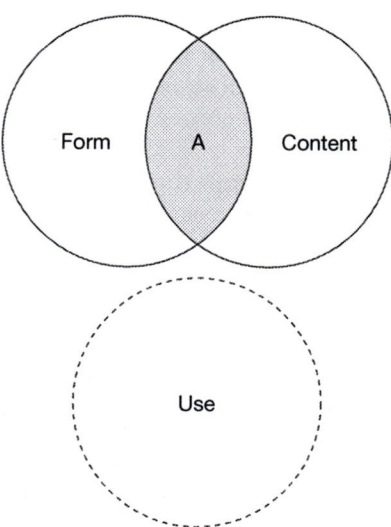

FIGURE 1–5. Bloom and Lahey's model of use disorders. (From *Language Disorders and Language Development*, by M. Lahey. © 1988, Allyn and Bacon.)

and syntax. Often the child with a pragmatic deficit has poor communication fluency, poor conversational skills, and poor nonverbal social skills.

Deficits in the Interaction Among the Components of Language

Occasionally, a child has some development of each component of language but incompletely developed or distorted interactions among the components (Figure 1–6). That is, he or she has failed to integrate form, content, and use completely during the acquisition of language.

According to Bloom and Lahey, the child will use forms to communicate ideas, but the forms he or she uses may be inappropriate to the content and meaning intended to be conveyed. Typically, this child will use very little meaningful speech; in fact, it may be limited to **stereotypic speech**. On occasion, the child may use what appear to be appropriate utterances; but, most likely, these are complete utterances that the child has learned to use in response to certain situations or ideas, even though he or she may not know the semantic-syntactic relations that are represented within the sentences (Bloom & Lahey, 1978).

Stereotypic speech. The unintentional use of a real or invented word or phrase that has little meaning.

With regard to differential diagnosis, unlike children who have a form deficit, these children might produce sophisticated examples of the conventional language structures. They differ from children with semantic deficits because they may have complex ideas about the world, but they do not have the ability to appropriately code the ideas they have. Finally, they differ from

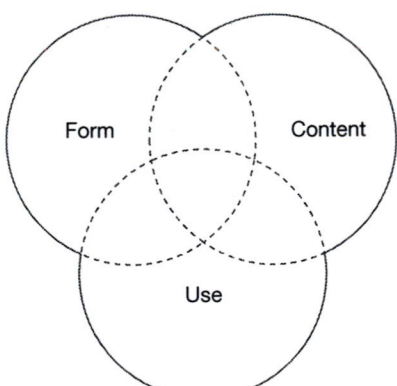

FIGURE 1–6. Bloom and Lahey's model representing disordered interactions between the components of language. (From *Language Disorders and Language Development,* by M. Lahey. © 1988, Allyn and Bacon.)

children with more isolated pragmatic disorders because they do use forms for personal interaction. When a child has distorted interactions among form, content, and use, messages are well formed and used for specific purposes in the situation; however, there is a mismatch between the content of a message and its use and between the content and its form, even though some element of the content is related to the message or the situation in which it occurs.

Lack of Interaction Among the Components

Even more rare is the child who has incomplete development of each component of language and no interaction among the components (Figure 1–7). Children in this category will use stereotypic speech utterances that have little or no relation to the situation at hand. No apparent function is evident for speech, other than possibly to maintain some form of communication contact. The child may recite TV or radio commercials or repeat utterances heard previously that are, in some idiosyncratic way, associated with the present context. It is important to note that, in this example, as well as in all of the disorders based on features of language, isolated instances are not a basis for determining the existence of a problem. The use of commercial jingles and idiosyncratic utterances must be prevalent in the child's communicative exchanges. A few years ago, one of my son's friends came to the door and inquired as to whether or not my son could go to the movie with the friend's

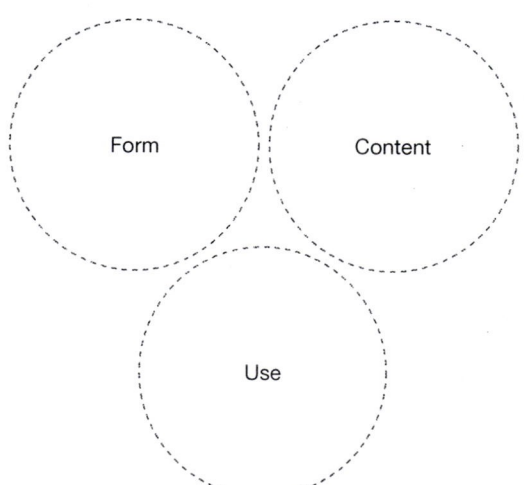

FIGURE 1–7. Bloom and Lahey's model of distorted interactions and incomplete development of the components. (From *Language Disorders and Language Development,* by M. Lahey. © 1988, Allyn and Bacon.)

family. My husband asked where the movie was playing, and the child responded, "At theaters everywhere!" This child could not be labeled as having a lack of interaction of his form, use, and content based on this one utterance. However, if this statement were made randomly, frequently, and without any relation to the existing context, and if it were the standard mode of communication, there would be reason for concern.

LANGUAGE DIFFERENCES

A **speech community** is a group of people who routinely and frequently use a shared language to interact with each other (Fasold, 1990). A communication difference exists when communication behaviors meet the norms of the primary speech community but do not meet the norms of standard English (Shames et al., 1994). This difference can exist whether the person in question is a child from a different country or simply a different neighborhood in the same city. The slight variations that occur in a language are systematic, patterned, and rule-governed and constitute a **dialect**. Dialects often develop along lines of geographic separations or social differences (Fasold, 1990). Dialects may be distinguished from each other by word choices and/or variations in how a sound or word is pronounced.

Speech community. A group of people who routinely and frequently use a shared language to interact with each other.

Dialect. Systematic, patterned, rule-governed variations in a language.

Regardless of the degree of variation, all dialects are considered to be linguistically valid and legitimate. They develop as a result of the mixing of a variety of languages of different cultural groups. When the minority language mixes with the language of the native speakers, dialects emerge. Frequently, the distribution of political and economic power plays a role in determining which language will become the dominant one, with the language of those in power becoming the primary language and the application of the cultural differences developing the dialect. Thus, regional dialects and cultures emerge based on geographical boundaries, social and legal boundaries, and political and economic power.

Culture is defined by Nelson (1993) as a combination of values, beliefs, and survival systems used by members of a specified group to perpetuate their accepted quality and philosophy of life. The study of culture can be based on an ethnography of the communication or on sociolinguistics.

Culture. The philosophies, ideas, arts, and customs of a group of people that are passed from one generation to the next.

Ethnography is the study of language use for communicative purposes, considering social and cultural factors. It tends to be descriptive in nature.

Ethnography. The study of language use for communicative purposes, considering social and cultural factors.

Sociolinguistics is the study of social and cultural influences on language structures. Sociolinguists study the communicative interactions of people in social situations. The field of sociolinguistics is relatively new in the social sciences. It developed at the end of the first Head Start program in 1965 when psycholinguistics and anthropologists met in an attempt to explain why some

TABLE 1–2. Seven areas of concentration that need to be considered when studying the issue of dialectal variations in individuals.

Race and ethnicity
Social class, education, and occupation
Region
Situation or context
Peer group association and identification
First language community or culture
Gender

Source: Adapted from *Human Communication Disorders: An Introduction* (4th ed.), by G. H. Shames, E. H. Wiig, and W. A. Secord, 1994, pp. 143–144. New York: Macmillan Publishing Company.

children had problems in school and others did not (Nelson, 1993). Together, the professionals in these two sciences initially approached the topic from a psycholinguistic viewpoint. That is to say, they looked at the "interrelationships between the structures and processes underlying the ability to speak and understand language" (Nelson, 1993, p. 26). Eventually, the sociolinguistic viewpoint developed. Instead of looking for psycholinguistic problems within children, they came to the conclusion that they needed to look at language differences between the homes and schools of children who succeeded and of those who did not succeed in school (Nelson, 1993).

Ethnographic and sociolinguistic researchers have studied several factors that influence language acquisition, language behavior, and communication and discourse rules. Together, these social scientists identified seven areas of concentration that need to be considered when studying the issue of dialectal variations in individuals (Table 1–2).

The first domain of study is race and ethnicity, based on cultural attitudes and values, not on biology and genetics. Samovar and Porter (1994) summed up the issue as follows:

> Language is the primary vehicle by which a culture transmits its beliefs, values, norms, and world views. Language gives people a means of connecting and interacting with other members of their culture and a means of thinking. Language thus serves as a mechanism for communication and as a guide to social reality. (pp.16–17)

The second domain is based on the study of social class, education, and occupation. To address these issues, it was necessary to evaluate the effects of the home environment, child-rearing practices, family interaction patterns, travel, and experiences. It would be expected that children who have stable homes with consistent parenting would do better in school than those who do not. However, it is critical that children not be labeled as deficient in their cognition or language because of personal biases related to a specific social group or speech community. Some children have the opportunity to travel and learn about regional dialects firsthand, whereas others have few opportunities to go beyond their hometowns and neighborhoods. An enriched environment is one in which children are exposed to a variety of experiences, and these experiences do not need to be of epic proportions! Taking a child to a grocery store and letting the child feel and smell fresh produce is a wonderful experience that dovetails with events that occur in the daily lives of families.

Regional issues constitute the third domain that needs to be addressed when studying language. As stated earlier, many dialects emerge as a result of geographic boundaries. In the lower 48 states, at least 10 regional dialects are recognized (Nist, 1966). These dialects consist of phonological features, word choices, idioms, and characteristic patterns in syntax, prosody, and pragmatics. Speech-language pathologists need to analyze their own dialects to see if they could impact the intervention process!

The social context of a situation often influences a person's choice of a language or dialect. With regard to situation or context, peer group associations, and the first language community, it is sometimes necessary to speak a more standard dialect; at other times the native dialect emerges. The ability of an individual to switch dialects or languages depending on the situation is called code-switching. Teenagers may speak in one dialect when they are with their peer group and in another dialect when they are with their families. Frequently, these dialectal variations are semantic in nature. For example, a teenager came home from school and announced that she had a boyfriend and that they were going steady. The mother assumed that this meant they were dating only each other (based on the definition of "going steady" when she was in school), only to find out that "going steady" meant you held hands in the halls at school.

The effects of gender are topics of much interest to those who study the sociolinguistic aspects of language. However, this aspect of dialectal variations does not play a role in most patients seen by the speech-language pathologist. Nonetheless, an astute speech-language pathologist will need to study the gender-related and/or age-related issues of clients who are from a different culture. For example, one culture does not allow a woman to establish eye contact with a male or permits a child to speak only when spoken to first. Another culture may focus on loudness, with women being very soft-spoken in comparison to the men in their environment. It is important to understand the effects of gender in different cultures in order to effectively plan diagnostic and therapeutic services.

Topic-centered narrative. A tightly structured discourse on a single topic or a series of closely related topics and events.

A major impact on language use comes from the cultural influences on storytelling. In some cultures, stories are primarily topic-centered narratives, whereas in others topic-associated narratives take precedence. In addition, an oral storytelling tradition, as opposed to a written storytelling tradition, is a cultural factor that affects language development and language use. Storytelling facilitates the development of critical cognitive functions, such as conceptualization, social interaction, and problem-solving skills. A **topic-centered narrative** is characterized by a tightly structured discourse on a single topic or a series of closely related topics and events. Such narratives tend to have a temporal organization or a thematic focus that prevails throughout the story. Frequent exposure to storybooks helps a child to understand topic-centered narratives, which can eventually influence the development of cognitive and language foundations. Most storybooks assume that the reader has little information about the subject. Typically, storybooks have an orientation section that sets up the story and introduces the characters, an elaboration that develops the story, and a resolution that completes the story.

Topic-associated narrative. A series of narratives linked to a topic with no particular theme or point to the narrative.

In contrast, **topic-associated narratives** are more traditional in countries where stories are told orally but are usually not written down. A topic-associated narrative consists of a series of narratives linked to a topic, with no particular theme or point to the narrative. Rather, the stories are a source of entertainment, with the details frequently altered as the stories are passed through the oral tradition. The listener must make the shifts and links in the story on the basis of presumed knowledge about the topic, which typically has no temporal or focal connections between the segments of the story. Often the temporal aspects and segmental shifts are provided by pitch and tempo changes instead of by words. Topic-associated narratives usually are more common among children of working-class parents whose families may not have money available for many storybooks (Payne & Taylor, 2006).

■ SUMMARY

As clinicians, we need to determine what the individual knows about language and how adept he or she is at using knowledge in a functional manner. In other words, the question guiding the assessment of language must be based on the concept of functional application of the person's knowledge of his or her language. Can this individual integrate the rules that govern language use and language knowledge in a manner that will allow him or her to be understood in interactions with others?

Throughout this book, the term "language disorder" is used as a diagnostic entity to refer to any disruption in the learning of language in the absence of primary intellectual, sensory, or emotional deficits (Bloom & Lahey, 1978). The term "language delay" is used as a description of qualitative differences from normal with regard to time of onset, rate of development, actual behavior learned, or the sequence in which the behavior was learned. By taking this view of language delays and disorders, we are forced to describe what the child can do without difficulty, what the child can do with some degree of difficulty, or what the child cannot do. This enables us to have a better understanding of possible disruptions in the child's language development and to design more appropriate plans of intervention.

CASE STUDY

History

J is a 4-year-old child who presents in the clinic with problematic speech intelligibility. He was born at 37 weeks gestation by C-section following a high-risk pregnancy. J's mother started premature labor at 13 weeks gestation and remained on bed rest for the remainder of the pregnancy. She received terbutaline and morphine to slow down contractions throughout the pregnancy. J has two older sisters who both attend public school and are doing well. Both of J's parents have master's degrees. His father is a biologist and his mother is a teacher. J attends a church preschool program that focuses on socialization, preschool readiness, and perceptual motor skills from 8:00 A.M. to 5:00 P.M. daily. His teachers report that he is very social, well behaved, and adapted well to the preschool setting. He gets along well with his peers. He does have difficulty with fine motor tasks and shows little interest in coloring and puzzles. Reports from school testing using the Weschler Intelligence Scale for Children-IV (Weschler, 2003) indicate that J has a verbal IQ of 114 and a performance IQ of 94.

When J was 3 years old, he was referred to a pediatric neurologist by his pediatrician due to delayed gross motor milestones and difficulty with fine motor control. J's mother also reported that he had difficulty as an infant coordinating his sucking patterns when drinking from a bottle and continues to have an uncoordinated chewing motion when eating solid foods. The neurologist diagnosed J as having mild cerebral palsy (static encephalopathy). J was referred to this clinic for evaluation of his speech.

Evaluation

In the preassessment interview, J's mother described his sound acquisition pattern as being unique to him and not following a standard acquisition sequence or rate. When J began talking around 15 months of age, he used the sound /h/ in place of all consonants and also had some vowel distortion. When he learned a new sound, such as /p/, he would drop the /h/ and use /p/ in place of all consonants. When he figured out where to appropriately use a /p/, he would revert to using the /h/ for all consonants other than /p/. This pattern continued until J had acquired most of the consonants. Vowel distortion remained a consistent problem.

J's speech was evaluated using the Assessment of Phonological Processes–Revised (APP-R) and a spontaneous language sample. On the APP-R, J had a phonological deviancy score of 33. Based on J's performance, the clinician concluded that J had a moderate phonological disorder that consisted of fronting (cat ➤ tat), liquid gliding (red ➤ wed; lock ➤ wock), consonant deletion, and vowel distortions. In spontaneous speech he was approximately 40% unintelligible. His intelligibility is compromised not only by his phonological patterns, but also by a rapid rate of speech that borders on cluttering.

He was tested for apraxia using an informal battery and it was determined that he had mild oral apraxia. He had difficulty puckering his lips on command, and with lateral movement of the tongue. These difficulties also interfered with his intelligibility in connected speech.

J tested within normal limits on a hearing screening.

On language testing using the Test of Language Development–P:3, J scored in the 91st percentile with a composite score (quotient) of 120. The Word Articulation subtest was the only subtest that was problematic. J has an excellent command of sound-symbol correspondence, and he reads at a first-grade level. It should be noted that when J reads aloud, he has an accelerated rate just as he does in spontaneous speech. Content and use of language are intact.

Summary

J is a bright young man who presents with speech difficulties that interfere with his intelligibility. A review of his speech and language development reveals that J had an unusual pattern of sound acquisition that impacted the ability of others to understand him. At the single word level, J has fronting, liquid gliding, and consonant deletion. He also has distortion of the vowels. He has mild oral apraxia that also interferes with speech clarity. J has no difficulties with semantics and pragmatics, and the only aspect of form that is affected is his phonology.

	Strengths	Weaknesses
Communicative	Oral decoding and segmentation abilities	Phonological processes that interfere with intelligibility
	Hearing WNL	Rapid rate of speaking that interferes with intelligibility
	Pragmatics	Oral apraxia
	Semantics	
Noncommunicative	Good home environment	Mild frustration when he cannot make himself understood
	Good preschool program	
	Positive personality	Poor eye-hand coordination
		Weak fine motor skills

Recommendations

It is recommended that J receive phonological therapy using the cycles approach two times a week. Therapy should also include oral-motor strengthening and coordination activities. Following 10 weeks of therapy, it is suggested that he be reevaluated.

■ REVIEW QUESTIONS

1. Cross-cultural studies suggest that
   a. Early semantic rules are universal.
   b. Early phonological rules are not universal.
   c. There are no similarities in grammar across cultures.
   d. Early semantic rules are not universal.

2. Sociolinguistics is defined as the study of
   a. Social institutions.
   b. Language assimilation.
   c. Causes of language disorders.
   d. Social and cultural influences on language structure.

3. Which of the following "-isms" (McLaughlin) support the nature philosophy of language development?
   a. Empiricism and behaviorism
   b. Interactionism and nativism
   c. Mentalism and nativism
   d. Mentalism and behaviorism

4. Which of the following set of "red flags" is most typical of a disruption of content/semantics?

   a. Slow acquisition of first words, slow in understanding temporal and spatial relationships, lack of understanding of antonyms and synonyms

   b. Slow acquisition of first words, delayed understanding of category words, difficulty maintaining a topic

   c. Slow acquisition of first words, slow in understanding temporal and spatial relationships, normal communication

   d. Slow acquisition of first words, slow in temporal and spatial relationships, frequent word reversals

5. Use of "cocktail party speech" could be indicative of which of the following?

   a. Disruption in interactions between content and form

   b. Incomplete development of content

   c. Disruption in interactions between use and content

   d. Incomplete development of use

6. A child who has knowledge and ideas about events and objects, can communicate ideas, but often uses gestures because he has difficulty learning conventional codes for expressive language has a disruption in

   a. Form

   b. Content

   c. Use

7. Plante and Beeson define late talkers as children between the ages of 16 and 30 months whose language skills fall below 80% of their age peers.

   a. True

   b. False

8. Topic-centered narratives are traditional in countries where stories are told orally but usually not written down.

   a. True

   b. False

9. Students who exhibit a language difference are considered to be language disordered.

   a. True

   b. False

10. Use of limited functions of language would be indicative of a pragmatic disorder.

    a. True

    b. False

■ REFERENCES

American Speech-Language-Hearing Association(ASHA) (1993). Definitions of communication disorders and variations. A report by the Ad Hoc Committee on Service Delivery in the Schools. *Asha, 35*(Suppl. 10), 33–39.

American Speech-Language-Hearing Association (ASHA) Committee on Language (1983, June). A definition of language. *Asha, 25*(6), 44.

Bloom, L., & Lahey, M. (1978). *Language development and language disorders.* New York: John Wiley and Sons.

Chafe, W. (1970). *Meaning and the structure of language.* Chicago: University of Chicago Press.

Chomsky, N. (1965). *Aspects of a theory of syntax.* Cambridge, MA: MIT Press.

Fasold, R. (1990). *The sociolinguistics of language.* London: Basil Blackwell.

Fillmore, C. (1968). The case for case. In E. Bach & R. Harmas (Eds.), *Universals in linguistic theory.* New York: Holt, Rinehart & Winston.

Hulit, L. M., & Howard, M. R. (2002). *Born to talk: An introduction to speech and language development.* Boston: Allyn and Bacon.

Lahey, M. (1988). *Language disorders and language development.* New York: Macmillan Publishing Company.

McLaughlin, S. (1998). *Introduction to language development.* San Diego: Singular Publishing Group, Inc.

Nelson, N. W. (1993). *Childhood language disorders in context: Infancy through adolescence.* New York: Merrill.

Nicolosi, L., Harryman, E., & Kresheck, J. (1996). *Terminology of communication disorders* (4th ed.). Baltimore, MD: Williams & Wilkins.

Nist, J. (1966). *A structural history of English.* New York: St. Martin's Press.

Owens, R. E. (1984). *Language development: An introduction.* Columbus, OH: Charles E. Merrill.

Parker, F., & Riley, K. (1994). *Linguistics for non-linguists: A primer with exercises* (2nd ed.). Boston: Allyn and Bacon.

Payne, K. T., & Taylor, I. L. Multicultural differences in human communication and disorders. In Human Communication Disorders: An Introduction (7th ed.) by N. Anderson & G. H. Shames. Boston: Pearson Education, Inc.

Plante, E., & Beeson, P. M. (2004). *Communication and communication disorders: A clinical introduction* (2nd ed.). Boston: Allyn and Bacon.

Rossetti, L. M. (1986). *High risk infants: Identification, assessment, and intervention.* Boston: College-Hill Press.

Samovar, L. A., & Porter, R. E. (1994). *Intercultural communication: A reader* (7th ed.). Belmont, CA: Wadsworth Publishing Company.

Schaffer, S., Dyson, A., & Vinson, B. (1989). *Phonological development: A case study.* Unpublished master's thesis. Gainesville, FL: University of Florida.

Shames, G. H., Wiig, E. H., & Secord, W. A. (1994). *Human communication disorders: An introduction* (4th ed.) New York: Macmillan College Publishing Company.

Thal, D. J., Bates, E., Goodman, J., & Jahn-Samilo, J. (1997). Continuity of language abilities: An exploratory study of late- and early-talking toddlers. *Developmental Neuropsychology, 13*, 239–274.

Thal, D. J., & Tobias, S. (1992). Communicative gestures in children with delayed onset of oral expressive vocabulary. *Journal of Speech and Hearing Research, 35*, 1281–1289.

Weschler, D. (2003). Weschler Intelligence Scale for Children = IV. San Antonio, TX: Harcourt Assessment, Inc.

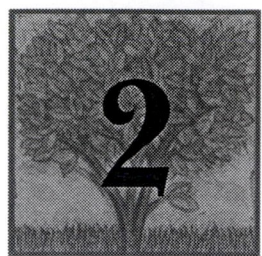

Classification of Language Abnormalities Based on Etiology and Diagnostic Labels

■ LEARNING OBJECTIVES

After completion of this chapter, the reader will be able to

1. Identify the primary characteristics of a variety of pediatric language disorders, including, but not limited to, Robin sequence, Stickler syndrome, Down syndrome, fetal alcohol syndrome, fragile X syndrome, Apert syndrome, velo-cardio-facial syndrome, mental handicaps, multidrug babies, and those often associated with hearing loss and cerebral palsy.

2. Argue the philosophical stance as to whether cognition precedes language.

3. Differentiate between a sequence and a syndrome.

4. Describe the speech and language characteristics of a child with Stickler syndrome, and list three other defining characteristics.

5. Describe the effects of hearing loss on a child's development of form, content, and use of language.

6. List the diagnostic criteria for autism, and describe the speech and language behaviors associated with autism.

■ INTRODUCTION

As defined by the American Speech-Language-Hearing Association, a language disorder is

> the abnormal acquisition, comprehension, or expression of spoken or written language. The disorder may involve all, one, or some of the phonologic, morphologic, semantic, syntactic, or pragmatic components of the linguistic system. Individuals with language disorders frequently have problems in sentence processing or in abstracting information meaningfully for storage and retrieval from short and long term memory. (ASHA, 1980, p. 318)

Although it certainly is preferable to address a language disorder in terms of the language abilities and disabilities that the child demonstrates within his or her linguistic system, it often becomes a legal and financial necessity to officially "label" a child's disorder with a diagnostic descriptor on the basis of etiological considerations. Funding for special education and related services in the public schools often hinges on the diagnostic label which has been used to classify the disorder with regard to the child's abilities and disabilities. Eligibility for Medicaid and other reimbursement programs also requires the application of a diagnostic label. Therefore, whether the clinician philosophically supports or opposes the concept of labeling, it is a necessity in many settings. Together, the professionals and the family must consider the benefits and drawbacks of labeling a child's disorder, and act accordingly. Actually, it is not the act of labeling that is the major problem; rather, it is the *assumption* of the presence or absence of specific skills and traits that often accompanies a label that is problematic. In instances such as this, even though it is the condition that is labeled, the clinician should not forget that it is the *child* who is being assessed and treated, not the disorder. If the child's speech and language patterns do not interfere with the message being understood, the problem may not be labeled a communication disorder. However, if interference occurs with the message being received by the listener, it is most likely that some professional such as a teacher or speech-language pathologist may label the problem a communication disorder. For purposes of discussion, the remainder of this chapter will address the language aspects of a communication disorder.

Cognition. The process of thinking, using information gained through perception, memory, discrimination, judgment, and other thought processes.

Another philosophical stance on labeling is brought forth by the argument as to whether language precedes **cognition** or cognition precedes language. This is an important consideration, particularly when planning treatment strategies. For years, researchers have concluded that cognition precedes language and designed intervention programs accordingly. With the increased emphasis on functional outcomes in a limited amount of time, some clinicians are deviating from the historical plan of developing the cognitive skills to form a basis from which language can then develop. However, research indicates that language and cognition develop in concert with each other. A study by Bates, Benigni, Bretherton, Camaioni, and Volterra (1979) looked specifically at the relationship between cognition and language and found that intentional language develops earlier than previous research had indicated. Children represent their intentions through gestures prior to using speech to communicate the same intentions. Both are complex systems, but these authors' research suggests that a set of common symbols exists in the environment of a child from which language and cognition develop simultaneously. Tiegerman-Farber summed it up best when she wrote, "Language represents the child's most critical accomplishment during the early childhood years; *all* academic subjects, *all* educational instruction, *all* later acquisitions are based on the language learning system" (Tiegerman-Farber, 1995, p. 5). Therefore, it is important that a clinician understand this relationship and the effects that various **etiological** factors can have on a child's language development during the preschool years.

Etiology. Causative factors that lead to a developmental delay disorder.

■ GENETIC AND CHROMOSOMAL SYNDROMES

Genetic. The denoting of specific characteristics or traits passed from one generation to the next.

Frequently, the terms "genetic" and "chromosomal" are used as if they are synonymous. **Genetic** disorders refer to those that are carried on genes. Genetic disorders may be acquired, as when a gene undergoes a mutation, or they may be inherited. **Chromosomal disorders** refer to deviations of the genes that are located on the chromosomes, and they also may be inherited or acquired.

A chromosomal disorder is defined as "a disorder of the number or structure of the chromosomes as they are distinctively arranged for a particular individual" (Johnson, 1996, p. 80).

Two other terms that are frequently misapplied are "sequence" and "syndrome." According to Shprintzen (1997), a sequence is "a disorder where many of the anomalies are actually secondary disorders, caused by a single anomaly which sets off a chain reaction of changes in the developing embryo that result in other anomalies" (p. 75). Robin sequence is discussed in the next section. A syndrome is defined as "the presence of multiple anomalies in the same individual with all of those anomalies having a single cause" (Shprintzen, 1997, p. 53). It is possible for a child to have a syndrome and a sequence, such as having the Stickler syndrome in the Robin sequence. Down syndrome, fragile X syndrome, and velo-cardio-facial syndrome are discussed in this chapter.

Robin Sequence/Stickler Syndrome

Historically, Robin sequence has been called Pierre Robin syndrome. Based on the definition previously discussed, it should be called Pierre Robin sequence, or Robin sequence. These babies have a very small jaw and a U-shaped cleft palate (see Figure 2–1). Both of these characteristics compromise the upper airway system. They are obligatory mouth breathers, so that interferes with feeding and the more natural nasal breathing. This is an example of a sequence in which the child's tongue cannot be positioned anteriorly due to the small jaw. Thus, the pharynx (breathing space) does not expand because when the child's mouth is closed, the tongue falls back into the oropharynx. This, in turn, causes an obstruction to the upper airway and the child cannot breathe nasally. This condition is called **glossoptosis** which is secondary to the inherited genetic trait of **micrognathia** (very small jaw) (Shprintzen, 1997).

Stickler syndrome is the most common cause of the Robin sequence. In fact, one-third of the patients diagnosed with Robin sequence are also diagnosed as Stickler syndrome. Stickler syndrome shares the characteristics of Robin sequence in addition to skeletal anomalies such as a club foot and eye problems. Stickler syndrome is "a common genetic form of connective tissue **dysplasia** and perhaps the second most common syndrome associated with cleft palate in the absence of cleft lip" (Shprintzen, 1997, p. 84).

The Robin sequence is typically classified as either the Robin deformation sequence, or the Robin malformation sequence. In the Robin deformation sequence, the causes of the abnormality are extrinsic to the fetus. That is to say,

Chromosomal disorders. A disorder in the structure or number of chromosomes, or both.

Glossoptosis. Displacement of the tongue into a downward position.

Micrognathia. A very small lower jaw that is frequently paired with a recessed chin.

Dysplasia. Abnormal tissue development.

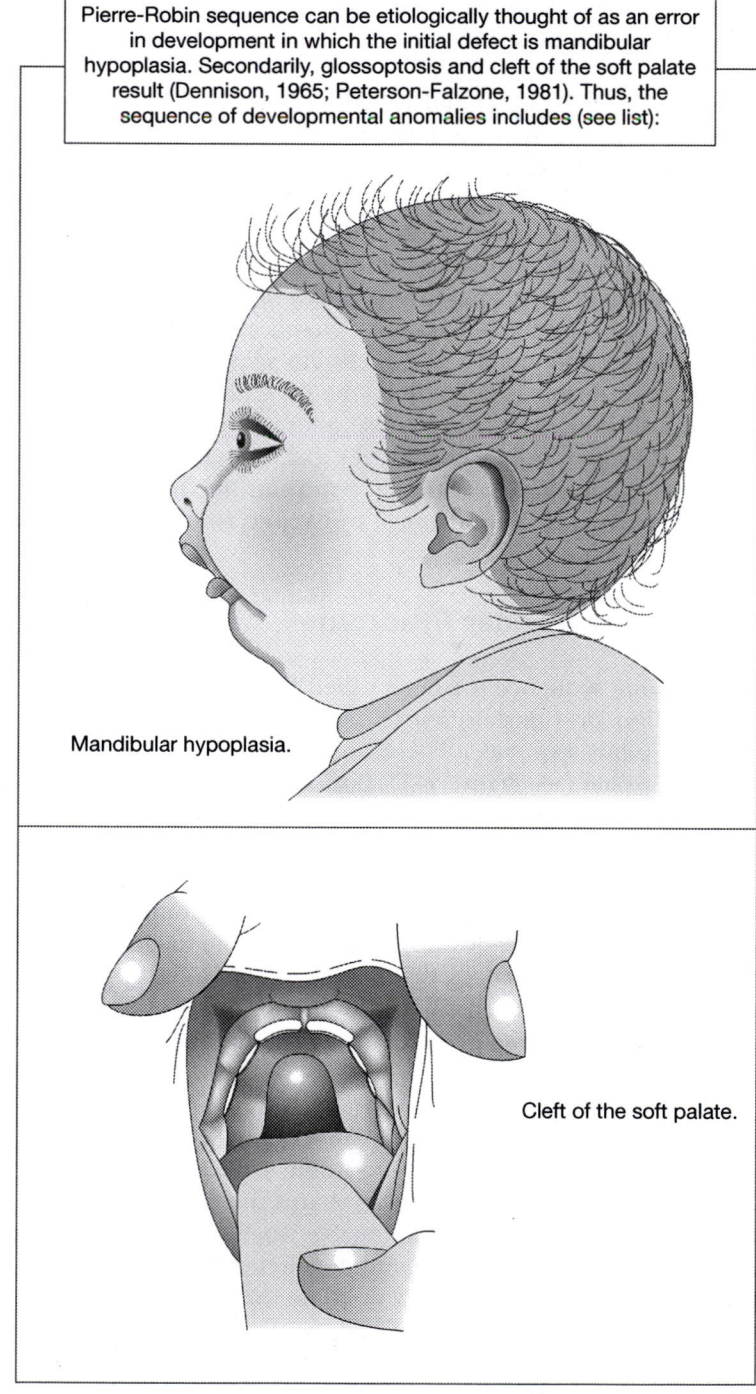

Pierre-Robin sequence can be etiologically thought of as an error in development in which the initial defect is mandibular hypoplasia. Secondarily, glossoptosis and cleft of the soft palate result (Dennison, 1965; Peterson-Falzone, 1981). Thus, the sequence of developmental anomalies includes (see list):

Mandibular hypoplasia.

Cleft of the soft palate.

FIGURE 2–1. Characteristics of children with Stickler syndrome/Robin sequence. Adapted from *Genetic Syndromes in Communication Disorders* (Austin, TX: Pro-Ed, 1988).

the anomalies are caused by positional deformities that are not likely to be repeated in subsequent pregnancies. The child may inherit a familial trait such as a small jaw, which is exacerbated by compression problems that would occur if the mother's uterus and/or pelvis were too small, resulting in compression of the baby. In Robin malformation sequence, the cause(s) of the problems are intrinsic to the baby. The baby could have a malformation such as a small mandible that could result in the tongue's abnormal positioning that results in poor palatal growth (Shprintzen, 1997).

Speech and Language Characteristics of Stickler Syndrome/Robin Sequence

Speech and language problems can result from the cleft palate and hearing loss exhibited by many individuals with Robin sequence and Stickler syndrome. As mentioned previously, the child with Robin sequence will have a cleft palate, and possible cleft lip, and the speech will be hypernasal. Hyponasality is sometimes seen when the nasal cavity is extremely small. The posterior location of the tongue may contribute to feeding and breathing problems that would result in failure to thrive, dysphagia, and apnea.

The child will typically have dentition abnormalities that could contribute to poor articulation. Lingual protrusion distortions and backing are common. The child may develop abnormal compensatory articulation patterns. Mental retardation, possibly due to a lack of oxygen to the brain and upper airway obstruction, sometimes occurs (Jung, 1989; Pore & Reed, 1999; Shprintzen, 2000).

Other Characteristics of Stickler Syndrome/Robin Sequence

Approximately 15% of patients with Stickler syndrome will exhibit a sensorineural hearing loss that typically affects the high frequencies. In those with cleft palate, chronic middle-ear effusion may lead to a conductive loss. The child with Robin sequence often has anomalies of the middle and external ears. These anomalies include low-set ears, an abnormally angled external auditory meatus, deformed outer ears, and structural defects of the middle ear ossicles (Jung, 1989; Shprintzen, 2000). Eye problems include retinal detachment, occasional cataracts, myopia, and vitro-retinal degeneration. Thus, is it essential the child diagnosed with Robin sequence and/or Stickler syndrome receive frequent eye examinations (Pore & Reed, 1999; Shprintzen, 2000).

Down Syndrome (Trisomy 21)

Down syndrome is a chromosomal disorder that is caused by the presence of three copies of chromosome 21 rather than the usual two, and this disorder also is labeled trisomy 21. The most prevalent of the chromosomal anomalies, Down syndrome occurs once in approximately every 600 to 800 live births (Nyhan, 1983). Historically, children with Down syndrome were assumed to have moderate to severe mental retardation. However, more recent evidence does not support that assumption, and the range of mental deficits in children with Down syndrome is documented as mild to severe. The more contemporary findings may, in part, reflect the greater availability of early intervention and increased understanding of the importance of structuring a rich and redundant language environment to facilitate the development of nonlinguistic and linguistic language and communication in children with Down syndrome.

Speech and Language Abilities in Preschool Children with Down Syndrome

Prognathism. Abnormal facial construction in which the upper and/or lower jaws project forward.

Down syndrome is recognizable by its common features that are generally well known. The children typically have a round face with abnormal development (dysplasia) of the midface area with a prominent jaw (**prognathism**). The oral cavity is relatively small which limits movement of the tongue and affects speech intelligibility. Also, these children tend to be mouth breathers with a habitually open mouth. The "mouth breathing" is also due to the fact that the nasopharyngeal area is underdeveloped. Due to hypotonia, the tongue is typically carried forward in the oral cavity and may protrude. Teeth are late to develop and are frequently incompletely developed or missing. Submucous clefts are fairly common in individuals with Down syndrome, and the hard palate may be high and narrow and may also be a cleft (Jung, 1989; Shprintzen, 1997). See Figure 2–2.

Although the degree of disability varies quite a bit, all Down syndrome babies show a developmental delay with regard to their motor, speech, and language development. After reviewing several studies, Stoel-Gammon (1981) concluded that there was little difference in terms of the quality and quantity of vocalizations in babies with Down syndrome up to age 12 months. However, as they reach the age of 1 year, the delay begins to become evident as many Down syndrome children do not begin to use words until 24 to 36 months of age, with some beginning vocalization as late as age 7 to 8 years (Stoel-Gammon, 1981).

Articulatory errors tend to be inconsistent when compared to normal children and children with other forms of retardation. The vocal quality is characterized as being lower pitched than normal, breathy, and husky (Jung, 1989). Stuttering is fairly common, along with prosody and phrasing problems (Shprintzen, 2000).

In Italy, Caselli, Vicari, Longobardi, Lami, Pizzoli, and Stella (1998) conducted a study to investigate the development of language and communication in

Down syndrome is one of the most common chromosomal abnormalities, with an estimated incidence of one in every 700 live births (de Grouchy & Truleau, 1984). The diagnosis can be made clinically on the basis of characteristics that may include (see list):

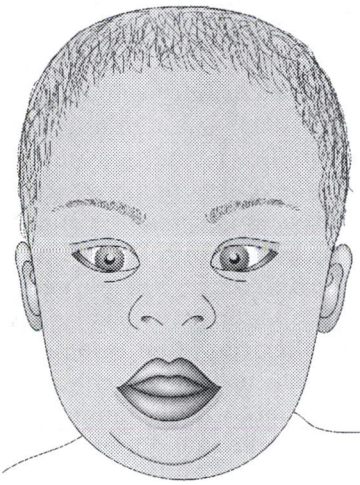

Typical Down syndrome facies. The eyes demonstrate the epicanthal folds. The tongue is relatively large with a tendency to protrude. This is accentuated by a small chin.

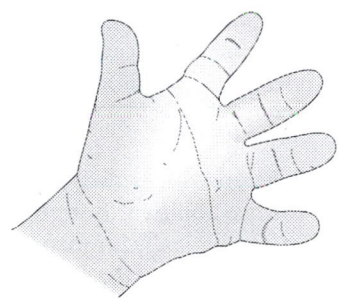

Relatively short fingers and altered palmar creases. Here, a classic transverse palmar crease (Simian crease) is demonstrated. There is also mild incurving of the fifth finger (clinodactyly) secondary to dysplasia of the fifth middle finger bone.

Epicanthal fold and Brushfield spots of iris.

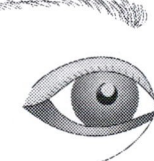

FIGURE 2–2. Characteristics of children with Down syndrome. Adapted from *Genetic Syndromes in Communication Disorders* (Austin, TX: Pro-Ed, 1988).

children who had Down syndrome. They studied 40 children between the ages of 10 to 49 months who had Down syndrome, and 40 normally developing children aged 8 to 17 months in order "to examine the relations among verbal comprehension, verbal production, and gesture production in the very early stages of development" (p. 1125). Specifically, Caselli and colleagues wanted to determine if a dissociation between comprehension and production exists, and if so, did it affect speech only, or speech and gestures. The Italian version of the MacArthur Communicative Development Inventory (CDI) (Fenson et al., 1993) was administered to each child, and they found that the children with Down syndrome were severely delayed in reaching the developmental milestones compared to the normally developing children. Although differences in semantics and syntax between normally developing children and children with Down syndrome appear to be minimal in the early stages, the differences become more pronounced as the children get older. This is true particularly in relation to phonology and morphosyntactic abilities, with lexicon often being spared. The older children with Down syndrome typically use simple sentences with words such as articles, pronouns, and prepositions being omitted (Fowler, 1990; Chapman, 1995; Rondal, 1993; Fabbretti, Pizzuto, Vicari, & Volterra, 1997). The results of the Caselli study concluded that "a dissociation emerged in children with DS between verbal comprehension and production, in favor of comprehension, whereas synchronous development was found in vocal lexical comprehension and gestural production" (Caselli et al., 1998, p. 1132). The dissociation between comprehension and production is similar in normally developing children and children with Down syndrome when the children are matched based on lexical comprehension, but children with Down syndrome use more gestures, especially when comprehension of the lexicon exceeds 100 words.

In general, the communication skills of children with Down syndrome fall below what would be expected based on cognitive ability, although these children are typically very social. Receptive language typically is more intact than expressive language, and the language abilities frequently plateau around the 3-year-old developmental level. Auditory and short-term memory are also impacted (Pore & Reed, 1999; Shprintzen, 2000).

Another confounding factor that occurs when the child with Down syndrome approaches adulthood is the early occurrence of senility and Alzheimer's disease (Shprintzen, 1997).

Other Characteristics of Down Syndrome

Hypotonia. Abnormally low muscle tone that is sometimes referred to as athetosis.

Another factor to consider in looking at language development and use in preschool children with Down syndrome is that their motor development is delayed, and they are hypotonic and hyporeflexive owing to immature development of the central nervous system (Sparks, 1984). **Hypotonia** refers to abnormally low muscle tone, which leads to a characteristic description of Down syndrome babies as "floppy." Hyporeflexia refers to an abnormally low response when the reflexes are stimulated. Therefore, babies with Down syndrome may not do as much environmental exploration as a normal baby would. This decreased exploration of the environment will impact the child's ability to have experiences that help in language development.

Another factor is the frequent occurrence of hearing impairment in children with Down syndrome. Small auricles and congenital malformations of the Eustachian tube and of the nasopharynx typically are present. It is not uncommon for children with Down syndrome to suffer from impacted wax (Jung, 1989). **Conductive hearing loss** coupled with frequent middle ear infections also can affect language development. Pueschel (1987) reported that over 75% of children with Down syndrome suffer from a hearing loss, with the majority of these individuals having mild to moderate losses in the 15- to 40-dB range. These losses may be conductive, sensorineural, or mixed, although the conductive hearing loss is the most common.

Conductive hearing loss. A breakdown in the ability of the middle ear to receive the acoustic signals from the environment and then to transmit the acoustical information to the inner ear.

Generally speaking, the individual with Down syndrome has the following major systems affected: central nervous system, craniofacial system, cardiac system, gastrointestinal system, hematologic system, limbs, and ocular systems (Shprintzen, 2000). The occurrence of cancer is higher in individuals with Down syndrome, and they frequently have congenital heart and respiratory disorders. Obesity, blood disorders (particularly, leukemia), and immune deficiencies are common. All of this has the potential to reduce life expectancy to 30 to 40 years (Shprintzen, 1997; Pore & Reed, 1999; Shprintzen, 2000).

Fragile X Syndrome

The second most common genetic syndrome is fragile X syndrome with the cause being "a fragile site on the long arm of the X chromosome" (Pore & Reed, 1999, p. 80). It is also referred to as Martin-Bell syndrome (Shprintzen, 1997). Figure 2–3 is a drawing depicting the facial characteristics of a boy with fragile X syndrome is an easily missed. . . . An easily missed abnormality that is believed to account for one-third to one-half of all X-linked cases of mental handicaps (Sparks, 1984). Articulation delays are common, as are language problems. Typically, children with this syndrome demonstrate deficits in auditory reception, visual and **grammatic closure**, and **auditory sequential memory** (Sparks, 1984).

Grammatic closure. The ability to determine the missing elements in a sentence.

Auditory sequential memory. The ability to remember sounds, words, phrases, and sentences in a specified sequence.

Disorders in speech and language range in degree from very mild to very severe, and the speech and language deficits often are the first sign that something is wrong with the child (Johnson, 1996). The diagnosis of fragile X syndrome hinges on the presence of mental retardation of unknown

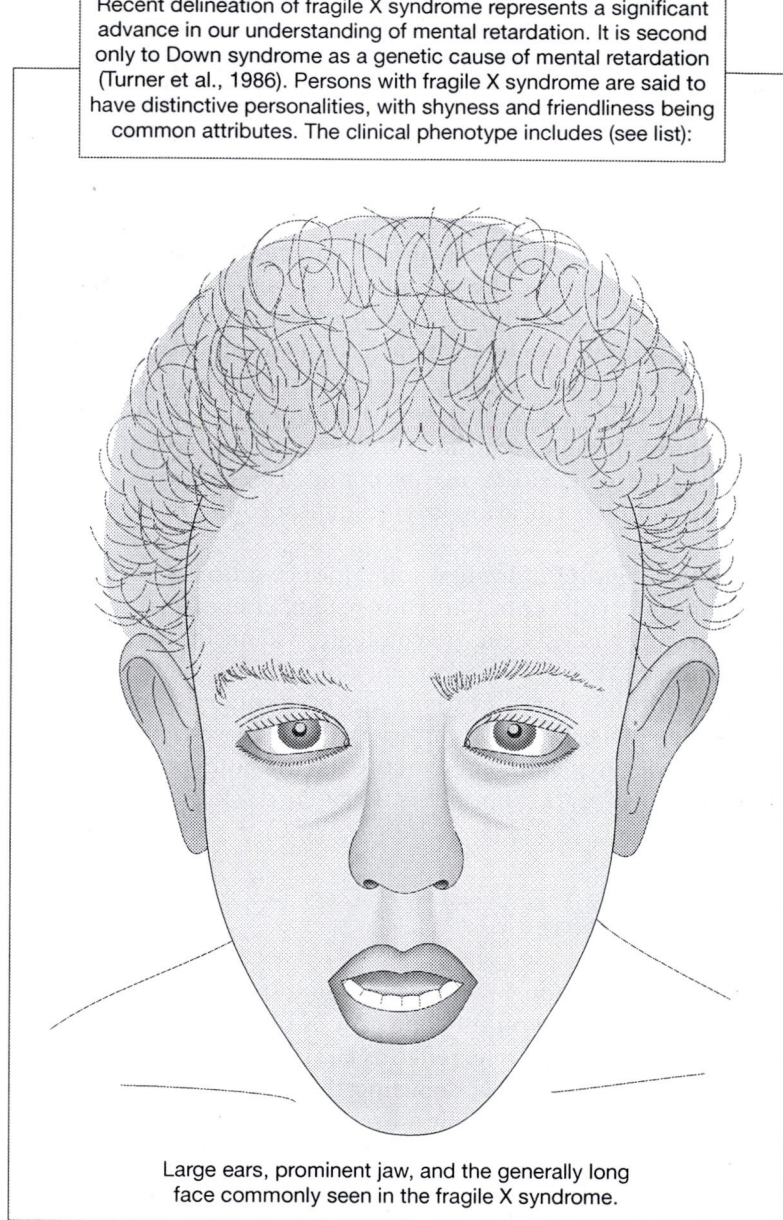

Recent delineation of fragile X syndrome represents a significant advance in our understanding of mental retardation. It is second only to Down syndrome as a genetic cause of mental retardation (Turner et al., 1986). Persons with fragile X syndrome are said to have distinctive personalities, with shyness and friendliness being common attributes. The clinical phenotype includes (see list):

Large ears, prominent jaw, and the generally long face commonly seen in the fragile X syndrome.

FIGURE 2–3. Characteristics of children with fragile X syndrome. Adapted from *Genetic Syndromes in Communication Disorders* (Austin, TX: Pro-Ed, 1988).

cause, autism, or four or more of the following characteristics: mental retardation, perseveration in speech, hyperactivity, short attention span, negative reaction to physical contact, hand flapping, hand biting, poor eye contact, hyperextensive finger joints, large and prominent ears, large testicles, simian crease, and family history of mental retardation (Johnson, 1996).

Also, associated with fragile X syndrome is a prominent forehead and chin and flat feet. The syndrome is more prevalent in males than in females, with incidence figures of 1:1000 male births and 1:2000 female births (Pore and Reed, 1999).

Speech and Language Characteristics of Children with Fragile X Syndrome

Although the language symptoms can range from mild to severe, there is not a direct relationship between the severity of the retardation and the degree of the language impairment. Children with fragile X syndrome exhibit intellectual impairment, along with a variety of speech, language, and learning deficits such as poor eye contact, hyperactivity, social deficits that mimic autism, social withdrawal, and a limited attention span (Roberts et al., 2002). When comparisons are made between male children with fragile X syndrome and male children with Down syndrome who have the same cognitive levels, those with fragile X syndrome have more depressed language skills. The development of expressive language skills frequently lags significantly behind the development of receptive language skills. Some children with fragile X syndrome may show a strength in their lexicon but have poor abstract reasoning skills; others may have poor development of their lexicon. A poor short-term memory and the presence of an auditory processing disorder are also characteristic.

In an effort to further study the communication and symbolic behaviors of boys with fragile X syndrome, Roberts et al. (2002) studied the language of 22 males diagnosed with fragile X syndrome. The boys ranged in chronological age from 21 to 77 months and developmentally were younger than 28 months. Each boy was tested using the Reynell Developmental Language Scales and the Communication and Symbolic Behavior Scales. All of the boys demonstrated significant delays, and there was substantial individual variability. Generally speaking, the testing indicated that the boys had weaknesses in the use of gestures, reciprocity, and symbolic play skills. The boys had specific weaknesses in "the use of repair strategies, conventional gestures (i.e., pushing away), distal gestures (pointing at a distance), and complex action schemes" (pp. 300–301). Strengths were found in vocal and verbal communication, specifically in using a wide variety of words, sounds, and word combinations. On repeat assessment after one year had passed, "children who (initially) scored higher in communicative functions, vocalizations, verbalizations, and reciprocity scored higher in verbal comprehension. Children with higher scores in verbal communication also scored higher in expressive language development" (p. 295).

Speech is usually delayed, and the more severely affected child may be non-verbal. Articulation errors, stuttering and cluttering are frequent symptoms and these individuals typically have a hoarse and breathy quality of voice.

A high-arched palate and/or cleft palate and feeding problems are also common (Pore & Reed, 1999; Shprintzen, 1997). Boys with fragile X syndrome do not use as many gestures to support their verbal attempts at communication. Rather, they use more jargon, and they tend to have more **echolalia** and **perseveration** than their counterparts with Down syndrome. In fact, their communicative behaviors are more typical of children with autism (Wolf-Schein et al., 1987).

Echolalia. The unintentional repetition of words spoken by others.

Perseveration. Unintentional repetitive movements or vocalizations.

Retardation is more common in males than females, with the females having mild to severe learning disabilities and males having moderate to severe mental retardation (Pore & Reed, 1999).

Other Characteristics of Children with Fragile X Syndrome

According to Pore and Reed (1999), approximately 63% of boys who have fragile X syndrome also have otitis media. Seizures are seen in approximately one-fifth of the afflicted individuals. It is not unusual to see attention deficit disorders (ADD), or attention deficit disorders with hyperactivity (ADHD). Motor development is typically delayed, partially due to possible hypotonia, and sensory integration skills are also deficient (Pore & Reed, 1999). Another characteristic found in individuals with fragile X syndrome (and coincidentally, also in Down syndrome) is late-onset psychosis (Shprintzen, 1997).

Apert Syndrome

The incidence figure for Apert syndrome is 1 per 160,000 live births (Gorlin & Pindborg, 1976). It is an example of a progression of facial phenotype, with the facial malformations becoming more evident as the child gets older. Physical characteristics include an open bite and, frequently, cleft palate. In the absence of a cleft, one would expect to see an abnormally thick and long soft palate that, when combined with a small nasopharynx, mouth breathing, and forward carriage of the tongue, leads to hyponasality (see Figure 2–4). However, the child also may demonstrate hypernasality or mixed resonance. Individuals with Apert syndrome will present with abnormal oral resonance secondary to reduced dimensions of the pharyngeal cavity. In addition, they may have calcification of the larynx leading to a hoarse and breathy vocal quality. There is usually a high arched hard palate with or without a cleft, and a class III malocclusion. Other facial features include prognathism, **exorbitism**, **hypertelorism**, and maxillary and midfacial hypoplasia due to the **craniosynostosis**.

Exorbitism. Bulging of the eyes beyond the socket of the orbit.

Hypertelorism. Wide placement of the entire bony orbit surrounding the eye.

Craniosynostosis. Premature fusion of the bones of the cranium.

Chronic upper airway obstruction is also typical in these individuals. Hydrocephalus associated with craniosynostosis leads to cognitive deficits that range from learning disabilities to severe retardation. The child has short upper

Apert syndrome is a distinctive acrocephalosyndactyly syndrome initially reported by Wheaton (1894) and more recently reviewed by Blank (1960). It is characterized by (see list):

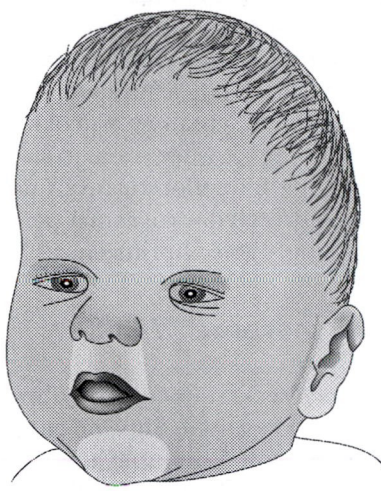

Abnormally tall head shapes secondary to premature cranial synostosis. The midfacial region is also underdeveloped.

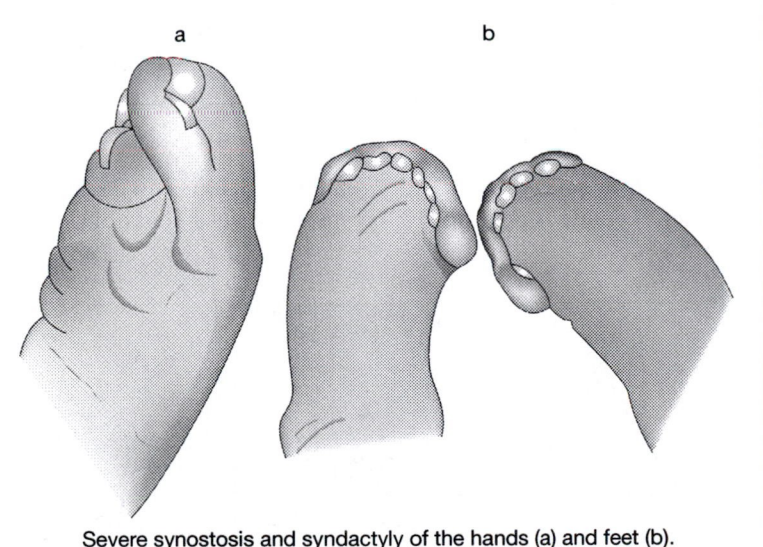

a   b

Severe synostosis and syndactyly of the hands (a) and feet (b).

FIGURE 2–4. Characteristics of children with Apert syndrome. Adapted from *Genetic Syndromes in Communication Disorders* (Austin, TX: Pro-Ed, 1988).

arms, and syndactyly (fusion) of the fingers and toes. Anomalies of the skin (severe and prominent acne lesions) are common. There is conductive hearing loss with "middle ear space slightly reduced in size, but the major contributor to conductive hearing loss is fixation of the footplate related to the synostosis, which also occurs in the cranium and other joints of the body" (Shprintzen, 1997, p. 183). Middle ear effusion also contributes to conductive hearing loss. Typically, the child has speech delays associated with the cognitive impairments. He or she may have compensatory articulatory patterns due to the oral-facial anomalies, including possible cleft palate. Language delays are common, but some children will develop relatively normal receptive and expressive language, although speech disorders may persist due to the structural anomalies (Sparks, 1984; Jung, 1989; Shprintzen, 1997; Shprintzen, 2000).

Velo-Cardio-Facial Syndrome (VCFS)

Velo-cardio-facial syndrome was first documented in 1978 and has received additional attention in recent research. Shprintzen (2000) reports that it "is probably the second most common multiple anomaly syndrome in humans with an estimated population prevalence of 1:2000 people and a birth incidence that is higher because some babies do not survive the neonatal period" (p. 411). It affects multiple systems: central nervous system, the craniofacial system, the digestive system, the genitourinary system, the immune system, the limbs, the mental system, the metabolic system, the renal system, the respiratory system, and the skeletal system. Drawings depicting characteristics in a girl with VCFS can be found in Figure 2–5.

Speech and Language Characteristics of Children with VCFS

Typically, there is severe velopharyngeal insufficiency in individuals with VCFS, and cleft palate is common. They have severe articulatory impairment

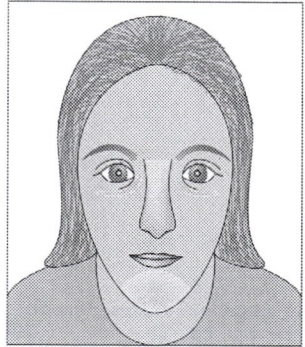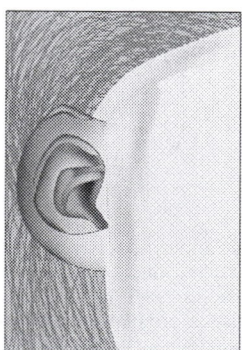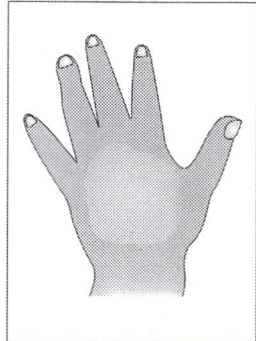

FIGURE 2–5. Characteristics of children with velo-cardio-facial syndrome (VCFS).

that is usually characterized by a preponderance of glottal stop substitutions. Unlike other children with cleft palate, children with VCFS usually do not develop other abnormal substitutions, pharyngeal stops, pharyngeal fricatives, or middorsal stops. The voice is high pitched, hoarse, and breathy, and they are typically highly hypernasal (Shprintzen, 1997; Shprintzen, 2000). Riski (1999) identifies VCFS as the most common cause of clefting associated with syndrome manifestation. However, with extensive speech therapy and surgical reconstruction of the velopharyngeal valve, the individual with VCFS can achieve normal sounding speech.

Children with VCFS typically demonstrate a mild language delay but catch up with their normally developing peers between 36 to 48 months of age. They frequently have learning disabilities and difficulty with abstract thinking. ADD/ADHD may be evident, and occasionally, mild retardation is noted. Deficits in auditory memory and processing have also been documented (Shprintzen, 1997; Shprintzen, 2000).

Other Characteristics of Children with VCFS

Individuals who are diagnosed with VCFS often have hearing loss. Although the loss may be sensorineural (15% of the VCFS population), a conductive loss is more common, with the conductive loss occurring with secondary to middle ear effusion. The external canals are usually narrow, and the helix is overfolded. Ears may be small and/or cup shaped with attached auricular lobules. The hearing loss is usually mild to moderate and unilateral. The individual may demonstrate an exaggerated startle response (Shprintzen, 2000).

The craniofacial system is characterized by upper-airway obstruction during infancy, an anterior laryngeal web, a large pharyngeal passageway, absent or small adenoids, asymmetrical movement of the pharyngeal walls, and a unilateral vocal cord paresis. The infant may have difficulty feeding, leading to the baby's failing to thrive. Gastroesophageal reflux, nasal vomiting and regurgitation, and constipation are problematic (Shprintzen, 2000).

Behavioral problems in individuals with VCFS are common. During infancy, these babies may be irritable and have poor bonding (although frequent illnesses and hospitalizations may contribute to this).

■ MOTOR AND SENSORY DEFICITS

Motor and sensory deficits can contribute to language deficits in children because they affect the degree to which children can explore their environment and, hence, learn language through this exploration. Children who have motor deficits have limited abilities to move about in their environment. The limited mobility may, in turn, restrict some of the environmental exploration that helps them learn about the various properties of specific objects. Similarly, children with sensory deficits will face limitations in their ability to explore all properties of an object. For example, a child with a hearing impairment may not be able to hear the music from a music box or be able to hear and process spoken language. A child with a visual deficit will not be able to distinguish between objects based on appearance alone. These issues are expanded on in the following sections.

Static Encephalopathy

Historically referred to as cerebral palsy, static encephalopathy is not consistently associated with any particular or specific language disorders. Because of abnormal muscle tone and reflexes, it is expected that a child who has moderate or severe static encephalopathy will experience his or her environment in a different way than a child who does not have mobility, motility, and sensory deficits. For example, if a child has hypotonic musculature and hypotonic reflexes (a low-tone, "floppy" baby), it is likely that he or she will not be as responsive to tactile stimulation as would a child without such deficits. Thus, concepts based on kinesthetic feedback, such as hot-cold and smooth-rough, may be more difficult to learn because tactile sensation is not as intact. Likewise, a child who has hypertonia and hyperreflexia (a high-tone, "tight" baby) may exhibit an abnormal startle response to noise, leading his or her parents to create a more subdued acoustic environment and limiting the child's exposure to noise. For example, if the child startles and becomes neurologically disorganized when exposed to a vacuum cleaner, the parent is more likely to use the vacuum cleaner when the child is not at home. Therefore, it is possible that the child would not correctly identify certain specific sound sources when listening to tape recordings of common environmental sounds. In such a case, it is not anticipated that every child with static encephalopathy will have the same difficulty with language concepts based on kinesthetic and auditory input; rather, the child has an altered experience of these sensations depending on (1) the degree of sensorimotor impairment and (2) how the environment was structured specific to his or her needs.

Hearing Impairment

Depending on the degree of the hearing loss and the age at which the child becomes hearing impaired, the language disorders associated with hearing impairment are quite variable. Other hearing factors associated with the degree of language impairment are (1) whether or not the hearing loss is stable or progressive, (2) whether it is unilateral or bilateral, (3) what type of hearing loss the child demonstrates, (4) how much intervention the child has had, and (5) the attitude of the family members. Most of these questions and concerns are best addressed by an audiologist who evaluates the hearing of the child and determines if a disorder is present. Audiologists are the best qualified individuals to determine if hearing amplification (using hearing aids or an FM system) is a viable alternative for the child and, if so, what type of amplification is best.

Types of Hearing Loss

The deficits in the auditory system are categorized in a number of ways. Based on a child's ability to process linguistic information, and taking into account audiometric findings, a child is diagnosed as hard of hearing or deaf. Hearing is typically measured at 500, 1000, 2000, and 4000 Hz. The hearing level of pure tones at 500, 1000, and 2000 Hz (the speech frequencies) is averaged in the better ear. If the loss is 70 dB or more, the individual is considered to be deaf. If the loss is in the 35- to 69-dB range in the better ear, the individual is considered to be hard of hearing (Northern & Downs, 1984).

Conductive hearing losses are those that occur due to a breakdown in the ability of the middle ear to receive the acoustic signals from the environment and then to transmit the acoustic information to the inner ear (Figure 2–6). **Sensorineural hearing losses** refer to those that occur in the inner ear. Sensorineural losses are divided into those that occur due to damage to the inner ear (sensory loss), and those due to damage to the eighth cranial nerve (neural loss).

Another method used to categorize hearing loss is through the use of the terms **peripheral hearing loss** and **central deafness**. Conductive hearing losses and losses related to malfunction of the inner ear make up the losses associated with peripheral hearing loss. Damage to the eighth nerve in the brain stem or to the cortex is frequently referred to as central deafness. A child also may demonstrate a mixed hearing loss, which means that the child has components of a conductive and of a sensorineural hearing loss, both peripheral deficits.

Prelingual and Postlingual Hearing Loss

It is not unusual for a child with prelingual hearing impairment to exhibit disorders of language content, use, and form, as outlined in Table 2–1. **Prelingual hearing impairment** means the hearing loss was acquired before the child developed language. Early detection is absolutely critical because it enhances the opportunity to provide early intervention to help the child use any residual hearing that may be present. Crystal and Varley (1993) reported that 95% of babies born deaf have some residual hearing, and their prognosis for development of speech increases with early detection. This figure certainly supports the need for routine screening of hearing in all neonates. The extent of the handicap, particularly in the area of the form of his or her

Conductive hearing loss. Hearing loss due to inability of the middle ear to receive or transmit acoustic information.

Sensorineural hearing loss. Hearing loss due to malfunctioning of either the inner ear, or due to damage to the acoustic nerve.

Peripheral hearing loss. Conductive hearing losses and losses related to malfunction of the inner ear.

Central deafness. Damage to the eighth nerve, in the brain stem, or in the cortex.

Prelingual hearing loss. The acquisition of a hearing loss prior to the development of speech and language.

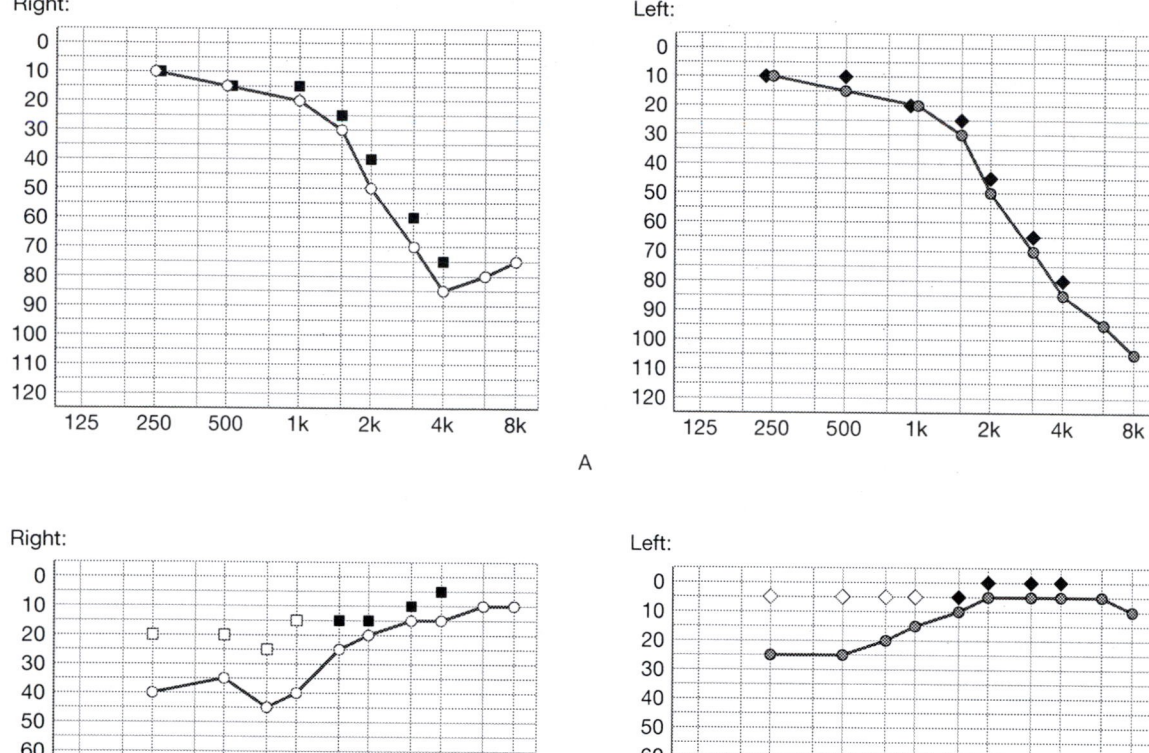

FIGURE 2–6. Audiograms illustrating two types of hearing loss. **A.** Sensorineural hearing loss. **B.** Conductive hearing loss.

Postlingual hearing loss. The acquisition of a hearing loss after the development of speech and language.

Otitis media. Inflammation of the middle ear.

language, may be affected by the child's use of the residual hearing, appropriate stimulation in the environment, and use of the proper amplification systems. Typically, children with **postlingual hearing loss**, who acquire their hearing loss after they develop language, are expected to do better than do prelingually deaf children.

Levels of Hearing Loss

If a child has a mild hearing loss, it is particularly important to determine if the loss is permanent or fluctuating. Children who are prone to repeated occurrences of **otitis media** and **otitis media with effusion** will experience

TABLE 2–1. Impact of hearing loss on language development and use.

Amount of Loss	Degree of Impact	Characteristics
15–30 dB	Mild	Can still hear all vowels and most voiced consonant sounds; may miss voiceless consonants, which will have an impact on morphology
30–50 dB	Moderate	Vowels heard more clearly than consonants; has difficulty understanding spoken language; misses word endings and unstressed words; form is the most severely impacted feature of language
50–70 dB	Severe	Will not hear most speech sounds, and conversational speech is delayed; hears own voice and loud noises in environment; content, form, and use of language are disrupted
70 dB+	Profound	Cannot hear spoken language; may hear own vocalizations, rhythmic patterns, and extremely loud noises; form, content, and use are significantly disrupted

Source: Adapted from *Hearing in Children.* (4th ed.), by H. L. Northern and M. P. Downs (1991). Baltimore, MD: Williams & Wilkins. Copyright 1991 Williams and Wilkins.

fluctuating hearing losses depending on the presence of fluid in the middle ear system. These children should be followed to be sure they are acquiring all their speech sounds and language concepts as expected, but it is rare that extensive intervention is needed. However, if a child has a permanent mild hearing loss, it is worth doing some level of intervention, which may range from environmental manipulation to parent training to direct speech and language therapy. These children may be missing some of the subtleties in our speech and language, so early prevention intervention is warranted.

A child with a moderate hearing loss is very likely to benefit from amplification to facilitate the understanding of conversational speech. It is expected that a child with a moderate hearing loss will have trouble with auditory perception, auditory discrimination, and auditory memory, as many speech signals are distorted or absent. **Auditory perception** refers to the child's ability to hear specific environmental and speech sounds.

Auditory discrimination is the child's ability to identify specific sounds by their source or their acoustical features, or by both. **Auditory memory**

Otitis media with effusion. Inflammation of the middle ear accompanied by the accumulation of infected fluid.

Auditory perception. The ability to hear specific environmental and speech sounds.

Auditory discrimination. The ability to identify specific sounds by their source and/or acoustical properties.

Auditory memory. The ability to remember sounds in their proper sequence.

refers to the child's ability to remember sounds in their proper sequence. Auditory memory deficits will affect a child's capabilities with regard to remembering how sounds are sequenced in particular words, a deficit that will certainly hinder a child's speech and language abilities.

Speech and language skills are likely to be delayed or disordered (or both) in children with severe hearing loss, even when identified at an early age and the child is provided with adequate and appropriate amplification. It is likely that the child will experience differences in vocal quality and have trouble with the production of all speech sounds, as he or she will have trouble discerning the acoustic qualities of speech. None of these problems is insurmountable as long as the hearing loss is identified early, appropriate amplification is provided, and speech and language intervention is implemented.

For children with a profound hearing loss, the ability to discriminate speech will be greatly hindered, even with amplification. They will continue to rely on tactile and visual cues and will most likely benefit from a Total Communication approach, particularly if they are very young.

Regardless of the level of hearing impairment, there is no doubt that it can have an effect on the child's use of the features of language. These effects are summarized in Tables 2–2 through 2–4. Table 2–2 lists the effects of hearing impairment on form, including phonology, syntax, and morphology.

TABLE 2–2. Effects of hearing loss on form (phonology, syntax, and morphology).

Impaired intelligibility

Consonant deletions, particularly final consonants

Impaired production of vowels

Reduced speech rate

Slow articulatory transitions

Frequent pauses

Poor coordination of breathing patterns and syntactic phrasing

Inappropriate use of stressed and unstressed syllables

Delay in developmental syntax

Use of innovative syntactical structures by deaf children

Difficulty with verbs and pronouns

Decreased use of unstressed, final inflectional morphemes (plurals and verb endings)

Decreased use of some parts of speech, including adverbs, prepositions, quantifiers, and indefinite pronouns

Receptive and expressive delays in acquisition of morphological rules

Receptive and expressive delays in acquisition of syntactical rules

---

Source: Adapted from *Childhood Language Disorders in Context: Infancy Through Adolescence,* by N. Nelson, 1993, New York: Merrill.

TABLE 2–3. Effects of hearing loss on semantics (vocabulary comprehension and production).

Difficulty understanding and using concept words

Difficulty with figurative meanings of words and phrases

Difficulty with multiple-meaning words

Difficulty with connected discourse in oral language

Difficulty with connected discourse in written language

Source: Adapted from *Childhood Language Disorders in Context: Infancy Through Adolescence,* by N. Nelson, 1993, New York: Merrill.

TABLE 2–4. Effects of hearing loss on use (pragmatics).

Communication skills which exceed their semantic abilities

Use of gestures, some invented, to convey linguistic function

Better response to questions than comments

Lack of complexity in discourse

Source: Adapted from *Childhood Language Disorders in Context: Infancy Through Adolescence,* by N. Nelson, 1993, New York: Merrill.

The information in Table 2–3 is a review of the effects of hearing loss on semantics, or the content of language. It is expected that children with hearing loss would have more difficulty extrapolating meaning associated with words. Curtiss, Prutting, and Lowell (1979) found that hearing impaired children tend to use more talk about location than do hearing children.

In Table 2–4, the effects of hearing loss on the use domain, or pragmatic domain, of language are described. Infants and toddlers will use a greater variety of pragmatic methods than do many school-age children. In fact, Curtiss et al. (1979) found that pragmatic skills were not as delayed or disordered in hearing impaired preschoolers as were semantic skills (Nelson, 1993).

■ LANGUAGE DISORDERS ASSOCIATED WITH PREMATURITY AND/OR HIGH-RISK INFANCY

"Failure to Thrive" Babies

Some infants are diagnosed as "failure to thrive" babies because they are physically small or delayed in their overall development. Although this syndrome is due to a variety of factors, emotional or physical abuse (or both) and neglect are often responsible for the developmental defects. Often, these children are the babies of teenage parents, many of whom have their own physical and emotional needs unmet for a variety of reasons. In such instances it is difficult to isolate one factor that is responsible for the developmental delays. Malnutrition before and after birth can lead to decreased neurological development, with some babies having undersized brains. In fact, lack of stimulation in an otherwise healthy brain also can lead to brains with less intricate neural connections (Fewell, personal communication, 1996). The clinical criteria used to diagnose children who fail to thrive include weight below the third percentile followed by weight gain in the presence of normal nurturing. Also, the failure to grow has to be present in the absence of evidence of systemic diseases or other abnormalities based on physical examination and laboratory studies. Initially, babies who fail to thrive may show signs of developmental retardation, although acceleration in subsequent development may occur with appropriate stimulation (Barbero, 1982).

Prematurity

Premature babies may be classified primarily into one of three categories: appropriate for gestational age (AGA), small for gestational age (SGA), and very low birth weight (VLBW) (Rossetti, 1986), with differing outcomes with regard to physical, cognitive, and language development. Normally, children are born after 38 weeks of gestation and weigh more than 2,500 grams. Full-term infants who do not weigh at least 2,500 grams are considered SGA babies, and they may be at risk for developmental disabilities. Even though some of these SGA babies may have relatively normal IQs, research indicates that they frequently have major neurological deficits and have an increased frequency of placement in special education or related services when they reach school age (Rossetti, 1986).

Babies who are born too early (i.e., those who are preterm and SGA) are frequently categorized as VLBW babies. These babies vary in their development, with those who weigh more than 1,500 grams doing significantly better than those who weigh less than 1,500 grams (Rossetti, 1986). In 1973, Fitzhardinger and Ramsey found that 15 to 35% of VLBW infants had delayed speech and language development when they were 24 months old.

■ PRENATAL EXPOSURE TO ALCOHOL AND OTHER DRUGS

Fetal Alcohol Syndrome (FAS) and Fetal Alcohol Effects (FAE)

Although recent news reports have focused more on the effects of drugs such as cocaine on a fetus, research clearly shows that alcohol is the worst drug in terms of pervasive, lifelong effects on the fetus (Trace, 1993). Statistics indicate that fetal alcohol syndrome affects one in every 500 to 600 live births annually; fetal alcohol effects are found in one of every 350 live births (Owens, 2004). Fetal alcohol syndrome occurs almost 10 times as often in the Native American and Alaskan American populations, two populations that are known to drink excessively (Trace, 1993).

Fetal alcohol syndrome is one of the leading causes, and the most preventable cause, of mental handicaps in the United States (Gerber, 1998). It is estimated that one-third to two-thirds of all children in special education settings have been affected by alcohol in some way. They often have other associated birth defects, including facial anomalies and growth retardation. The estimated cost of treating a child with fetal alcohol syndrome over the course of a lifetime is $1.4 million.

In order to be diagnosed as having fetal alcohol syndrome, a child must exhibit three primary symptoms: growth retardation, facial anomalies, and central nervous system deficits. If a child does not exhibit symptoms in all three categories, he or she may be diagnosed as fetal alcohol effects, which is diagnosed three times as often as fetal alcohol syndrome. In fetal alcohol effects, the child will usually exhibit signs of central nervous system dysfunction but may not have signs of growth retardation and facial anomalies.

Numerous physical characteristics are associated with fetal alcohol syndrome. Both prenatal and postnatal growth deficiencies are present, including insufficient development of the head circumference. This is particularly significant because it has been documented that if head circumference is below the 5th percentile, a child is at high risk for developmental disabilities. Other physical anomalies include short stature (from birth), small fingers and toes that are bent or webbed, abnormal palmar creases, hip dislocations, and kidney defects. Club feet, minor genital abnormalities, abnormal pigmentation ("strawberry" birthmarks), heart defects, and generalized failure to thrive also have been noted. Drawings depicting the physical characteristics of FAS are found in Figure 2–7.

As stated earlier, a child with full-blown fetal alcohol syndrome also exhibits characteristic facial features. These features include eyes that appear slanted, small, or squinty, with short eye slits and droopy eyelids. Typically, the eyes are widely spaced or crossed. The upper lip is usually narrow, with no groove between the lip and nose. The nose is flat, and, during infancy, the child usually has a flat midface with a small rounded chin and jaw. In later childhood, the face appears elongated. Mild to moderate hearing loss and large or malformed ears are frequent anomalies, particularly in fetal alcohol syndrome. Cleft lip and cleft palate also are common.

In addition to the facial and physical characteristics, central nervous system dysfunction is always present in fetal alcohol syndrome and is very common in children with fetal alcohol effects. With regard to mental functioning, a

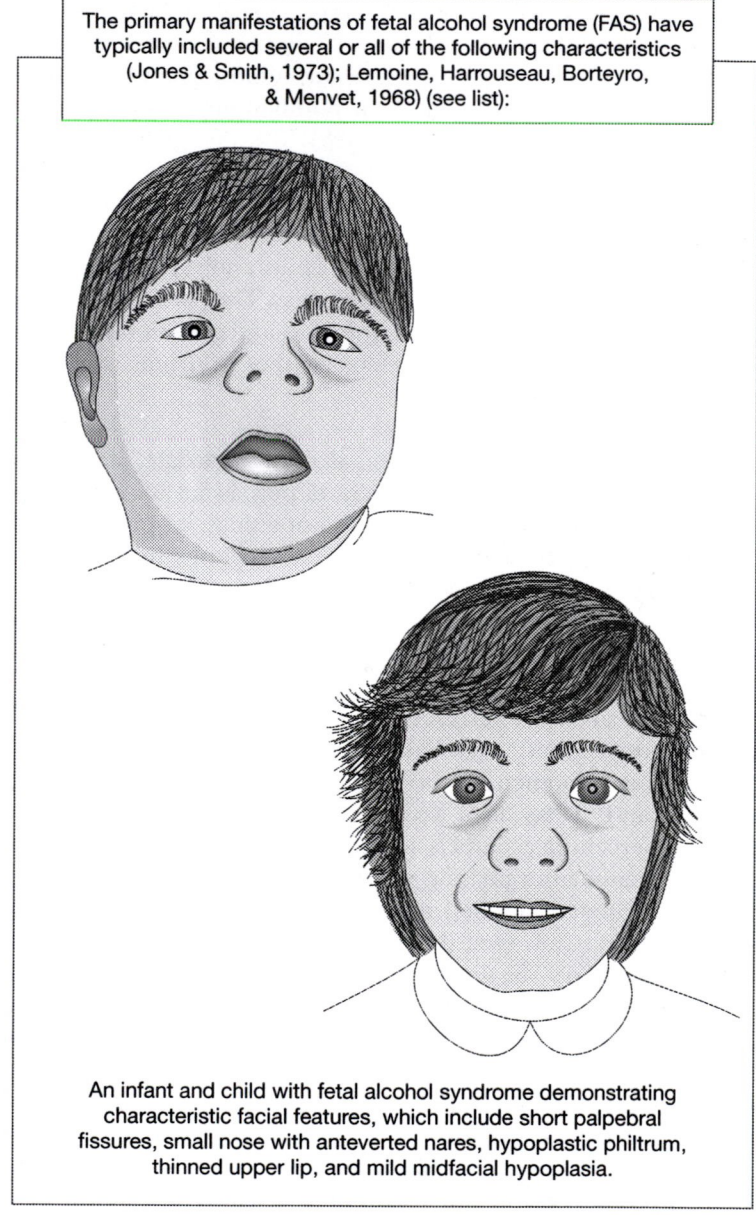

The primary manifestations of fetal alcohol syndrome (FAS) have typically included several or all of the following characteristics (Jones & Smith, 1973); Lemoine, Harrouseau, Borteyro, & Menvet, 1968) (see list):

An infant and child with fetal alcohol syndrome demonstrating characteristic facial features, which include short palpebral fissures, small nose with anteverted nares, hypoplastic philtrum, thinned upper lip, and mild midfacial hypoplasia.

FIGURE 2–7. Characteristics of children with fetal alcohol syndrome. Adapted from *Genetic Syndromes in Communication Disorders* (Austin, TX: Pro-Ed, 1988).

child with fetal alcohol syndrome typically functions in the mild to moderate range of intelligence, with an average IQ around 70. Behavioral problems, including attention deficit disorder, are also common. Subtle learning problems due to cognitive deficits often are exhibited by children with fetal alcohol effects, including poor attention skills, poor judgment, and memory deficits. These characteristics often carry over to adulthood, and children and adults with either of these disorders frequently are considered underachievers. The picture is further complicated by the frequent presence of impulsivity and hyperactivity, tremors, restlessness, and frequent temper tantrums.

Cocaine or Polydrug-Exposed Infants

It is a difficult task to separate the effects of specific drugs on developing babies because, in numerous cases, the mother may be abusing a variety of drugs, including alcohol. Therefore, it is probably more correct to talk about polydrug-exposed babies than about specific drugs. Environmental factors also must be considered because many of these women live in substandard situations. Drug-exposed babies are more vulnerable to other developmental deficits and disorders owing to undesirable conditions such as prematurity, poor nutrition, lack of prenatal health care, and poor to no environmental stimulation. In fact, Griffith (1992) points out that there are three erroneous assumptions about babies exposed to drugs: "(1) That all cocaine-exposed children are severely affected, (2) that little can be done for them, and (3) that all the medical, behavioral, and learning problems exhibited by these children are caused directly by their exposure to cocaine" (p. 30). In actuality, not enough long-term data are available to determine how severely or extensively affected the children are. Also, as pointed out previously, because it is likely that the mothers of these children do not limit their drug use to cocaine, it is a misnomer to call these children "cocaine babies."

Prenatal drug exposure causes some changes in the function and organization of the central nervous system. Typically, babies who have been exposed to cocaine or other drugs have poorly organized nervous systems, resulting in a state of physiological disorganization. In these babies, basic functions such as body temperature and arousal states become disorganized and erratic. The infants also tend to have low thresholds of tolerance for visual and auditory stimulation. In fact, they spend so much time and energy trying to maintain some level of internal organization that they have no stamina with which to interact or react to healthy stimulation from the environment (Griffith, 1992).

This disorganized state is often misinterpreted as an apparent inability to form attachments. In reality, it may be that one of the most important stimulations a mother shares with her baby—eye contact—is too much stimulation for a baby with a low threshold for sensory input. The complexity of the human face may be more input than a physiologically disorganized baby can handle. Thus, at feeding time, the child may not be able to use a coordinated sucking pattern to receive adequate nutrition. In a state of frustration, the mother may interpret the child's attempts to avoid eye contact and physical closeness as signs of rejection (Griffith, 1992).

By 1 month of age, most babies can learn to control the environment, and the mother and baby work in synchrony to recognize the meaning behind different vocalizations. For example, a mother quickly learns to interpret her baby's cries as indicating hunger, loneliness, or discomfort. Accordingly, the mother learns what response to make and how to grade the amount of stimulation the baby needs according to the baby's reaction.

An intervention program conducted by Griffith and his colleagues at the National Association for Perinatal Addiction Research and Education studied the interactions between mothers who had abused cocaine with or without other drugs and their infants. As part of their findings, Griffith points out that the differences between babies who were and were not exposed to drugs prenatally are greatest during the first few weeks of life (Griffith, 1992). The investigators found that very simple interventions helped the babies to become neurologically organized and improved the interactions between the mothers and their babies. For example, simply patting the baby at the rate of one pat per second (approximately the same rate as a normal heart beat) helped the baby to coordinate his or her sucking pattern. If this were paired with having the mother divert her face from the baby, the infant's internal organization continued to improve. Gradually, the mothers were able to reintroduce the stimulation associated with eye contact without having the baby react in a negative manner. Vertical (as opposed to the more typical horizontal) rocking also was shown to improve the babies' physiological states.

We cannot ignore the fact that other factors exist that may prolong or aggravate the long-term effects of drug use during pregnancy. For example, it is likely that the mother will continue to abuse drugs after the birth of the baby. This may be part of a cyclical pattern that interfaces with the baby's disorganized state. It is also possible that the mother's childhood experiences may affect her own child-rearing practices. Other environmental factors common in the homes of mothers who abuse drugs include poor postnatal nutrition and lack of postnatal health care for the baby and the mother.

Triggers for Behavioral Withdrawal or Increased Impulsivity

Clearly, the environment will play a role in the development of any child. For the child in an inconsistent environment, the amount of stimulation that is provided may be too little to facilitate cognitive, emotional, and social growth. Yet the same degree of stimulation might be too much for a baby with a disorganized nervous system.

Lack of structure in the home environment can lead to inappropriate and ineffective stimulation for a newborn baby. In an attempt to develop self-regulation, the infant is likely to express numerous signals of distress that can exacerbate the mother's feelings of distress and frustration. One way the baby will try to cope with his or her physiological distress is through gaze aversion. By shifting his or her own gaze away from the mother, the baby is systematically decreasing the amount of stimulation he or she is receiving from the mother. However, in addition to this behavioral phenomenon, the baby can exhibit a number of physiological distress signals, such as yawning, hiccoughing, sneezing, color changes, increased movement, crying, and increased rate of respiration.

As the baby gets older, he or she will have difficulty adjusting to new environments, with much the same type of difficulty as in the initial months of life. At a time when he or she should be learning basic cognitive processes through developmental tasks, the infant may have trouble learning through environmental stimulation, particularly those skills that lead to the ability to master complex tasks at the later stages of development. Finally, it is possible that babies who are not able to organize themselves in a disorganized environment will also have difficulty shifting tasks and handling change as they get older. This is particularly important when we consider that many babies born to addicted mothers may experience numerous shifts in their environments if they have to be moved from one care setting to another. The good news is that numerous techniques can be used to help the baby organize internal systems so he or she can benefit from normal environmental stimulation. These techniques are discussed in Chapter 4.

■ CYTOMEGALOVIRUS INFECTION

Cytomegalovirus (CMV) infection is a viral disease that results in brain damage to babies who become infected during childhood. The infection can lead to destruction of brain tissues and result in mental handicapping conditions. CMV infections can be contracted prenatally and postnatally, with the more devastating effects being seen when it is contracted prior to birth. It is the most common viral disease in fetuses and newborn babies, with approximately 3,000 infants being affected annually (Johnson, 1996). Infants who are born with CMV infection and survive have a high rate of mental handicaps, sensory deficits, motor disabilities, and seizure disorders (Johnson, 1996). The drawing in Figure 2–8 shows physical characteristics of a child with CMV. In developed countries where rubella has been eradicated, CMV is probably the most common causative factor of nonhereditary congenital hearing loss, and the loss is usually sensorineural. Jung (1989, p. 261) writes that otoneurological complications secondary to CMV include "extensive invasion of the cochlea and semicircular canals as well as structures of the central auditory nervous system, including the cochlear nuclei, brainstem nuclei, and cerebral cortex."

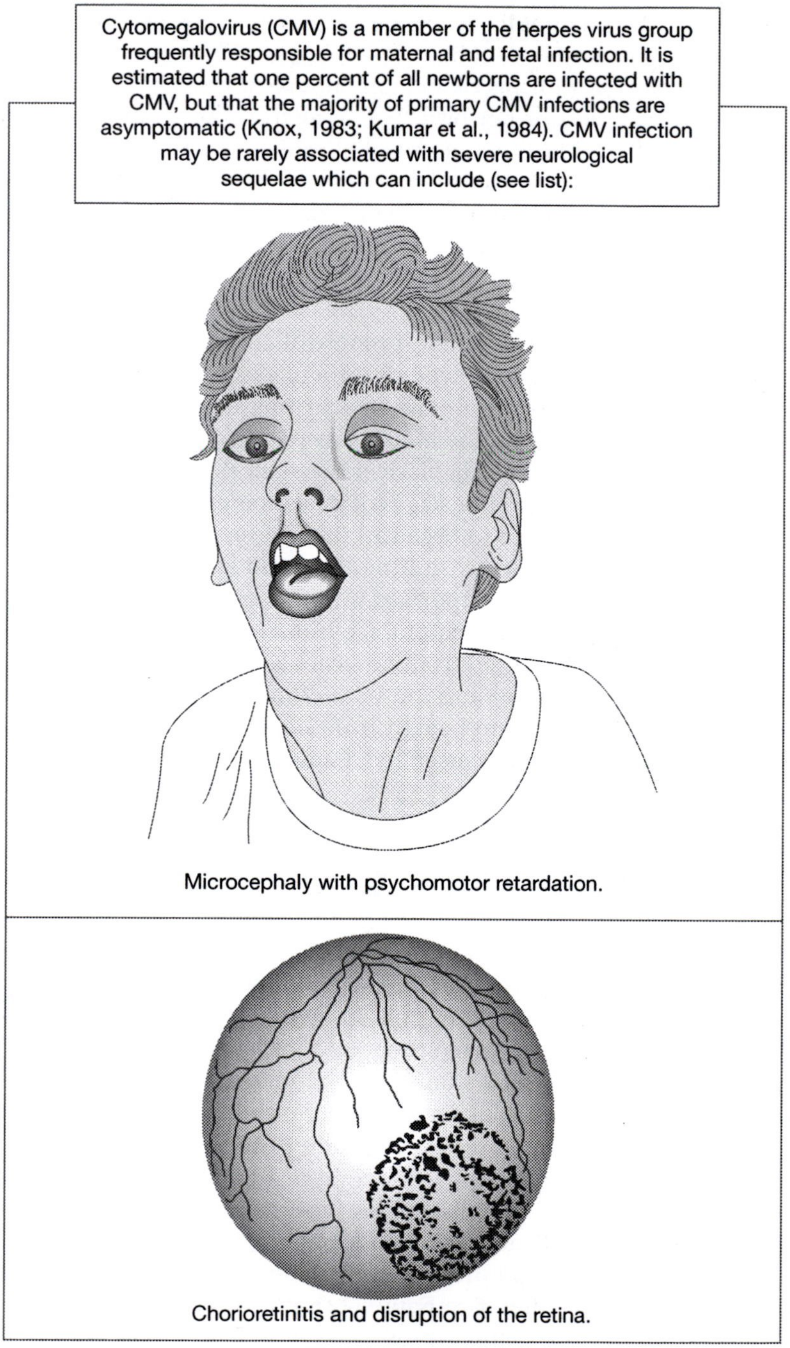

Cytomegalovirus (CMV) is a member of the herpes virus group frequently responsible for maternal and fetal infection. It is estimated that one percent of all newborns are infected with CMV, but that the majority of primary CMV infections are asymptomatic (Knox, 1983; Kumar et al., 1984). CMV infection may be rarely associated with severe neurological sequelae which can include (see list):

Microcephaly with psychomotor retardation.

Chorioretinitis and disruption of the retina.

FIGURE 2–8. Characteristics of children with fetal cytomegalovirus syndrome. Adapted from *Genetic Syndromes in Communication Disorders* (Austin, TX: Pro-Ed, 1988).

■ SPECIFIC LANGUAGE IMPAIRMENT

Children who have a specific language impairment (SLI) exhibit significant linguistic deficits that cannot be explained by sensory or motor deficits. In other words, they have normal hearing, normal vision, normal motor development, and normal nonverbal intelligence, but they have a deficit in their ability to understand and use language. Children with this condition may be frustrated communicators, but otherwise they are emotionally healthy. In addition, they may be variously identified as any of the following:

1. Language deviant (because their language is different from that of normally developing children)

2. Language delayed (because language development can be normal but slower than usual)

3. Developmentally aphasic (because, in many children with this disorder, the language problem has a neurological basis)

4. Severely language impaired

5. Language disordered (because their language often contains compensatory or unusual elements)

Numerous factors have been associated with children who have SLI. Some children with SLI demonstrate deficits in perceptual skills, often revealing behaviors and skills consistent with those seen in children with **auditory processing** deficits.

Auditory processing. A set of skills including auditory discrimination, auditory analysis, auditory attention, and auditory memory that integrate what is heard with language.

In other cases, impaired processing of information, either auditorily or visually (in the presence of normal auditory and visual acuity), has an impact on the child's understanding and interpretation of language experience in his or her daily environment. Furthermore, many children diagnosed as having SLI have difficulties in learning to read.

The presence or absence of specific brain damage in children with SLI has been contested in the literature for decades. Typically, the research has not supported the presence of brain damage in the absence of other deficits. However, the capabilities of **magnetic resonance imaging (MRI)** have greatly enhanced our ability to detect subtle changes in brain symmetry, which may or may not have significance with regard to language processing (Gauge, Lombardino, & Leonard, 1997). Bedore and Leonard summarize the literature in saying that "immediate family members of children with SLI are from two to seven times more likely than family members of normally developing children to have had language problems themselves" (Bedore & Leonard, 1998, p. 1186).

Magnetic resonance imaging (MRI). The use of large electromagnets that manipulate the spin of the hydrogen molecules to differentiate between white matter (which is composed primarily of neurons and related processes) and gray matter (bundles of nerve fibers).

Typically, children with SLI are characterized by language delay, although the amount of delay between different linguistic features may vary greatly. For example, if two features are acquired in a normally developing child at ages 12 months and 15 months, feature number 1 may be acquired in the language delayed child at 24 months, later than the normal 3-month span, but the second feature will not necessarily be acquired until much later. Syntactic deficits are the primary defining feature. In addition, many, but not all, of the children will have pragmatic deficits, which would affect their ability to interact appropriately with their peers. Bedore and Leonard also found that the verb morpheme composite may also be a clinical marker for SLI, but further studies are needed (Bedore & Leonard, 1998).

It is possible that children may have receptive language deficits due to a variety of etiological factors, such as hearing impairment or damage to the auditory processing centers of the brain. These receptive language deficits are sometimes labeled language disorders. A receptive language disorder will interfere with a child's ability to understand language, which will, in turn, affect the child's expressive ability. That is to say, if the child does not understand the language with which others communicate, it is possible that he or she will not develop the content and form of language that is critical to effective communication of ideas. The lack of language comprehension can be due to a variety of reasons, including sensory and physical impairments, trauma, cortical damage, and environmental deprivation of experiences that facilitate language development. However, these types of factors would not explain the presence of SLI.

McNamara, Carter, McIntosh, and Gerken (1998) summarize the literature about the comprehension and use of grammatical morphemes by children with SLI. Grammatical morphemes include copulas, auxiliary verbs, third-person singular inflections, regular past inflections, and articles, and they are rarely used by children with SLI. It is evident "that children with SLI produce fewer grammatical morphemes than age-matched children with normal language (NL), that they produce them with less consistency, and that their limited production of grammatical morphemes persists even as they produce complex syntactic constructions" (McNamara et al., 1998, p. 1147). In their study, McNamara and colleagues hoped to determine if children with SLI are sensitive to grammatical morphemes, and to delineate differences in receptive language between children with SLI and children who are developing language normally. The subjects in their study were 12 children aged 2:6 to 4:8 who were being treated by speech-language pathologists for language impairments. The children with SLI were matched with a control subject, controlling for gender and chronological age, with the normals being ± 15 days of age. In a spontaneous language sample, all of the children with SLI had mean length of utterances below expected based on normative data with 10 of the children having a MLU at least one standard deviation below what would be predicted for children their age. In addition, the children with SLI had a mean of 18% usage of grammatical morphemes, while the controls had a mean of 47%. McNamara's findings include the following:

1. Children with SLI appear to be sensitive to grammatical morphemes because they performed better on sentences that were grammatical than on sentences that were ungrammatical when choosing pictures to represent what they heard;

2. This improved performance on grammatical items is evident even though they may not produce the morphemes in their spontaneous speech;

3. There was no significant difference in the performance of the subjects and the controls on the frequency with which they chose the correct picture representing a grammatical sentence;

4. Poor memory of the target morpheme may play a role in the comprehension and production of grammatical morphemes, but it is not the sole factor.

■ COGNITIVE DISABILITIES

The American Association on Mental Retardation defines mental retardation as "significantly subaverage intellectual functioning resulting in or associated with concurrent impairments in adaptive behavior and manifested during the developmental period." This definition is in contrast with the Developmental Disabilities Assistance and Bill of Rights Act of 1984 (P.L. 98-527) in which a developmental disability is defined as

> a severe chronic disability of a person which (a) is attributable to a mental or physical impairment; (b) is manifested before a person attains age 21; (c) is likely to continue indefinitely; (d) results in substantial limitations in three or more of the following areas of major life activity: (i) self-care, (ii) receptive and expressive language, (iii) learning, (iv) mobility, (v) self-direction, (vi) capacity for independent living, (vii) economic self-sufficiency; and (e) reflects the person's need for a combination and sequence of special, interdisciplinary, or generic care, treatment, or other services which are of lifelong or extended duration and are individually planned and coordinated.

Regardless of the preferred definition, children who are cognitively challenged (or any related term such as mentally challenged, mentally retarded, or mentally disabled) demonstrate intellectual functioning, personal independence, and social responsibility that are below those expected on the basis of their chronological age. If a child does not demonstrate deficits in each of these three areas, the term mentally handicapped is inappropriate. However, we also must look at the age of the person when determining the

TABLE 2–5. Classification by IQ level (Based on and determined by President's Committee on MR, 1977).

Scale	Level	IQ Range
Wechsler Scale	Mild	55–69
	Moderate	40–54
	Severe	25–39
	Profound	0–24

appropriateness of the diagnosis. Developmental scales that delineate the skills and expectations of children beyond age 6 years are quite sparse and inconsistent in their content.

Generally speaking, speech acquisition by children with mental handicaps may parallel that of children with SLI in that they acquire the linguistic features in a normal sequence, but at a slower rate, and may plateau before all are acquired. Also, the children may have multiple handicaps that interfere with the coordination of oral motor skills for speech production.

Traditionally, cognitive handicaps are classified by severity according to the child's IQ status (Table 2–5). Children with profound or severe cognitive handicaps will typically have an etiological history of genetically inherited disabilities, chromosomal deficits, brain injury (either pre-, peri-, or postnatally), head injury, infections, prematurity, gestational disorders, or drug or alcohol abuse by the birth mother. Etiologically, individuals considered to be mildly or moderately cognitively handicapped can trace their deficits to cultural and environmental deprivation, familial patterns, or nutritional deficits, or a combination of these.

With regard to expectations associated with severity classifications, mildly cognitively handicapped (also called educably mentally handicapped) preschoolers would typically have delayed social and communication skills, and minimal retardation in sensorimotor areas of functioning. Many children in this category may not have deficits that are recognized until they reach school age.

During the preschool years, the child who has moderate cognitive handicaps will experience delays in learning to talk and communicate but, as a rule, will eventually develop adequate language skills. The child typically displays poor social awareness and fair motor development (Nelson, 1993).

In contrast, the child who has severe cognitive handicaps will typically have minimal speech development during the preschool years and will continue to have severely limited communication skills as he or she matures. Children at this level of functioning typically have difficulty acquiring self-help skills and poor motor development.

Children who are profoundly cognitively handicapped will show very little development of communication, sensorimotor integration, or self-help skills. These children will have complete dependence on adults. Sensorimotor skills include cognitive concepts such as object permanence, visual pursuit, object relations, spatial relations, means-end, causality, imitation, and gestures. Table 2–6 lists the developmental stages and an explanation of each of these domains is given in Table 2–7. Examples of activities used to assess the domains are listed in Appendix B. An explanation of sensorimotor assessment is given in Chapter 3.

TABLE 2–6. Sensorimotor stages of development.

Stage/Age	Skill	Description
Stage 1 Birth–1 month	Use of reflexes	Organizes motor and perceptual responses to the environment
Stage 2 1–4 months	Primary circular reactions	Use of motor schemes without intention
Stage 3 4–8 months	Secondary circular reactions	Use of motor schemes with intention
Stage 4 8–12 months	Coordination of secondary circular reactions	Can organize and sequence behaviors to achieve a desired response
Stage 5 12–18 months	Tertiary circular reactions	Discovery of new means to accomplish a given objective
Stage 6 18–24 months	Representation and foresight	Mental problem-solving skills

Source: Adapted from *Ordinal Scales of Psychological Development,* by I. C. Uzgiris and J. M. Hunt, 1978. Urbana: University of Illinois Press.

TABLE 2–7. Domains assessed in sensorimotor testing of preschool language disorders.

Assessment Domain	Description
Visual pursuit and object permanence	Ability to maintain perceptual contact with an object that undergoes various transformations
Means-ends	Ability to use own body and objects to obtain goals in the immediate environment and to use foresight in simple problem-solving
Causality	Strategies used to reactivate objects which create an interesting spectacle
Object relations	Ability to use and understand spatial relationships
Schemes	Use of complex behaviors and discriminative use of objects, with recognition of their functional and socially appropriate use

■ AUTISM/PERVASIVE DEVELOPMENTAL DELAY

Autism is defined according to the presence or absence of a variety of behaviors. The *Diagnostic and Statistics Manual of Mental Disorders* (American Psychiatric Association, 1994) lists the following criteria for a diagnosis of autism:

1. Impairment in social interaction: This would include impairment in the use of nonverbal behavior, lack of spontaneous sharing, lack of social/emotional reciprocity, and failure to develop peer relationships;

2. Impairment in communication: The child with autism typically has a delay or lack of development of spoken language and gestures, is impaired in the ability to initiate and/or maintain a conversation, lacks pretend play, and repetitive and idiosyncratic use of language;

3. Restricted repertoire of activities and interest: Preoccupation with restricted patterns of interest, inflexible adherence to routines, repetitive movements, and preoccupation with parts of objects (for example, the wheels on a toy car).

Oftentimes, autism/PDD is not diagnosed until a child is 2 ½ to 3 years of age (Sigman & Capps, 1997). Because of this, there is very little research on children with autism under the age of 2.

Much confusion exists regarding the etiology of autism. Cortical dysfunctions that influence speech and language processing are hypothesized by researchers to be at the root of autism and its related syndromes. Other suspected/associated etiological factors include tuberous sclerosis, maternal rubella, fragile X syndrome, perinatal trauma, and seizure disorders (Hewitt, 1992). Other less specific research points to a malfunctioning of some aspects of the neurologic system. One theory published in 1994, based on results from a small study by DeLong and colleagues at Duke University (Trace, 1996), holds that nonneurologic autism may be an inherited, early onset form of manic depression. The researchers at Duke University studied 40 children diagnosed as having autism or autism spectrum, of which 14 had normal neurologic examinations. In those 14 children there was a strong family history of depression, manic depression, or both. The prevalence of these two disorders in the general population is 1% for manic depression and 8 to 10% for depression. However, in the families of the 14 children, a 26.8% prevalence was found across three generations of parents, grandparents, aunts, uncles, and cousins. In these children with higher level autism, also known as Asperger's syndrome, the researchers were able to isolate a neurochemical disorder in the absence of physical signs of brain damage. They concluded that autism in higher functioning children with apparently normal brains is an inherited psychiatric disorder—probably a neurochemical imbalance—rather than a destructive brain disorder. This is certainly an interesting finding and deserves further study with larger numbers of children to learn more about this perplexing disorder that causes so much distress in families with afflicted children.

Owens (1995) states that symptoms of autism often become more pronounced around 18 months of age. These early symptoms include frequent tantrums and extreme reactions to certain stimuli. The child may exhibit a lack of social play and will have communication deficits. He or she may also start to demonstrate ritualistic play and repetitive movements.

Speech and Language Characteristics in Autism

Many children with autism exhibit frank echolalia. Historically, echolalia was considered to be a symptom of autism that served no meaningful purpose. In 1981, in studies by Prizant and Duchan, a hypothesis was put forth that echolalia actually serves a variety of communicative purposes. The echolalia may serve to acknowledge and/or validate the speaker's input, even if the input is not adequately processed by the child. Imitation by children with autism can be differentiated from that of normally developing children in that the children with autism typically imitate fully phrased and familiar words, while normally developing children tend to imitate new and unfamiliar words. Also, children with autism have more pervasive echolalia than do children with specific language impairment or mental retardation.

Owens (1995) describes language impairment in children with autism as consisting of the following characteristics:

1. Limited range of communication functions

2. Perseverations

3. Overuse of questions

4. Word-retrieval deficits

5. Morphological difficulties

6. Less complex sentences

7. Pragmatic and conversational deficits (lack of initiation, lack of topic maintenance, lack of turn-taking, poor conversational repair)

Rollins (1999) studied the development of pragmatic skills (focusing on the development of communicative means and intents) in five children via a longitudinal parallel case study. She writes that "children with autism have pragmatic deficits both in how they communicate (i.e., communicative means) and how they express intentions (i.e., communicative intents)"

(p. 181). Not all children with autism are verbal, but in those that are there is a preponderance of echolalia (immediate and delayed), neologisms, and use of metaphors (American Psychiatric Association, 1994). Delays in the development of communicative intents include the later development of social intentions ("look at me") than the development of regulatory or instrumental intentions ("give me"). In her study, Rollins analyzed the social interchange level of children with autism. She defined social interchange as "one or more rounds of communication, all of which serve a unitary interactive function, implicitly agreed on by the interlocutors" (p. 184). Rollins cites several studies that indicate that shared attention between an adult and an object is a precursor to the development of early language skills, with regulation and maintenance of shared attention having a strong impact on outcomes of language learning in young children. The development of shared attention and preverbal intentions are problematic for children with autism.

Results of Rollins's study suggest that the children who increased their lexicon exhibited the following skills following intervention:

a. Decreased use of behavioral regulations to less than 40% of the communicative activity

b. Decreased use of unconventional means to less than 30% of the communicative activity

c. Increased use of different communicative contexts (p. 188)

The children with the greatest vocabulary development also developed direct attention and joint focus for more than 40% of their communicative exchanges. Thus, there is a need to use techniques of intervention with children with autism that focus on social-pragmatic devices during the development of a child's lexicon.

Rollins's findings are in keeping with those of Wetherby, Prizant, and Hutchinson (1998), who studied two groups of preschool children: one group of children with a diagnosis of pervasive developmental disorder (PDD), and a second group who had developmental delays in language, but who were not diagnosed with PDD (the DL group). A total of 44 children were assessed, with 35 of them being males. All children were tested using the Communication and Symbolic Behavior Scales (CSBS) (Wetherby & Prizant, 1993), and the examiners did not know to which group each child had been assigned. The CSBS consists of 22 scales that yield seven cluster scores. The first six cluster scores profile communication (communicative functions, gestural communicative means, vocal communicative means, verbal communicative means, reciprocity, and social/affective signaling), and the seventh score addresses symbolic play. The results of their study are listed in Tables 2–8 and 2–9.

TABLE 2–8. Summarization of results for DL group in study by Wetherby, Prizant, and Hutchinson.

Strengths	Communicative functions (behavioral regulation, joint attention, and sociability of functions)
	Reciprocity (respondent acts, rate, repair strategies)
	Social/affective signaling (gaze shifts, shared positive affect, episodes of negative affect)
	Symbolic behavior (language comprehension, inventory of different action schemes, complexity of action schemes, constructive play)
	Social communication skills even if having trouble using sounds and words
Weaknesses	Vocal communicative means (vocal acts without gestures, inventory of different consonants, syllables with consonants, and multisyllables)
	Verbal communicative means (inventory of different words, inventory of different word combinations)

Source: From Wetherby, A. M., Prizant, B. M., and Hutchinson, T. A. (1998, May). Communicative, social/affective, and symbolic profiles of young children with autism and pervasive developmental disorders, *American Journal of Speech-Language Pathology,* 7(2) (May 1998), pp. 79–91. © ASHA, 1998. Reprinted by permission.

TABLE 2–9. Summarization of results for PDDL group in study by Wetherby, Prizant, and Hutchinson.

Poorer scores than the DL group on the following

Communicative functions (behavioral regulation, joint attention, and sociability of functions)

Gestural communicative means (conventional gestures, distal gestures, coordination of gesture, and vocal acts)

Reciprocity (respondent acts, rate, repair strategies)

Social/affective signaling (gaze shifts, shared positive affect, episodes of negative affect)

Symbolic behavior (language comprehension, inventory of different action schemes, complexity of action schemes, constructive play)

Comparable scores to DL Group

Vocal communicative means (vocal acts without gestures, inventory of different consonants, syllables with consonants, and multisyllables)

Verbal communicative means (inventory of different words, inventory of different word combinations)

Weak in sounds and words plus weaknesses in social communicative domains

Source: From Wetherby, A. M., Prizant, B. M., and Hutchinson, T. A. Communicative, social/affective, and symbolic profiles of young children with autism and pervasive developmental disorders, *American Journal of Speech-Language Pathology,* 7(2) (May 1998), pp. 79–91. © ASHA, 1998. Reprinted by permission.

Wetherby and colleagues (1998) summarize several studies in identifying impaired symbolic abilities and social aspects of communication as falling into three primary categories: communicative means, communicative functions, and symbolic play. The primary purpose of communication by a child with autism is to regulate the behavior of others such as requesting others to perform or stop performing a specific action. Their study supports these descriptions and has implications for early identification and early intervention. Some early indicators of autism/PDD include the following:

1. Lack of joint attention

2. Lack of complex gestural communication

3. Lack of reciprocal interaction

4. Poor rate of communication

5. Lack of repair strategies in communication

6. Absence of gaze shifts

7. Poor language comprehension

8. Deficits in symbolic play

Implications for intervention planning based on the work of Wetherby et al. (1998) is that the easiest skill to teach to children with autism/PDD is behavior regulation, and the most difficult to teach is joint attention. "Communicating for social interaction to draw attention to self may be viewed as a transition between communication for behavior regulation to achieve an environmental end and joint attention to draw attention to an object or event" (Wetherby et al., 1998, p. 89). The use of contact gestures should be stressed as a way to enhance communication. Finally, the use of constructive play as a means to develop language and functional use of objects should be incorporated into therapy for children with autism/PDD.

The disruptive behavior most characteristically associated with autism is the failure to develop normal responsivity to other persons (varying degrees of social withdrawal). The emotional devastation felt by family members is compounded by the typical failure to develop normal verbal and nonverbal communication (i.e., an inability to interact appropriately with the environment). Failure to use objects functionally and abnormal fixations on inanimate objects are also widely described characteristics. Under- or overreaction to certain sensory stimuli may be observed, leading clinicians and researchers to believe that the sensory thresholds of children with autism are significantly different from those of people in the general population. Other characteristics frequently observed in children who are diagnosed with autism are listed in Table 2–10.

TABLE 2–10. Characteristics frequently observed in autism and related syndromes.

Failure to develop normal responsivity to other persons

Social withdrawal in varying degrees

Failure to develop normal verbal and nonverbal communication

Failure to use objects functionally and/or appropriately

Abnormal fixations on inanimate objects

Abnormal sensory thresholds (over- or underactive)

Cyclical behavioral extremes

Obsessive traits such as fixations on strange objects

Special abilities to calculate numbers or remember facts

Regression of social and language skills after an early period of normal development

Reluctance or difficulty in forming interpersonal relationships

Preference for being left alone

Use of echolalia (unsolicited imitative verbal behavior)

Monotone speech

Pronoun confusions (particularly I, you)

Articulatory skills exceeding vocabulary, syntax, and social language use (not the case with children who have SLI or MR)

Source: From *Essentials for Speech-Language Pathologists,* by B. Vinson, 2001, p. 172. San Diego: Singular Publishing Group. Copyright 2001 by Singular Publishing Group.

■ ACQUIRED LANGUAGE DISORDERS

Acquired language disorders are due to a variety of reasons, with the most frequent being illnesses such as **meningitis**, convulsive disorders, and head trauma. It is difficult to describe a typical language pattern in children with acquired language disorders because the damage is not consistent across patients owing to variations in the area of the brain that is injured by the trauma or illness. Common after-effects of traumatic brain injury that can influence the degree of damage and subsequent recovery include edema, hypoxia, hemorrhage, and seizure activity (Blosser & DePompei, 1994). The causes of trauma in infants are most frequently reported as accidental dropping of the baby, the infant's rolling off the changing table, and physical abuse. In toddlers and preschoolers, motor vehicle accidents, falls, and physical abuse are the major causes of injury (Blosser & DePompei, 1994). Regardless of the cause, the long-term impact of the injury or illness must be considered, including cumulative effects that develop as heavier developmental demands are placed on the child. In these cases, failure to fully

Meningitis. An inflammation of the meninges lining the brain and/or spinal column.

recover some of the basic cognitive skills may eventually lead to an overtaxing of the system as the child progresses through school. Thus, a deficit may not become apparent until the child reaches school age (Blosser & DePompei, 1994).

Generally, the younger the child, the better the chance for recovery. If the injury or illness occurs before 3 years of age, the child may seem to regress to a point of being mute and unresponsive, then regain his or her linguistic ability, progressing back through normal development. If the damage occurs after 3 years of age, the child will regress, but not as drastically as a younger child. However, the recovery will be slower and less complete and the child typically will have residual word-finding problems.

■ SUMMARY

To understand language disorders in the preschool population more fully, a clinician must develop a sense of what constitutes age-appropriate language behavior. That is to say, a clinician should have a thorough understanding of language development before beginning to assess and treat language disorders. If he or she does not understand the depth and breadth of normal language development, it will be impossible to provide effective and accurate diagnosis and treatment. In the preschool population, this understanding will influence a clinician's own bias with regard to whether or not language precedes cognition or cognition precedes language. It will also affect the clinician's approach to labeling a disorder without understanding the impact of doing so. It is critical to remember that the child is at the center of the philosophical pull, and that it is his or her life that will be most affected by the clinician's decisions.

CASE STUDY

History

L is a 5-year-old boy with Down syndrome. He lives at home with his mother (age 39), who is a nurse, and his father (age 42), who is a salesman. He also has two older brothers (ages 8 and 10) who live in the home. His mother reports no problems with the pregnancy. She took daily prenatal vitamins, but no other medications during the pregnancy.

From 18 months of age until this year, L attended school at the Early Intervention Program. This year he is in a self-contained varying exceptionalities kindergarten class. He receives occupational therapy for one

30-minute session a week at school. He also receives group speech therapy for two 30-minute pull-out sessions a week. The speech-language pathologist also spends two hours a week with L in the classroom as part of a collaborative approach encompassing his goals from speech, occupational therapy, and education.

L has all the physical characteristics typically associated with Down syndrome. He has hypotonic musculature, and he is a mouth-breather. L has had recurrent ear infections since he was 6 months old. He had PE tubes inserted when he was 26 months old. An audiological evaluation revealed a mild (25-dB) hearing loss in the right ear, and normal hearing in the left ear.

Evaluation

L has an expressive vocabulary of approximately 15 single words. He does not combine words. L's cognitive and language skills were assessed using the *Communication and Symbolic Behavior Scales—Developmental Profile* (Wetherby & Prizant, 2002). The results yielded a receptive language age score of 21 months. L takes turns when playing with toys. He demonstrates the concept of object permanence by looking for an item that has been hidden under one of three screens. He enjoys looking at a picture book with an adult and will attend to this activity for about two minutes. Occasionally L will imitate a sound produced by the clinician, and he imitates gestures such as "so big," pointing, and clapping hands, and signs such as "more," "eat," "drink," and "play." He will engage an adult in communication by hand-leading the adult to obtain an object or action and declaring an intent to communicate by giving the adult an object. L understands and responds appropriately to simple commands such as "Go find Daddy."

Summary

L has a receptive language age equivalent of approximately 21 months, and an expressive language age of 15 months.

A summary of L's strengths and weaknesses is a follows:

	Strengths	Weaknesses
Communicative	Pragmatic skills (turn-taking, eye contact, joint attention)	Delayed and limited vocabulary development (expressive and receptive)
	Means-end and causality	Does not combine words

	Likes books	Mild unilateral hearing loss
	Attempts to communicate using single words and gestures; engages adult in communication	
	Sound imitation emerging; imitates gestures and signs	
Noncommunicative	Supportive family	Hypotonia
	Has had early intervention	Poor eye-hand coordination
	Personable	Attention span limited to 2–3 minutes on most tasks
	Feeds and dresses self and is toilet trained	

Recommendations

L should continue to receive speech-language therapy in the school, and additional 1:1 therapy outside the school setting with the school-based clinician and the private therapy clinician sharing goals and procedures to facilitate language and communication growth. Therapy should focus on expanding his receptive language skills and facilitating communication through speech and sign.

■ REVIEW QUESTIONS

1. An etiological classification of language disorders is
   a. Often used when it is necessary to "label" a child for educational placement
   b. Based on defining a language disorder in terms of causative factors
   c. Focuses on the specific features of language in order to define the disorder
   d. b and c
   e. a and b

2. Lack of normal responsivity, failure to use objects functionally, and abnormal fixations on inanimate objects are characteristic of
   a. Being cognitively challenged
   b. Being autistic
   c. Having acquired language disorders
   d. Exhibiting developmental aphasia

3. Which of the following signs must be present for a child to be diagnosed as having fetal alcohol syndrome?

   a. Growth retardation
   b. Central nervous system deficits
   c. Facial anomalies
   d. a, b, and c
   e. b and c
   f. a and b

4. The number one cause of congenital hearing loss, as well as brain damage, in babies who become infected during childhood (prenatally or postnatally) is

   a. Autism
   b. Cytomegalovirus
   c. Fragile X syndrome
   d. Encephalitis

5. The primary etiological factors for children who are mildly to moderately cognitively challenged are environmental and cultural deprivation, familial patterns, and/or nutritional deficits.

   a. True
   b. False

6. In Robin deformation sequence, the problems are intrinsic to the baby.

   a. True
   b. False

7. Children with velo-cardio-facial syndrome usually have a mild language delay but typically catch up with their peers by 36 to 48 months of age.

   a. True
   b. False

8. A sequence is defined by Shprintzen as "the presence of multiple anomalies in the same individual with all of those anomalies having a single cause."

   a. True
   b. False

9. In children with Down syndrome, expressive language is usually more intact than receptive language.

   a. True
   b. False

10. All children with cerebral palsy will have some type of language deficit.

    a. True
    b. False

■ REFERENCES

American Psychiatric Association (1994). *Diagnostic and statistical manual of mental disorders* (4th ed., rev.). Washington, DC: Author.

American Speech-Language-Hearing Association. (1980). Definitions for communicative disorders and differences. *Asha, 22*(4), 317–318.

Barbero, G. (1982). Failure to thrive. In M. H. Klaus, T. Leger, & M. A. Trause (Eds.), *Maternal attachment and mothering disorders: Pediatric round table: 1.* Skillman, NJ: Johnson & Johnson Baby Products Company.

Bates, E., Benigni, L., Bretherton, I., Camaioni, L., & Volterra, V. (1979). *The emergence of symbols: Cognition and communication in infancy.* New York: Academic Press.

Bedore, L. M, & Leonard, L. B. (1998, October). Specific language impairment and grammatical morphology: A discriminant function analysis. *Journal of Speech, Language, and Hearing Research, 41*(5), 1185–1192.

Blank, C. E. (1960). Apert's syndrome (a type of acrocephalosyndactyly). Observations on a British series of thirty-nine cases. Annals of Human Genetics, 24, 151–164.

Blosser, J. L., & DePompei, R. (1994). *Pediatric traumatic brain injury: Proactive intervention.* San Diego: Singular Publishing Group.

Caselli, M. C., Vicari, S., Longobardi, E., Lami, L., Pizzoli, C., & Stella, S. (1998, October). Gestures and words in early development of children with Down syndrome. *Journal of Speech, Language, and Hearing Research, 41*(5), 1125–1135.

Chapman, R. S. (1995). Language development in children and adolescents with Down syndrome. In P. Fletcher & B. MacWhinney (Eds.), *The handbook of child language* (pp. 641–663). Oxford: Blackwell.

Crystal, D., & Varley, R. (1993). *Introduction to language pathology* (3rd ed). San Diego: Singular Publishing Group.

Curtiss, S., Prutting, C. A., & Lowell, E. L. (1979). Pragmatic and semantic development in young children with hearing impairment. *Journal of Speech and Hearing Research, 22,* 534–552.

de Grouchy, J., & Turleau, C. (1984). 21 trisomy. Clinical Atlas of Human Chromosomes (p. 338). New York: John Wiley and Sons.

Fabbretti, D., Pizzuto, E., Vicari, S., & Volterra, V. (1997). A story description task in children with Down syndrome: Lexical and morphosyntactic abilities. *Journal of Intellectual Disability Research, 41,* 165–179.

Fenson et al. (1993). *MacArthur Communicative Development Inventories: User's guide and technical manual.* San Diego: Singular Publishing Group.

Fewell, R. (1996). Personal communication.

Fitzhardinger, P., & Ramsey, M. (1973). The improving outlook for the small prematurely born infant. *Developmental Medicine and Child Neurology, 15,* 447.

Fowler, A. E. (1990). Language abilities in children with Down syndrome: Evidence for a specific syntactic delay. In D. Cicchetti & M. Beeghly (Eds.), *Children with Down syndrome: A developmental perspective* (pp. 302–328). Cambridge: Cambridge University Press.

Gauge, L. M., Lombardino, L. J., & Leonard, C. M. (1997). Brain morphology in children with specific language impairment. *Journal of Speech, Language, and Hearing Research, 40,* 1272–1284.

Gerber, S. E. (1998). *Etiology and prevention of communicative disorders* (2nd ed.). San Diego: Singular Publishing Group.

Gorlin, R., & Pindborg, J. (1976). *Syndromes of the head and neck.* New York: McGraw-Hill.

Griffith, D. R. (1992, September). Prenatal exposure to cocaine and other drugs: Developmental and educational prognoses. *Phi Delta Kappan,* pp. 30–34.

Hewitt, L. E. (1992, March). *Facilitating narrative comprehension: The importance of subjectivity.* Paper presented at the Conference on Pragmatics: From Theory to Therapy, State University of New York, Buffalo.

Johnson, B. A. (1996). *Language disorders in children: An introductory clinical perspective.* Albany, NY: Delmar Publishers.

Jonews, K. L., & Smith, D. W. (1973). Recognition of the fetal alcohol syndrome in early infancy. *Lancet, 2,* 999–1001.

Jung, J. H. (1989). *Genetic syndromes in communication disorders.* Boston: College-Hill.

Knox, G. E. (1983). Cytomegalovirus: Patient counseling. *Seminars in Perinatology, 7*(1), 43–46.

Kumar, M., Nankeris, T. G., Jacobs, I., Ernhart, C., Glasson, C., McMillan, P., & Gold, E. (1984). Congenital and postnasally acquired cytomegalovirus infections: Long-term follow-up. *Journal of Pediatrics, 104,* 674–679.

Lemoine, P., Harrousseau, H., Borteyro, J. P., & Menvet, J. C. (1968). Les enfants de parents alcoholoques: anomalies observees, a propose de 127 cas. Archives Francaise de Pediatrie, 25, 830–832.

McNamara, M., Carter, A., McIntosh, B., & Gerken, L. (1998, October). Sensitivity to grammatical morphemes in children with specific language impairment. *Journal of Speech, Language, and Hearing Research, 41*(5), 1147–1157.

Nelson, N. W. (1993). *Childhood language disorders in context.* New York: Merrill Publishing Company.

Northern, H. L., & Downs, M. P. (1984). *Hearing in children* (3rd ed.). Baltimore, MD: Williams and Wilkins.

Northern, H. L., & Downs, M. P. (1991). *Hearing in children.* (4th ed.). Baltimore, MD: Williams and Wilkins.

Nyhan, W. L. (1983). Cytogenetic diseases. *Clinical Symposia, 35*(1). West Caldwell, NJ: Ciba.

Owens, R. E. (1995). *Language disorders: A functional approach to assessment and intervention* (2nd ed.). Needham Heights, MA: Allyn and Bacon.

Owens, R. E. (2004). *Language disorders: A functional approach to assessment and intervention* (4th ed.). Needham Heights, MA: Allyn and Bacon.

Papolos, D. F., Faedda, G. L., Veit, S., Goldberg, R., Morrow, B., Kucherlapati, R., & Shprintzen, R. J. (1996). Bipolar spectrum disorders in patients diagnosed with velo-cardio-facial syndrome: Does a hemizygous deletion of chromosome 22q11 result in bipolar affective disorder? *American Journal of Psychiatry, 153,* 1541–1547.

Pore, S. G., & Reed, K. L. (1999). *Quick reference to speech-language pathology.* Gaithersburg, MD: Aspen.

President's Committee on Mental Retardation (1977). *Mental retardation: Past and present.* Washington, D. C.: U. S. Government Printing Office.

Prizant, B. M., & Duchan, J. F. (1981). The functions of immediate echolalia in autistic children. *Journal of Speech and Hearing Disorders, 46,* 127–142.

Pueschel, S. M. (1987). Health concerns in persons with Down syndrome. In S. M. Pueschel, C. Tingey, J. E. Rynders, A. C. Corcker, & D. M. Crutcher (Eds.), *New perspectives on Down syndrome.* Baltimore, MD: Paul H. Brookes.

Riski, John (1999, October). VCF: Neurological findings impacting speech. *Proceedings from 12th Annual Symposium on Cleft Lip and Palate and Related Conditions,* Atlanta, GA.

Roberts, J. E., Mirrett, P., Anderson, K., Burchinal, M., & Neeve, E. (2002, August). Early communication, symbolic behavior, and social profiles of young men with fragile X syndrome. *American Journal of Speech-Language Pathology, 11*(3), 295–304.

Rollins, P. R. (1999, May). Early pragmatic accomplishments and vocabulary development in preschool children with autism. *American Journal of Speech-Language Pathology, 8*(2), 181–190.

Rondal, J. A. (1993). Down's syndrome. In D. Bishop & K. Mogford (Eds.), *Language development in exceptional circumstances.* East Sussex, UK: Lawrence Erlbaum Associates, Ltd.

Rossetti, L. (1986). *High risk infants: Identification, assessment, and intervention.* Boston: College-Hill Publications.

Sigman, M., & Capps, L. (1997). *Children with autism: A developmental perspective.* Cambridge, MA: Harvard University Press.

Shprintzen, R. J. (1997). *Genetics, syndromes, and communication disorders.* San Diego: Singular Publishing Group, Inc.

Shprintzen, R. J. (2000). *Syndrome identification for speech-language pathology: An illustrated pocket guide.* San Diego: Singular Publishing Group.

Sparks, S. N. (1984). *Birth defects and speech-language disorders.* San Diego: College-Hill Press.

Stoel-Gammon, C. (1981). Speech development of infants and children with Down syndrome. In J. Darby, Jr. (Ed.), *Speech evaluation in medicine* (pp. 341–360). New York: Grune & Stratton.

Tiegerman-Farber, E. (1995). *Language and communication intervention in preschool children.* Boston: Allyn and Bacon.

Trace, R. (1993, June 21). Fetal alcohol syndrome. *Advance for Speech-Language Pathologists and Audiologists.*

Trace, R. (1996, January 8). Research links infantile autism, manic depression. *Advance for Speech-Language Pathologists and Audiologists,* pp. 3, 14.

Turnerm G., Opitz, J. M., Brown, W. T., et al. (1986). Conference report: Second international workshop on fragile X and X-linked mental retardation. *American Journal of Medical Genetics, 23,* 11–68.

Uzgiris, I. C., & Hunt, J. M. (1978). *Assessment in infancy: Ordinal scales of psychological development.* Urbana: University of Illinois Press.

Vinson, B. P. (2001). *Essentials for speech-language pathologists.* San Diego: Singular Publishing Group.

Wetherby, A. M., & Prizant, B. M. (1993). *Communication and symbolic behavior scales.* Chicago: Riverside.

Wetherby, A. M., & Prizant, B. M. (2002). *Communication and symbolic behavior scales developmental profile.* Baltimore, MD: Brookes.

Wetherby, A. M., Prizant, B. M., & Hutchinson, T. A. (1998, May). Communicative, social/affective, and symbolic profiles of young children with autism and pervasive developmental disorders. *American Journal of Speech-Language Pathology, 7*(2), 79–91.

Wheaton, S. W. (1894). Two specimens of congenital cranial deformity in infants associated with fusion of the fingers and toes. *Transcriptions of the Pathological Society of London, 45,* 238.

Wolf-Schein, E. G., Sudhalter, V., Cohen, I. L., Fisch, G. S., Hanson, D., Pfadt, A. G., Hagerman, R., Jenkins, E. C., & Brown, W. T. (1987). Speech-language and the fragile X syndrome: Initial findings. *Asha, 29,* 35–38.

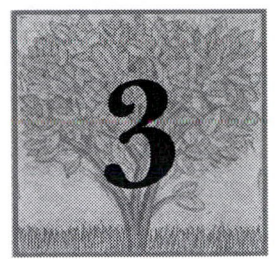

General Considerations in Assessment of Language Deficits in Infants and Preschool Children

▪ LEARNING OBJECTIVES

After completion of this chapter, the reader will be able to

1. Describe the etiological-categorical approach to assessment, and the descriptive-developmental approach.

2. Discuss the four basic assumptions for assessment on a social interaction theoretical perspective.

3. Discuss the application of the seven steps of the scientific model to the diagnostic process.

4. Identify and differentiate between the different types of validity and reliability with regard to language testing.

5. Describe the various types of receptive assessment tasks including the features of language that can be assessed with each type.

6. Describe the various types of expressive assessment tasks including the features of language that can be assessed with each type.

▪ INTRODUCTION

For many reasons, the identification of children under the age of 5 years who have language abnormalities is not the easiest job in the world. One of the biggest problems is that there is no universal screening of preschool children. Pediatricians do not routinely do screenings of speech and language. Most day-care centers and preschools do not have a regular means of screening and assessment, so even enrolling a child in a preschool or day-care setting does not guarantee that speech and language abnormalities will be identified prior to the child's attending school. A tendency exists to take a "wait and see" approach, hoping that any suspected problems will resolve by the time the child enters school. Both of these problems were partially remedied with the passage of P. L. 99-457, the Education of All Handicapped Children's Act Amendments in 1976. However, one major problem is the lack of uniformity in testing procedures and programming for preschool children.

Regardless of the age of the child being assessed and the nature of the assessment, specific questions need to be answered. Some of these questions will be directed toward the parents or primary caregivers, whereas others may be better addressed by the referral source if it is someone other than the child's family. Furthermore, the clinician or professional must be aware of his or her own personal biases regarding children from different cultural or socioeconomic backgrounds. Personnel associated with any educational institution, including preschool settings, must be careful about racial and cultural bias when considering children with nonstandard English as language-impaired.

> The issue of readiness, interlaced with the unquestioned assumption that the child must "fit" the classroom rather than the classroom made to "fit" the child, makes for a rigid, formalized curriculum and turns the developmental kindergarten into a training ground for compliance. More significantly, the developmental kindergarten seems to have become a receiving room for poor children whose economic disadvantage marks them as cognitively and socially deficient; they are being acculturated into monocultural passive learning norms in preparation for formal schooling. (Polakow, 1993, p. 135)

This is an important concept to keep in mind since one of the primary objectives of assessment of preschool children is to ensure that any absence of readiness skills is identified and remedied prior to having the child enter school.

In the previous chapter, the classification of disorders by etiology was presented. In this chapter, a descriptive/developmental approach is discussed. This is in keeping with the two approaches to language assessment outlined by Bernstein and Tiegerman-Farber (2002). Bernstein's and Tiegerman-Farber's two approaches are etiological-categorical and descriptive-developmental. The five causative categories Bernstein and Tiegerman-Farber suggest in the etiological-categorical approach are motor disorders, sensory deficits, central nervous system damage, severe emotional-social dysfunctions, and cognitive disorders. Similarly, these same two authors (2002) list five descriptors of language problems in the descriptive-developmental approach based on the work of Bloom and Lahey (1978):

1. Problems learning linguistic form, including rules of phonology, morphology, and syntax

2. Semantic difficulties, including conceptualizing and formulating ideas about objects, events, and relations

3. Pragmatic disorders including difficulty in using language for a wide variety of functions, and adapting language to different speakers or events

4. Difficulties integrating the form, content, and use of language

5. Delayed language development, with the usage of language resembling that of younger normally developing children

Regardless of whether one prefers the etiological-categorical approach or the descriptive-developmental approach, the process as described in the remainder of this chapter is essentially the same. How the outcome is expressed is where the process is different. Both approaches rely on essentially the same procedures in that language is assessed through case history information, observation, standardized and nonstandardized assessment tools (including language scales), and language samples (Shipley & McAfee, 1998).

■ OBJECTIVES OF THE ASSESSMENT AND DIAGNOSTIC PROCESS

As outlined in Table 3–1, Lund and Duchan (1988) list five major objectives of the assessment process.

Does the Child Have a Problem?

Assessment process. The process of interviewing, observing, and testing an individual to determine the nature, extent, and severity of his or her language disorder, delay, or difference.

The major objective of the **assessment process** is to determine whether or not the child has a language problem of any type. That is, is the child's language different, disordered, or delayed in comparison to that of his or her peers?

Typically, a child is referred for evaluation because someone (e.g., parents, teachers, neighbors, child-care workers) believes that the child's language does not compare favorably with the language used by his or her peers. Sometimes, a child is evaluated by a psychologist for possible behavioral or learning problems, who then refers the child to a speech-language pathologist for an evaluation. In those cases, children who have scored one or more standard deviations below their age group on standardized tests, or whose language performance falls at a level 6 months or more below his or her chronological age in language production, should be referred for testing.

Furthermore, any child who is at risk for developing language problems should also be referred for testing. This would include children who are born with handicapping conditions, such as hearing impairment, cerebral palsy, or a variety of syndromes and sequences, children who are born addicted to alcohol or other drugs, and children who are at risk due to poverty or trauma in their histories. A sample of a nonstandardized checklist of language development from birth through age 7 is provided in Appendix 3A.

TABLE 3–1. Five major objectives of the assessment process.

1. Determine whether or not the child has a language disorder, a language delay, or a language difference
2. Identify etiological factors
3. Identify weaknesses in the child's use of language
4. Describe the strengths in the child's language behaviors
5. Make the appropriate recommendations for the child

Source: Adapted from *Assessing Children's Language in Naturalistic Contexts,* by N. Lund and J. Duchan, 1988, Englewood Cliffs, NJ: Prentice Hall, as cited in *An Introduction to Children with Language Disorders,* by V. Reed, 1994, New York: Merrill.

What Caused the Problem?

A second objective is to identify the cause of the problem. Although this is not always important, it is helpful information if the child has a condition that will cause progressive deterioration such as muscular dystrophy, or a genetic condition such as fragile X syndrome (see Chapter 2), that may affect decision making in the family about future children. For example, a child who was enrolled in a local public school had pervasive developmental disabilities as well as unique facial characteristics and ataxia. It was eventually determined that she had Angelmann syndrome, a genetic condition that could be passed on to other biological siblings or to the children of her siblings who did not have the syndrome. In this case, the diagnosis did not change anything being done in therapy, but it did affect family planning decisions by her siblings.

What Are the Child's Deficits?

A third purpose of the assessment process is to identify deficit areas in the child's production and comprehension of language. In the preschool population, these deficits are described most frequently in terms of the features of language that the child exhibits, or does not exhibit, and relative to the child's level of cognitive functioning.

As expressed in Chapter 1, it is preferable to describe a child's language deficits in terms of the features of language that are affected or in terms of a comparison of the child's abilities and deficits in relation to normative development. In other words, it is critical to review the child's language in terms of content, form, and use in relationship to normative data. It is also important to review a child's cognitive and sensorimotor skills and how they affect the child's language.

What Are the Child's Abilities?

Closely tied to the third objective is a fourth goal of the assessment process. It is just as important to identify a child's abilities as it is to identify his or her deficits. This is particularly important when interpreting the assessment findings and deciding what to recommend for the child. A careful review of a child's abilities can be used to provide "stepping stones" to follow in remediation of the deficits. This process of comparing abilities and deficits is called **task analysis**, and it forms the foundation for effective therapy. The abilities the child demonstrates must be examined in order to build a task-analyzed program to help the child develop the areas that are revealed as deficits in the assessment process. Therapy should always be focused on a **functional outcome**, with treatment being provided in the most expedient and effective manner possible.

Task analysis. The breaking down of a task into small steps that must be accomplished individually before the whole task can be completed.

Functional outcome. Terminology coined to define environmentally based results of therapy that can be generalized to the patient's natural settings.

In order to plan therapy, the clinician needs to know the skills in the child's repertoire that can serve as a foundation for developing skills that are absent. Therefore, the need to know what the child can do as well as what he or she cannot do is of paramount importance.

What Are the Correct Recommendations?

It is critical for the beginning clinician to understand that diagnosis of a language disorder is a process, not an event. Too often, the assessment process is viewed as the two to three hours that a clinician spends giving a set of tests that were chosen to answer specific questions. However, should it be determined that the child needs intervention, assessment is an ongoing process that continues throughout the delivery of services to the child. The initial diagnostic meeting is only the first step in the assessment process.

Based on the research of Erickson, Nelson (1993) lists four basic assumptions that serve as an efficient and effective basis for assessment on a social interaction theoretical perspective:

1. Language is a symbolic, generative process that does not lend itself easily to formal assessment.

2. Language is synergistic, so that any measure of the part does not give a picture of the whole.

3. Language is a part of the total experience of a child and is difficult to assess as an isolated part of development.

4. Language use (quality and quantity) varies according to the setting, interactors, and topic. (p. 228)

Using these perspectives, the clinician is prepared for the fifth major purpose for a complete diagnostic process. The final step in the diagnostic process before beginning therapy is to make the appropriate recommendations for the child. In some cases, this may mean a referral to another professional, in others it is the beginning of the therapeutic relationship between the child and the clinician. Either way, a good referral will delineate the child's abilities and deficits in a clear, comprehensive manner.

■ APPLICATION OF THE SCIENTIFIC MODEL TO THE DIAGNOSTIC PROCESS

Nation and Aram (1984) put forth a model for the diagnostic process that likens the procedure to the scientific model taught in basic science courses. It is an excellent model for all clinicians to follow but is particularly useful for neophyte clinicians who are learning the diagnostic process. By following such a model, the clinician is prepared to implement the diagnostic process for any disorder. This approach is much more useful for the beginning clinician than disorder-specific approaches.

Step 1: Defining the Problem

In Step 1 (Table 3–2), the clinician is attempting to understand the subject matter. Some of this understanding comes about as a result of the preassessment discussion with the client or his caregivers, or both. During this stage, the clinician begins to assume the role of a diagnostician by asking questions that form the foundation for the other six steps of the process. This is the beginning of the application of academic knowledge in the clinical setting. After obtaining the child's developmental history, the clinician makes decisions as to what knowledge he or she has about the child's needs and how that information will be applied in a diagnostic manner.

The initial evaluation session usually is the first contact between a clinician and the client and his or her family, and it serves as the first step in the diagnostic process. Typically, the session will consist of a preassessment interview, observation and testing of the child, and a postassessment conference in which the initial findings are shared with the family.

Case History and Interview Questions

Every assessment should begin with an interview of the parent(s) or the person(s) designated to convey information about the child at the initial

TABLE 3–2. Step 1 in the diagnostic process based on the scientific model: Definition and delineation of the problem area.

What is the problem?

What is being diagnosed?

What fund of knowledge does the clinician need as a diagnostician?

How does the clinician acquire the knowledge needed to make the diagnosis?

How may this knowledge be organized by the diagnostician?

How much does theory rule the diagnostician's job?

Since the diagnostician is confronted with so many different speech and language disorders, does he or she need a broader base of knowledge than the researcher?

How does the diagnostician use his or her general fund of knowledge for the purpose of diagnosing an individual patient?

Source: Adapted from *Diagnosis of Speech and Language Disorders*, by J. E. Nation and D. M. Aram, 1984, San Diego: Singular Publishing Group. Copyright 1984.

Baseline. The preinter-vention measurement of a patient's skills.

assessment session. The first and most critical questions to be addressed are, "Why are you here?" and "What questions do you expect me to answer as a result of this session today?" These questions serve several purposes for the clinician. First, they give the clinician a good **baseline** of information for determining the family's understanding of a possible language deficit.

Second, these questions provide the clinician with a guideline to direct the testing so that the clinician can be sure to provide an answer to the family's most pressing questions. This is also an excellent time to empower the family to be a part of the diagnostic process. No matter how much knowledge a clinician has, it is important to remember that the clinician's knowledge relates to the disorder and the academic aspects of the process. Just as important is the fund of knowledge the family has about their child. The family needs to be encouraged to share as much information about the child and his or her environment as possible, so that the clinician can make the appropriate decisions as to what testing to use during the next phase of the diagnostic process. If the clinician is going to empower the family to be a part of the therapeutic process, a good first step is to answer the family's primary questions. It can be difficult to get information from the family, so active listening skills, clinical observations, and tactful questioning skills are critical. The clinician also should be prepared to explain the purpose of each question in case the family challenges the need for the information. A good rule of thumb is to ask only questions for which there is a clear use of the answer.

The hallmark of a good relationship between a clinician and his or her pediatric client's family is an ability to relate to the family. By understanding what the family wants to know, the clinician can be sure to include procedures in the diagnostic protocol that will provide an answer to the family's primary questions.

The third critical question is, "How does the child communicate now?" It is important to know this information before beginning the diagnostic session to improve the effectiveness of the communication exchanges between the clinician and the child. To answer this question fully and meaningfully, it is helpful to assess the environment using the questions outlined in Table 3–3. The family needs to be encouraged to share as much information about the child and his or her environment as possible so that the clinician can make the appropriate decisions as to what testing to use during the next phase of the diagnostic process. An example of a case history for a pediatric language patient is in Appendix 3B.

Step 2: Developing the Hypotheses

Table 3–4 delineates the questions to be addressed in Step 2 when the diagnostician begins to formulate the questions that will be tested throughout

TABLE 3–3. Questions to determine the communication environment and status of a child.

1. What are the child's communication abilities at this time?
2. For what purposes does the child communicate at this time?
3. What are the demands and expectations in the child's daily environments?
4. How does the child interact with his or her environments?
5. Is there any difference in how the child communicates in one environment as opposed to other environments?

TABLE 3–4. Step 2 in the diagnostic process based on the scientific model: Development of hypotheses to be tested.

What are the purposes of diagnosis?

How can hypotheses be formulated by the diagnostician that fit the concept of the use of the hypotheses in research or in the use of the method of science?

Are statements of hypotheses appropriate for studying the individual?

How is a clinical hypothesis stated?

How do hypotheses relate to the problem presented by the patient, by the referral source?

What relationships should be expressed in a clinical hypothesis?

Can clinical hypotheses be unbiased?

A researcher is generally free to study hypotheses of specific interest to him or her; hypotheses that are as narrowly defined as he or she feels warranted for predicting events in his or her field of knowledge. Does the diagnostician have this freedom?

Source: Adapted from *Diagnosis of Speech and Language Disorders,* by J. E. Nation and D. M. Aram, 1984, San Diego: Singular Publishing Group. Copyright 1984 by Singular Publishing Group.

the diagnostic process. At this point, the clinician begins to apply theoretical knowledge to form a preliminary supposition as to the nature of the child's language deficits. This hypothesis will become the foundation for the selection of tests to be used in Step 3.

Step 3: Planning the Diagnostic Process

When the clinician progresses to Step 3 (Table 3–5), the driving question is, "What tests and procedures will be used to determine the nature and extent of the child's language abilities and deficiencies?" Using the predetermined hypotheses, the clinician develops questions that must be answered and decides which tools will best provide those answers. In the scientific model,

TABLE 3–5. Step 3 in the diagnostic process based on the scientific model: Development of procedures for testing the hypotheses (research design).

What clinical tools are needed by the diagnostician?

How are the tools of diagnosis selected for the purposes of diagnosis for the individual patient?

How does the diagnostician evaluate the appropriateness of his or her tools?

Can the diagnostician exert control in testing sessions by selection of tools?

Do clinicians have tools for diagnosis that meet the requirements for measuring instruments that are so important for research? Do they have to be concerned about precision, reliability, and validity?

Since the diagnostician does not know his or her patient personally before the time of the diagnosis, how can he or she consider control over the variables that may be present?

How much time should be allotted for testing procedures?

Is there an order for presenting testing procedures in diagnosis? Are clinicians concerned about the effect one procedure may have on another?

Source: Adapted from *Diagnosis of Speech and Language Disorders*, by J. E. Nation and D. M. Aram, 1984, San Diego: Singular Publishing Group. Copyright 1984 by Singular Publishing Group.

these questions are the research design—how to find out what the researcher wants to know. In many ways, the diagnostician becomes a researcher at this point. It is critical to choose the correct tools to get the desired answers. Otherwise, at the conclusion of the diagnostic process, the hypotheses will remain untested and the questions will remain unanswered.

Based on the information gleaned from the case history and preassessment interview, the clinician has to identify a set of questions that need to be answered at the conclusion of the testing. In most cases, a combination of standardized and nonstandardized procedures is needed to adequately address all of the questions that have been identified. **Standardized tests** or procedures include formal tests that are based on data gathered from normative samples. Nonstandardized procedures include criterion-referenced tests and observations of the child in a variety of contexts.

Standardized test. A test that has been evaluated using a sample of individuals that represents a broad cross section of cultural groups. Standardized tests offer norms that allow a comparison of a child's performance on a test with those in the standardization sample.

In addition, a variety of developmental checklists can be used to organize observations. Some of these checklists can be completed by the parents or caregivers, whereas others are used by the clinician while interacting with the child. These developmental checklists are particularly useful in the preschool population because a variety of factors make formalized testing more difficult with children in this age group.

The clinician's job is to analyze the information gathered in the interview or case history stage of the process, decide which questions to address, and then determine the best tools to use to answer the questions in an efficient manner.

TABLE 3–6. Questions preceding test selection.

What is the purpose of the test?

Has the test been validated for this purpose?

What is the standardization group?

Are the characteristics of the patient similar to those of the sample group?

Are there any data or experiences to support differing performances across cultural groups (age, sex, socioeconomic status, geographic location)?

Would different values, experiences, behaviors, or other factors affect any of the responses?

Identifying the most important questions and the most appropriate tools is critical; asking the wrong questions, or using the wrong tools so that the needed answers are not achieved, destroys the value of the assessment process.

Questions Preceding Test Selection

As stated previously, the evaluation should consist of interviews, standardized tests, nonstandardized measurements, and observation. Literally hundreds of assessment devices are available, so, before giving any test, a clinician should ask the questions outlined in Table 3–6. It is very important that the clinician have the answers to these questions when selecting the tests and testing procedures to be used in the initial evaluation session.

Although Question 1 seems obvious, many tests that claim to test a person's language skills, test some aspect of cognition, but not necessarily a specific dimension of language. For example, a test that has the word "comprehension" in the title may be testing recognition, memory or identification skills, or both, rather than language comprehension per se.

Statistics related to the validity and reliability of a test are in the test's manual. The clinician should read the information in the test manual carefully to determine whether or not the tool tests what it claims to test and whether or not it gives reliable data.

Validity. A major mistake made with regard to standardized testing is ignoring the **validity** and reliability information on the test. Validity may be of different types, and it serves the clinician well to understand the differences among the types. Validity is concerned with what the test measures and how well it does so.

One type of validity is **content validity**, which is a "systematic examination of the test content to determine whether it covers a representative sample of the behavior domain to be tested" (Anastasi, 1968, p. 100). Content validity

Validity. The degree to which a test measures what it is designed to measure, and how well it does so.

Content validity. A systematic examination of the relevance of the responses given to the test items in order to ascertain how well the test covers a representative sample of the skills to be assessed.

looks at the relevance of the responses instead of the relevance of the test items in an attempt to answer two questions:

1. Does the test contain an adequate sampling of relevant items to assess the behavior?

2. Are the responses relatively free from the influence of irrelevant variables?

Face validity. How well test items represent what they claim to test.

A second type of validity is **face validity**, which addresses the relevance of the test items. For example, a test designed to assess adults with language impairments caused by a stroke (aphasia) may cover some skills and concepts the clinician desires to test in a child with learning disabilities. However, the vocabulary of the test items on the aphasia test may not be applicable for an elementary school-age child. Therefore, the test would not have face validity for the purpose of testing a child for learning disabilities. Face validity answers the questions, "Are the items relevant and applicable in the setting in which they will be used?"

Criterion-related validity. How effectively a test predicts an individual's behavior or abilities, or both in specific situations.

A third type of validity is **criterion-related validity**, which is sometimes called predictive validity. Criterion-related validity determines how effectively a test predicts an individual's behavior or abilities, or both, in specific situations. For example, the Graduate Record Examination (GRE) is used to predict success in graduate school.

Construct validity. The degree to which a test measures a theoretical construct or trait.

Finally, **construct validity** is the degree to which the test measures a theoretical construct or trait (Anastasi, 1968). Theoretical constructs include intelligence, fluency, anxiety, aptitude, and other similar concepts. Table 3–7 illustrates the concept of test validity.

TABLE 3–7. Illustrative examples to compare and contrast validation procedures.

Purpose of Testing	Illustrative Question	Type of Validity
Achievement test in elementary school language arts	How much has Jim learned in the past?	Content
Aptitude test to predict performance in middle school language arts	How well will Jim learn in the future?	Criterion-related: predictive
Technique for diagnosing brain damage	Does Jim belong in the normal group or in the group of children with neurological deficits?	Criterion-related: diagnostic
Measure of logical reasoning	How can we describe Jim's cognitive processes?	Construct

Source: Adapted from *Psychological Testing,* by A. Anastasi, 1968, New York: Macmillan. Copyright 1968 by Macmillan Publishing Company.

Reliability. A test's **reliability** coefficients define the consistency of the test in measuring what it claims to measure in the same individual on reexamination. Statistical measures that can be used to determine a test's reliability include the **correlation coefficient, test-retest reliability**, and **alternate-form reliability**. For example, the *Peabody Picture Vocabulary Test III* (PPVT III) (Dunn & Dunn, 1997) is available in two forms. The clinician could test reliability by having the child take each form and then compare the child's performance on each form (alternate-form reliability); alternatively, the same form could be administered on two separate occasions (test-retest reliability). Usually some fluctuations will occur in the performance due to random chance factors. However, these are accounted for through the test's standard error of measurement, which enables the clinician to factor in chance circumstances that may cause some variation in an individual's scores (Anastasi, 1968).

Third, the information on the standardization sample should be perused carefully to be sure that the child to be tested is represented in the standardization sample. Newer tests tend to have broader standardization samples, as professionals have become more aware of the effects of different cultures and backgrounds on testing children's language abilities. However, many older tests do not have representative samples and should be used cautiously with underrepresented groups of children. Examples of culturally biased responses include the response of a child who was shown drawings of four different facial expressions and asked to show the examiner the one that represents "delight." Instead of selecting one of the four pictures, the child pointed toward lights on the ceiling.

Be Clear About the Test's Objectives

A common mistake made by beginning, and some experienced, clinicians is to give a test without being clear about the objectives to be accomplished with the test data. This is why, when planning a testing session, the clinician's first job is to determine what questions need to be answered about the child. Then, the clinician should carefully review his or her arsenal of tests to determine which ones (whether standardized, nonstandardized, or observational checklists) will help to answer the questions. If a test does not contribute to answering a question about the child, it should not be used. Specifically, the clinician should ask, "What question does this test answer, and do I have any use for the answer?"

The clinician should also keep in mind that no one test is right for every situation. Also, there are problems inherent in almost all standardized testing. For example, on **identification tasks**, the child is asked to identify a picture or object that is named by the clinician. Typically, three or four choices are given from which the child must make a selection. The child could get the correct answer by guessing or through the process of elimination. Therefore,

---

Reliability. The consistency of a test in measuring what it claims to measure in the same individual on reexamination.

Correlation coefficient. A number that represents the degree of the relationship between two sets of scores.

Test-retest reliability. Evaluating the reliability of a test by having the child take the same test on two separate occasions (usually within a 6-month period) and comparing the child's performance on each test.

Alternate-form reliability. Evaluating the reliability of a test by having the child take two different forms of the same test, then comparing the child's performance on each form.

Identification tasks. Tasks in which the child is asked to identify a picture or object that is named by the clinician.

identification tasks could be as much a test of recognition as they are of an ability to identify specific language constructs.

Acting-out tasks. Tasks in which the clinician offers a set of instructions on what the child must complete; the clinician needs to ascertain that the child is truly responding to the examiner's questions and not performing tasks that he or she knows due to real-world familiarity with the item.

In **acting-out tasks**, the clinician offers a set of instructions on what the child must complete. However, the clinician needs to ascertain that the child is truly responding to the examiner's questions and not performing tasks that he or she knows due to real-world familiarity with the item. For example, the clinician may give the child a cookie and a figurine of a boy. If the clinician asked the child to show "The boy eats the cookie," possibly the child would not understand the task but would have the boy eat the cookie because that is what would be expected. In other words, the child could perform the most probable action without comprehending the word order in the test question. However, if the clinician asked, "Show me the cookie eats the boy," and the child responds by making the cookie eat the boy or saying, "That is silly," the clinician could feel more convinced that the child responded to the request instead of what would be expected to occur.

Judgment tasks. Tasks that require the child to make a determination of the accuracy or reasonableness of a statement made by the clinician.

Another factor in determining if a test is appropriate for a situation is to look at the level of the task. A **judgment task** requires that the child make a determination of the accuracy or reasonableness of a statement made by the clinician. To complete such a task, the child must have developed his or her metalinguistic skills because the clinician is asking the child to interpret the language. For children under age 4 years, this may be an inappropriate task because it requires processing of the word's or sentence's form independent of the meaning, and the metalinguistic skills needed to accomplish this task do not usually evolve in a child's language until sometime after 48 months of age. The uses and difficulties with different types of test tasks are listed in Table 3–8 (receptive language tasks) and Table 3–9 (expressive language tasks). In addition to the tables, Figure 3–1 depicts a continuum that ranks tasks used to assess receptive and expressive language requiring the most to the least contextual support.

Step 4: Collecting the Data—Testing and Observing

In the scientific model, collecting the data is the fourth step of the scientific process (Table 3–10). In the diagnostic model, this is the actual testing of the patient. However, many factors need to be considered in this stage of the process. It is imperative, particularly with children, to get the most responses possible in the least amount of time. Therefore, the diagnostician must plan the data collection phase carefully to minimize distractions and maximize responses. The diagnostician also needs to select behavioral procedures carefully, considering the timing of the presentation of the pertinent stimuli as well as what reinforcements and reinforcement schedules will be used to facilitate the testing process. Some children can be sustained throughout the session with verbal praise. Others may need more tangible reinforcement

TABLE 3–8. Types of receptive tasks.

Type	Used For	Potential Limiting Factors
Identification tasks (child selects a picture in response to the examiner's questions)	Lexicon Morphology	Child can use guessing or use a process of elimination; may be more a test of recognition than comprehension
Acting out using schemes, role play, and scripts; child manipulates toys and objects in response to the examiner's directions	Semantics Morphology Pragmatics Syntax Comprehension	Have to be careful that the child is truly responding to the examiner's questions, and not performing tasks that he knows due to real-world familiarity with the item (the monster scared the boy; the boy scared the monster)
Judgment tasks: child makes formal judgment of the suitability of a word or sentence— examiner makes a statement, and the child responds if the statement is wrong or right, silly or OK, and so forth	Semantics Syntax Lexicon Morphology	Very difficult for children under age 4 years as it requires processing of the word or sentence's form independent of the meaning (requires metalinguistic skills)

such as stickers. It is a good idea to avoid the use of food because it can be messy, and eating extends the length of the evaluation session because the clinician must wait for the child to finish eating before progressing to the next item.

Observation and Testing Using Standardized Measures

Evaluation of a preschool child should consist of standardized tests, non-standardized measurements, and observation. Most tests for children are norm-referenced, meaning that there is a standardization sample against which the child's performance can be measured. In other words, the abilities of the child being tested are compared to those from a normative sample of children with similar characteristics to those of the child being assessed. It is the norms that give meaning to the raw scores. By definition, a standardized test allows comparison of a child's performance against that of age-level peers in the standardization sample. Therefore, norm-referenced

TABLE 3–9. Types of expressive tasks.

Type	Used For	Potential Limiting Factors
Elicited imitation tasks: examiner says a sentence, and the child repeats it	Semantics Syntax Morphology Rule out auditory memory problems	Works on the assumption that if a child does not use a particular construction in his or her speech, he or she will omit it in imitation
Delayed imitation tasks: show child two pictures and say, "The man sees the boy; the man sees the boys. Which one is this?"	Semantics Syntax Morphology	Works on the assumption that if a child does not use a particular construction in his or her speech, he or she will omit it in imitation
Carrier phrase task: Child completes incomplete sentences spoken by the clinician	Semantics Morphology Lexicon	Child can fail if there is an auditory memory deficit
Parallel sentence production tasks: place two pictures in front of child. Examiner describes first one, and child describes second one using a similar format	Semantics Syntax Lexicon Morphology	Works on the assumption that if a child does not use a particular construction in his or her speech, he or she will omit it in imitation
Analysis of spontaneous language sample: child and clinician engage in spontaneous conversation which is recorded mechanically and later analyzed by the clinician	Semantics Syntax Lexicon Morphology	Getting a sample with an adequate number of utterances

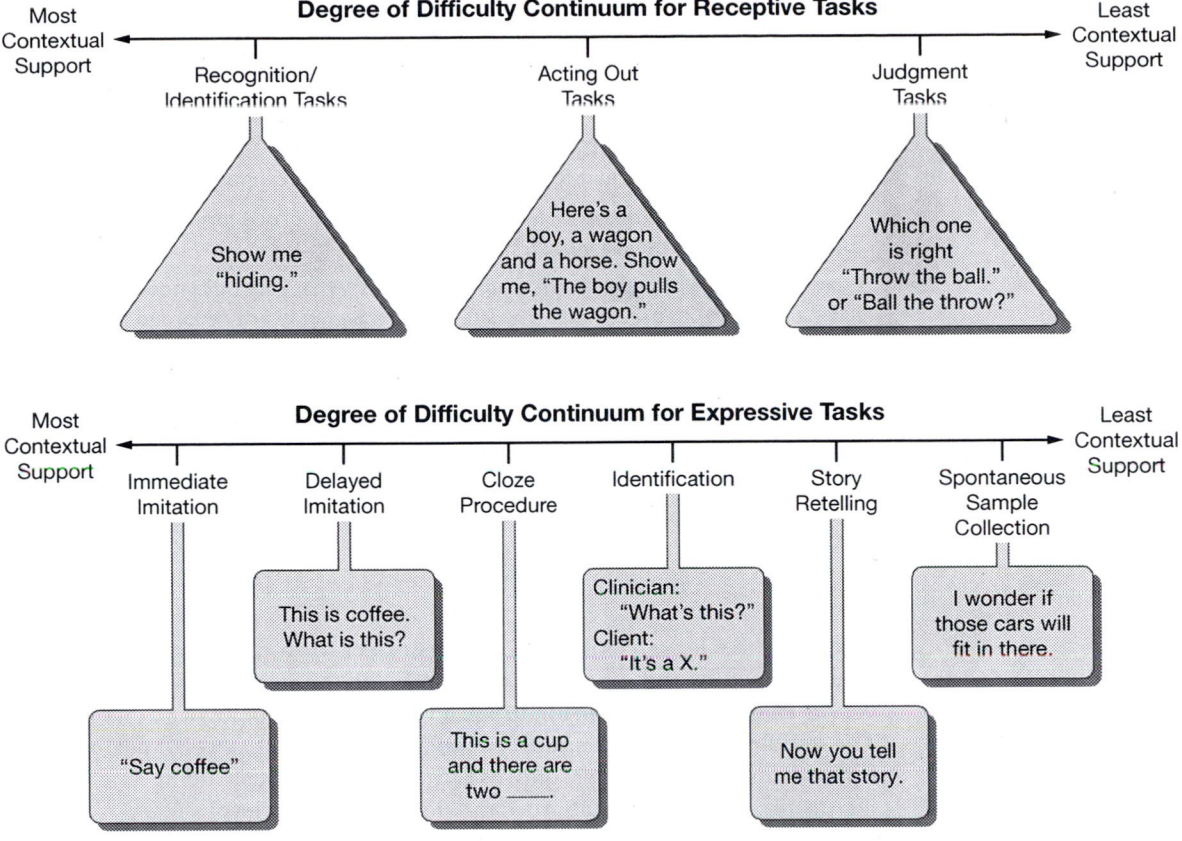

FIGURE 3–1. Tasks typically used to assess receptive and expressive language abilities depicted on a continuum representing most to least contextual support. (From *Diagnosis in Speech-Language Pathology*, by J. B. Tomblin, H. L. Morris, and D. C. Spriestersbach, 1994, p. 109. San Diego: Singular Publishing Company. Copyright 1994 by Singular Publishing Company, Reprinted with permission.)

tests frequently yield an Intelligence Quotient (IQ) or a Developmental Quotient (DQ).

Many times, a **screening** test is administered to a child as part of a routine assessment battery used to determine a child's possible deficit areas prior to beginning school. A screening test is a short test used to determine if a child may have a language deficit or difference. Screening tests are used to determine if a child's language is within normal limits. If the results are not within normal limits, the child should have a full evaluation. A screening test cannot be used to diagnose. It simply serves to determine if a child may be at risk for deficits in language development.

Screening. The administration of short tests in order to determine if a child's language is within normal limits or if he or she needs to be referred for a complete diagnostic process.

Most screening tests use cut-off scores, which can be percentile levels or raw scores. Most diagnostic tests provide this for each age level, with children

TABLE 3–10. Step 4 in the diagnostic process based on the scientific model: Collection of the data.

What are the clinical procedures of diagnosis?

Can the diagnostician control all the variables during the testing session?

How does he or she account for variables that he or she cannot control?

What happens if the diagnostician is not able to use the procedures initially selected? Does this invalidate the diagnosis?

Young children present significant testing problems. What can a diagnostician do during the testing to assure that the data that are obtained are recorded accurately?

Can the diagnostician be as systematically in collecting the data needed for diagnosis as the researcher who has control over his or her experiment? Can the word systematically be interpreted in such a way as to apply to the diagnostic process?

How can the diagnostician observe and record verbal information objectively?

Source: Adapted from *Diagnosis of Speech and Language Disorders,* by J. E. Nation and D. M. Aram, 1984, San Diego: Singular Publishing Group. Copyright 1984 by Singular Publishing Group.

scoring in the lower percentiles being suspect for a disorder in the area or areas assessed by that test. Percentiles indicate the percentage of children in the standardization sample for an age level who scored below a given raw score. The middle of the scale is usually anchored to an average level of performance for a particular normative group, with the units of the scale being a function of the distribution of scores above and below the average level.

Standard score. A score obtained by converting the raw score to a weighted raw score which takes into account the average score and the variability of scores of children that age.

Raw scores can be used to determine a **standard score** by converting the raw score to a weighted raw score, which takes into account the average score and the variability of scores of children that age. Using standard scores, a child who scores 1 **standard deviation** below the mean would be suspected of having a language deficit. A child who scores 2 standard deviations below the mean will, most likely, exhibit a language deficiency relative to his or her peers.

Standard deviation. A statistical measurement used to document the disparity between an individual's test score and the mean.

It is critical that any test used be administered, scored, and interpreted according to the directions for that particular test. Any deviation from the prescribed format can destroy the validity and reliability of the test and make the results meaningless.

Receptive and Expressive Tests. Many standardized tests assess either expressive or receptive language, whereas others have subscales that assess both dimensions of language and communication. Receptive tests measure a child's linguistic competence: what he or she knows about language. Expressive tests measure a child's linguistic performance: how well he or she uses the knowledge he or she has about language.

Evaluation Using Nonstandardized Measures

Developmental Checklists. Another type of test frequently used with infants and preschool children is the developmental checklist. Most checklists are ordinal, meaning that the behaviors are arranged in a developmental order and are dependent on each other, as in a hierarchy. The child's chronological age is compared to a developmental age based on the number of items passed on the checklist. The extent of the language deficit is based on the discrepancy between the child's chronological age and the developmental age (Dunst, 1980). Developmental checklists can be used to record observations, as a guide for a parent interview, or as a formalized method of assessing a child's developmental level based on behaviors and skills exhibited through play. In other words, some checklists are completed by observation, some are completed by interaction with the child, and some are completed by interaction with the primary caregivers.

Most checklists are descriptive in that they include items that should be passed by children at designated age levels. They can be used to describe the child's language, cognitive, and communicative behaviors, but they do not necessarily yield percentiles or standard scores. They simply provide information on specific skills that are present or absent in the child's repertoire. Many checklists are not limited to language functioning but tend to look at the overall development of the child. They provide excellent information, regardless of whether or not a child can be tested using more standardized measures.

The Receptive-Expressive Emergent Language Scale–2 (Bzoch & League, 1991) is a standard checklist used to guide the interviewing of parents about their child's speech and language capabilities. Another interview scale that is used in a variety of settings is the Vineland Social-Emotional Early Childhood Scale (Sparrow, Balla, & Cicchetti, 1998), in which the clinician checks off behaviors identified by the primary caregiver as typical of the child's communicative behaviors.

The Symbolic Play Assessment for Preschool Children (Lombardino & Kim, 1986) can be used for children from presymbolic through symbolic stages of play (12 to 16 months of age). The Symbolic Play Assessment for Preschool Children (Appendix 3C) and others similar to it are based on schemes or make-believe scenarios. The child may be asked to act out a doctor scenario or a cooking scheme. The independence the child demonstrates in imitating a variety of behaviors associated with each scheme is then recorded to determine the child's level of symbolic ability. This symbolic ability is critical to the development of metalinguistic and pragmatic skills that will guide much of the child's social development throughout the preschool and early elementary ages.

Play can be encouraged at many levels. The shy and withdrawn child should be approached using self-talk and parallel talk. In such a case, clinicians are often uncomfortable with silence in the room. However, it is critical that the clinician learn to wait silently for the child to respond. These periods of silence are needed periodically to give the child a chance to talk. When setting up play opportunities for diagnostic purposes, the clinician should sequence the interaction with the child. Initially, solo play may be the most effective. In the case of a cooking scheme, the clinician and the child could each have their own spoons and own pans to play with on the stove. Using self-talk, the clinician can comment on his or her own perceptions and activities ("I'm stirring my soup. It smells so good!"). After a period of solo play, tangential contact play can begin. During this phase, the clinician may add some food to his or her pan and also add some to the child's pan. Parallel talk in which the clinician comments on his or her own activities as well as those of the child should commence shortly after tangential contact play begins. This should be followed by intersecting play, during which the clinician's toys interact with the child's toys. For example, the clinician could take some food from his or her pan and put it in the child's pan. Finally, cooperative play should ensue in which the clinician assists the child in playing together. In the cooking scheme, this could involve setting the table and "eating" the good food that they have just cooked.

When working with an aggressive, hyperactive, or uncooperative child, the clinician must gain and retain control of the session. The setting should be structured to reduce stimulation and to help the child focus on the task at hand. Using a firm voice (firm, not loud or threatening), the clinician should let the child know that he or she is not threatened by the child's behavior. Do not reinforce the behavior by pleading, using rambling logic, or cajoling. Be matter of fact, and use self-talk. ("Well, if you want to scream, I'll just keep on with the work and I'll get the sticker for this set of words.") It also helps to do something you know the child likes to do. For example, if you know the child enjoys playing with cars and trucks, set up a garage scheme and use solo play to draw the child into the play.

Another checklist, the Early Communication Checklist (Lombardino, Stapell, & Gerhardt, 1987), can be used to evaluate communicative behaviors in infancy (Appendix 3D). Published in *The Journal of Pediatric Health Care*, this checklist was designed to assist nurses and other health care professionals in identifying suspected delays in the early development of communication and in making referrals to speech-language pathologists and audiologists when appropriate.

The Communication and Symbolic Behavior Scale (CSBS) was developed by Wetherby and Prizant (1993) and consists of normed developmental checklists that use parent interviews and naturalistic sampling procedures. They are designed not only to test language, but to also assess communication functions in children 8 to 24 months of age. They can also be used to assess the language and communication skills of children up to 72 months who have developmental delays. The communication skills that are assessed include gaze shifts, use of gestures, positive affect, and rate of communicating. The clinician interviews the primary caregiver(s) using the Caregiver Questionnaire and then videotapes an interaction between the caregiver and the child. The interaction is designed to include sharing books, setting up communication temptations, language comprehension tasks, constructive play activities, and symbolic play. There are 22 five-point scales that are divided into seven clusters: communicative function, communicative means—gestural, communicative means—vocal, communicative means—verbal, reciprocity, social-affective signaling, and symbolic behavior. The CSBS-Developmental Profile (CSBS-DP) (Wetherby and Prizant, 2002) is also norm-referenced and can be used as a screening and evaluation test. The CSBS-DP provides assessment of symbolic development and communicative behaviors. It is shorter than the CSBS and can be used for children who have a functional communication age of 6 to 24 months, and a chronological age of 9 months to 6 years.

Finally, the MacArthur Communicative Development Inventories (Fenson et al., 1993) are parent checklists based on normative data. There are two checklists: Words and Gestures and Words and Sentences. The Words and Gestures checklist is for use with 8- to 16-month-old infants, whereas the Words and Sentences checklist is designed to assess the language of children 16 to 30 months of age.

The MacArthur Communicative Development Inventory: Words and Sentences (CDI) (Fenson et al., 1993) is a parent report test tool that measures vocabulary development. The CDI includes an "extensive vocabulary checklist containing words that children typically produce in the second and third years of life" (Miller, Sedley, and Miolo, 1995, p. 1037). A study using the CDI was conducted by Miller et al. (1995) to determine the validity of the measure in reporting vocabulary development in children with Down syndrome who had a mental age of 12 to 27 months. The researchers measured the lexicon of 44 children with Down syndrome and 46 normally developing children in a clinical setting. They also evaluated predictive validity by comparing the lexicon of 20 of the children with Down syndrome and 23 of the typically developing children at a mental age of 20 months, then at a mental age of 28 months. The findings in the clinic were compared with those reported by the parents, and they concluded that parent report tools such as the CDI are valid for measuring a child's vocabulary. Miller and colleagues report that parent report tools are advantageous over clinical measures because they allow the clinician to tap into the parents' knowledge about their child's abilities with regard to language, the tools are cost-effective and efficient, and they record the child's language in a natural setting as opposed to formal testing that may be affected by the child's lack of familiarity with the setting and the examiner. In addition, tools such as the CDI can be completed by the parents prior to the clinical assessment, which enables the clinician to better plan subsequent testing, and they empower the parents to be a part of the assessment process.

TABLE 3–11. Scales of development assessed in the Uzgiris and Hunt Psychoedu-cational Battery.

Scale 1:	Visual Pursuit and the Permanence of Objects
Scale 2:	Means for Obtaining Desired Environmental Events
Scale 3A:	The Development of Vocal Imitation
Scale 3B:	The Development of Gestural Imitation
Scale 4:	The Development of Operational Causality
Scale 5:	The Construction of Object Relations in Space
Scale 6:	The Development of Schemes for Relating to Objects

Source: From *A Clinical and Educational Manual for Use with the Uzgiris and Hunt Scales of Infant Psychological Development*, by C. Dunst, 1980. Austin, TX: Pro-Ed.

Presymbolic language. The stage of communication that precedes the use of gestures, words, and actions to denote specific language concepts or words.

Ordinal Scales of Development. An example of an ordinal scale of development completed through interaction with the child is the Uzgiris and Hunt Scales of Infant Psychological Development (Uzgiris & Hunt, 1978). This scale is used to assess children at the **presymbolic level** of functioning, covering skills children normally develop between birth and 24 months of age. At the presymbolic level, the child does not use conventional words, gestures, or pictures for communication (Owens, 1995). In other words, it is most likely that the child does not use a recognizable communication system beyond a few words and gestures. The Uzgiris and Hunt checklist is divided into seven scales covering six domains that provide an overall picture of the child's cognitive functioning up to the age of 24 months, or during the presymbolic period of the child's life (Table 3–11). These domains can be tested through the establishment of play schemes in which the child is an active participant, as shown in Figure 3–2. Each domain is important in some manner to the assessment of cognitive skills needed for the child's future development.

The seven scales represent seven sensorimotor domains that develop parallel to each other. The Ordinal Scales of Psychological Development permits independent assessment of each domain, with the child's highest level of performance being determined for each scale by noting the highest item that is passed on each scale. This permits a clinician to develop knowledge about the child's weaknesses and strengths across several developmental domains (Dunst, 1980).

Criterion-referenced test. A nonstandardized probe used to study a language construct in more depth than is normally associated with standardized tests.

Criterion-Referenced Tests. By definition, a **criterion-referenced test** is a nonstandardized probe that is individualized for a child in order to examine a specific linguistic skill in greater depth. To use criterion-referenced tests, a clinician must rely on his or her own knowledge of normative data because the tests offer no comparison to children of similar ages. These types

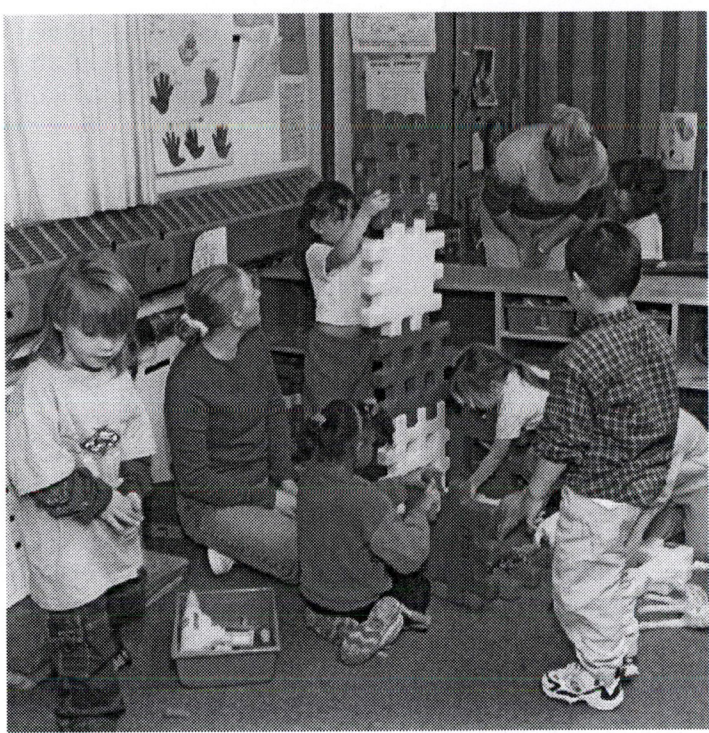

FIGURE 3–2. A preschooler's language can be assessed by having the child play with a variety of toys and observing his language and interactive behaviors while engaged in play activities.

of tests provide knowledge about the consistency of a child's problems and the contexts in which the problem occurs.

Reed (1994) offers three rationales for using criterion-referenced testing. First, they allow the clinician to examine in more detail features of language that appeared most troublesome for a child on a standardized instrument. For example, if a child demonstrates problems with the verb items on the PPVT, the clinician could construct a criterion-referenced test that would examine the child's understanding and use of verbs in a variety of contexts.

Second, Reed states that criterion-referenced testing examines aspects of language that may be omitted from standardized testing. This test can be used to determine the scope of a child's difficulty with a particular feature of language. Sometimes criterion-referenced testing can determine if it is the test stimulus that is creating the problem for the child, as opposed to the specific language feature.

Referring again to the PPVT, Penner and Vinson (1981) did a study that looked at performance of mentally handicapped adults on the PPVT after noticing that the individuals missed an inordinate number of verbs. On the PPVT, the verbs are actually presented as gerunds ("running"), the noun form of a verb. When the stimulus was presented as a verb ("somebody verb-ing"), the number of verbs missed decreased significantly. Therefore, in some of these cases, it was the stimuli, and not the verbs, that were problematic.

However, just as with standardized testing, problems occur associated with criterion-referenced testing. One problem is the choice of behaviors and items to be tested and selecting the criterion levels at which mastery will be determined. As a rule, it is not good to have 100% mastery as children will often miss an item owing to inattention or some other environmental reason, even though the child may know the item. Additional issues relate to validity, reliability, and problems associated with repeated testing, just as we find with standardized testing. Criterion-referenced tests are sometimes described as nonstandardized probes that are individualized for a child in order to examine a specific linguistic skill in greater depth. Many times, these tests are developed by the clinician who must rely on his or her own knowledge of normative data because no comparison to children of similar ages and abilities is available. Criterion-referenced tests can be useful in providing knowledge about the consistency of a child's problems and the contexts in which the problems occur.

Third, criterion-referenced testing can be used to answer the question, "Did the child fail to demonstrate a skill because of the manner in which the clinician tried to elicit the skill, or does the child not have the skill in his or her repertoire?" Thus, criterion-referenced tests provide an alternative means of assessing a child's language abilities and disabilities.

When developing criterion-referenced testing, care must be taken in deciding what criterion will be used to determine if the child has the skill, does not have the skill, or is developing the skill. Also, if using this type of testing to monitor progress in therapy, the clinician must take care to ensure that the skill is completely acquired and not just occurring in response to repeated administrations of the task.

A sampler of tests for language in preschoolers can be found in Appendix 3E. This list includes screening tools, normative tests, and criterion-referenced tests.

Step 5: Analyzing the Data

Test Scores: What Do They Mean?

The clinician should note the skills the child has, and their potential to serve as a foundation for the development of the absent skills. Of course, one of the objectives in using standardized testing is to find out how the child uses language in comparison with his peers (Table 3–12). The **percentile scores** that can be derived from standardized testing are a tremendous asset in this aspect of the diagnostic process. The percentile scores indicate the percentage of children in the standardization sample for an age level who scored below a given raw score. Most diagnostic tests provide percentile scores for each age level.

Percentile scores. The percentage of individuals in the standardization sample for an age level who scored below a predetermined raw score.

Another type of score available from standardized testing is a standard score. Using standard scores, a child's raw score (the actual number of correct and incorrect items) on a test is converted to a weighted raw score, which takes into account the average score and the variability of scores for children of that age. Thus, as with percentiles, a child's performance can be compared to that of children with similar characteristics. Children who score 1 standard deviation below the mean are suspected of having difficulties in language skills.

Any child who scores greater than 1.5 standard deviations below the mean should receive direct intervention. Using a four-box system, the skills that are present and absent in a child's repertoire can be divided easily into those that are communicative, those that are not communication related, those that are strengths, and those that are weaknesses. (Table 3–13). This information, along with the standard scores, can then be used to decide

TABLE 3–12. Step 5 in the diagnostic process based on the scientific model: Analysis of the data.

How is the information obtained for analysis?
How does the diagnostician score the information?
How is the information analyzed in the diagnostic process?
Are measures available that are descriptive and predictive?
Can the results obtained in diagnosis be quantified?

Source: Adapted with permission from *Diagnosis of Speech and Language Disorders*, by J. E. Nation and D. M. Aram, 1984, San Diego: Singular Publishing Group. Copyright 1984 by Singular Publishing Group.

TABLE 3–13. A four-box system to interpret findings from diagnostic tests and procedures.

	Strengths	**Weaknesses**
Communicative		
Noncommunicative		

whether to use direct intervention or whether to make some environmental manipulations and recheck the child at a later date.

Step 6: Interpreting the Data

Common Errors and Misconceptions

Beginning clinicians should be aware of the existence of many common errors and misconceptions about standardized tests.

First, although some clinicians believe that the way to demonstrate professional accountability is to give a standardized test, there are times when a situation does not warrant standardized assessment. For example, a child may not have the attention span needed to complete a standardized test. Also, it is usually recommended that a test not be repeated within a specified time period. Therefore, if a child has already taken specific standardized tests, the clinician may be better off to spend time using nonstandardized measures of assessment.

The second common error, particularly by new clinicians, is using tests with children not represented in the norming sample. If a speech-language pathologist is working in Montana, for example, there is a good chance that Native American children will be part of the population to be tested. Therefore, it is important for the clinician be sure that Native Americans are represented in the norming sample. If not, it might be necessary for the clinician to collect local norms in order to have a representative sample for comparison.

A third common error is the belief that, by reporting the scores a child receives on the standardized tests, the clinician has adequately informed the child's family about the meaning of the scores, the implications for placement in therapy, or the need for a referral to another professional. In actuality, reporting scores does little to help referral sources or the family understand the extent of a child's problems. Scores must always be derived in accordance with the directions in the manual, but the interpretation of these scores is not necessarily explained in the manual. Therefore, it is useful to spend some time analyzing the results in terms of what the child missed and what he or she got correct. This information is much more useful than a numeric score, particularly for preschool children. It is good to share with the parents the skills you believe the child has or has not developed, based on the items missed on the standardized test.

A fourth misconception is that standardized tests can be used as an end rather than as a means to an end in the diagnostic process. The administration of a standardized test is only the beginning of a process that includes scoring and interpretation before that test can be considered complete. Therefore, to administer a test just so a score can be reported is an injustice

TABLE 3–14. Step 6 in the diagnostic process based on the scientific model: Interpretation of the data (support or reject the hypothesis).

How does the diagnostician interpret the results obtained in the diagnosis?

How can clinicians know if their results are close to the true behaviors they set out to study?

When interpreting the findings of the diagnosis, do the clinicians rely only on the specific test findings?

How is the information organized in relationship to the hypothesis?

How is the information synthesized and summarized?

Source: Adapted with permission from *Diagnosis of Speech and Language Disorders*, by J. E. Nation and D. M. Aram, 1984, San Diego: Singular Publishing Group. Copyright 1984 by Singular Publishing Group.

to the child and to the persons waiting to hear the results of the assessment. Careful interpretation, as outlined in Table 3–14, is essential.

Step 7: Making Conclusions

The Postassessment Conference

After testing the child, the clinician should take the time to meet with the child's family to discuss some of the findings. The clinician is responsible for conducting the postassessment conference. Going into the postassessment conference, the family is likely to be concerned about the diagnosis and the prognosis. They will be grappling with assorted feelings including concern, fear, anxiety, and potential relief on finally having some answers. The clinician brings a body of knowledge gathered from the preassessment interview, the case history, and the individual's performance on the tests. Even though there may not have been time at this point to score and interpret the testing, there is still information that can be shared regarding the child's overall performance. The clinician should give the name of the test, describe what it is designed to test, and explain why he or she chose that particular test. The clinician should review some of the items that the child missed and passed and question the parents as to whether this is an accurate reflection of the child's typical abilities.

A description of the child's behavior and communication efforts should be offered to the family. Remember, during the preassessment interview, the family was empowered to be part of the team. Once the clinician has shared the results of the diagnostic session, it is helpful to ask the family, "What do you need to know from me at this point?" The answer to this question will guide him or her as to how much information they are willing and able to receive. The family and the clinician should use this time to share with each other all the knowledge they have about the child and to then decide the

TABLE 3–15. Step 7 in the diagnostic process based on the scientific model: Making conclusions from the data.

How does the diagnostician interpret and communicate the findings of the diagnosis?

What applications to other patients can be made from the interpretations made on the patient seen? Can this or should this be done?

In what forms is the information from the diagnosis communicated?

Does diagnosis stop at this point?

How does the diagnostician determine appropriate management plans?

Source: Adapted with permission from *Diagnosis of Speech and Language Disorders*, by J. E. Nation and D. M. Aram, 1984, San Diego: Singular Publishing Group. Copyright 1984 by Singular Publishing Group.

best follow-up procedures to implement in the future (Table 3–15). This is the time to reinforce to the family that they have been empowered to be part of the team, with the focus now moving from the diagnosis to the treatment. Keep in mind that the value of the diagnostic session may very well depend on the quality of the postassessment conference.

The Diagnostic Report

The diagnostic report is a written record that summarizes the relevant information obtained, why this information was obtained, and how this information was obtained. The diagnostic report has several functions. The first is to serve as an official document of the interaction with the child and the family. Information from the case history, the preassessment and postassessment conferences, and the testing session are all incorporated into the diagnostic report. Copies of this report are sent to the family and to any referral sources that the family would like to have notified.

Second, the report serves as an entry point into the clinical service delivery system for the client. The report contains baseline and pretherapy information that will be used to develop the goals and procedures for any subsequent therapy the child might receive. Thus, the report can be used to communicate the clinician's questions and findings to other professionals. Since this report may be the primary interaction with another professional, the clinician's professional credibility as a clinician may be established by his or her report writing. Finally, the diagnostic report serves as a document for research purposes.

A good diagnostic report should contain the most information in the fewest words possible. The author once asked a physician how much of a report he actually reads. The response was, "I read what would fit on the back of an envelope."

Typically, the first information in the report is the identifying information. This includes the child's name, his or her parents' names, and their address and telephone number. Background information should include a statement of the problem. Case history information is often critical in the formation of a diagnosis, so accuracy is paramount. The second primary area of focus in the report is the examination information. This includes a description of how the child approached the task, the tests that were used, the purpose of each test, and the results. Again, the results should not be limited to reporting the scores; rather, it should include information about what items the child missed, what items he or she answered correctly, and a description of the strengths and weaknesses exhibited by the child on the tests. Then the clinician should summarize behavioral observations made during the course of the session. This includes information about how the child approached the tasks, distractibility, and the child's ability to respond and maintain focus on the task.

The next section of the report should include the clinician's summary, conclusions, and recommendations. This consists of clinical impressions and formulation of the diagnosis. All of the information gained from the history, the assessment, and the conferences should be integrated and synthesized into this section of the report. It is very important in this section (and, indeed, throughout the report) to differentiate between clinical facts and clinical assumptions. **Clinical facts** are statements made about events that actually took place and were directly observed or measured by the clinician. **Clinical assumptions** are what clinicians judge to be true, although they may not observe or measure attributes related to these events directly.

Both clinical assumptions and clinical facts have their place in a report. However, clinical assumptions should be used only in the summary and conclusions section of the report. Also, clinical assumptions should be labeled as such to avoid any misconceptions by the reader. It is important to remember that the summary and conclusions are often the only section that many people will read. Thus, it should be concise, accurate, and the best written section of the report. Finally, the report should be signed by the clinician.

With regard to the ethics of report writing, the clinician must be honest about what he or she knows and does not know as a result of the assessment. If information was not gathered for whatever reason (e.g., the child was fatigued, the clinician inadvertently omitted it), assumptions cannot be made. Rather, the clinician needs to state honestly that the information was not obtained. Second, the clinician cannot guarantee results. The prognosis and recommendations must be written very carefully from an ethical viewpoint. Third, the clinician must not interpret causes of psychological symptoms and behaviors. To do so could lead to ethical and legal complications. A final warning is to be sure that a release of information has been obtained before sharing the evaluation results with anyone. A copy of the release should be sent with any report requested from or supplied to another individual.

Clinical facts. Statements made about events that actually took place and were observed or measured directly by the clinician.

Clinical assumptions. What clinicians judge to be true, although they may not observe or measure attributes related to these events directly.

■ SUMMARY

The assessment of preschool children presents a unique challenge for beginning and experienced clinicians. Regardless of the inherent difficulties, accurate determination of a child's abilities with regard to language and communication is critical. If a preschool child is already a frustrated communicator, it is possible that the child will abandon all attempts to communicate and regress to a point where communication intervention will be extremely difficult. It is also important to note if a child is using compensatory skills to accommodate deficits in language or communication skills. This, too, may indicate the level of ability and inability a child has in this critical area of development. For example, if a 36-month-old child relies primarily on gesturing to communicate, the clinician and family should carefully analyze the communicative environment of the child. Is the child gesturing because this is accepted as an adequate attempt without challenging the child to use speech? Or, if the child does not use speech despite adequate environmental stimulation and encouragement, is there an organic reason for this child not communicating as expected? The answers to these critical questions can be obtained only through a complete assessment process in which the child, the family, and the clinician all play a critical role.

CASE STUDY

History

R, a 3-year, 8-month-old boy, was initially seen at the University of Florida Speech and Hearing Clinic (UFSHC) on July 15, 1992 for a hearing evaluation. Reportedly, R has an ongoing history of serious otitis media that is treated with antibiotics. He has had three to four ear infections per year since birth. R's hearing was found to be within normal limits bilaterally for speech stimuli. However, his expressive language skills appeared to be below average for a child his age, and his parents advised the clinician that R was scheduled for a speech and language evaluation at Shands Hospital on July 17, 1992.

R's mother reported that his spontaneous speech was mostly jargon and babble rather than true speech, although occasionally he would produce two- to three-word sentences imitatively. She reported that R did not verbally respond appropriately when spoken to but rather babbled a response or repeated what he heard. R's mother believed that his language comprehension and language expression were delayed. R lives at home with his parents and one older brother. He attends a church-related preschool three mornings per week.

Previous Testing

R's speech and language were first evaluated by a speech-language pathologist in the Division of Child and Adolescent Psychiatry at Shands Hospital on July 17, 1992. The Preschool Language Scale-revised (PLS-R) was administered to assess auditory comprehension (receptive) skills as well as verbal abilities (expressive). No basal age was obtained for the receptive or the expressive portion of the PLS-R. The child's auditory comprehension skills were reported to be at the 27-month level and his verbal abilities to be at the 24-month level. The Bzoch-League Receptive Expressive Emergent Language Scale (REEL Scale) was completed through a parent interview. On the REEL scale, R's expressive language skills were estimated to be at the 12-month level, and his receptive skills were in the 20- to 26-month-old range.

Evaluation at UFSHC on November 9, 2002

Play Skills. Lombardino and Kim's Symbolic Play Assessment for Preschool Children (1986) was administered to assess R's level of nonverbal symbolic play development. During this assessment, R was presented with toys for a cooking scheme (i.e., cooking dinner script). Although R's play skills were limited, he demonstrated up to two different action schemes carried out in a logical sequence. For example, following a model by the clinician, R put play food on a plate and brought the food to his mouth. This corresponds to an approximate age range of 19 to 24 months. R demonstrated object substitution, which was modeled by the clinician, when he pretended to use a dowel to substitute for a spoon. R substituted a block for a telephone after a model was provided by the clinician. This corresponded to an approximate age range of 24 to 30 months. Agent play, during which the child ascribes agency to an object or assumes another person's role, was modeled by the clinician but not observed during R's play. The clinician pretended a doll was crying by imitating crying sounds and pretended the doll could walk and talk. R's optimal and modal level of play, which was modeled by the clinician, was object substitution with multistage combinations.

The Uzgiris and Hunt Scales of Infant Psychological Development (1975) assess an infant's cognitive development during the first 24 months of life. The integration and refinement of sensory and motor behaviors to produce adaptive responses during the first 24 months is referred to as sensorimotor intelligence. The acquisition of sensorimotor abilities affords children the critical skills necessary for achieving higher level thought and adaptive processes. Although R's chronological age exceeded 24 months, the clinicians used the Uzgiris and Hunt to better document R's status on cognitive and language skills that serve as a foundation for future language development. R attained Stage VI, representation and foresight, which is the highest developmental level within this assessment.

Receptive Language

The Peabody Picture Vocabulary Test-III (Dunn, & Dunn, 1997) was administered to assess R's receptive vocabulary. A basal level was not established because R would not point to the pictures the examiner named. However, he spontaneously labeled four pictures.

Expressive Language

The Expressive One Word Picture Vocabulary Test (Gardner, 1981) was administered to assess R's expressive vocabulary. Again, a basal level could not be established. However, R correctly identified six of the nine pictures in the age range of 3 to 3.5 years old. During interactions, R demonstrated the ability to produce utterances of two words, which were primarily echolalic. Most of his spontaneous speech consisted of single-word utterances such as "ball" and "shoe." Articulation was subjectively judged to be within normal limits.

Behavioral Observations

R easily separated from his mother and engaged cooperatively with the clinician during the evaluation session. He demonstrated very little spontaneous speech and limited imitation of conversation was observed. R did not play interactively with the clinician, and he made no verbal requests to obtain toys and snacks that were placed out of his reach. He rarely made eye contact with the clinicians and did not express curiosity when one of the clinicians left the room.

Summary and Conclusions

Based on the observations made during R's symbolic play assessment, his symbolic play behaviors were limited. Following a model, R demonstrated the ability to combine two schemes.

One instance of object substitution was observed following a model. These behaviors correspond to an approximate age range of 19 to 24 months. Results of the Uzgiris and Hunt Scales of Infant Development revealed that R has attained sensorimotor stage VI. On receptive and expressive language tests, R did not achieve a basal score. During conversational interactions, R produced single-word and two-word utterances that were often echolalic. He responded better to the clinicians' requests for action when the verbal requests were augmented with gestures.

R has an expressive and receptive language disorder that affects the content and use domains of language. He also demonstrates some autistic-like behaviors. Therapy is recommended, with emphasis on developing naming behaviors and pragmatic skills. Therapy should employ experiential language activities to facilitate contextually appropriate language.

	Strengths	Weaknesses
Communicative	Hearing WNL	Developmentally approx. 24–28 month delayed
	Responds to model of play	Unable to attain basal on PPVT, PLS, or EOWPVT
	Responds to model of speech	Does not point to pictures
	Spontaneously labeled some pictures (verbally)	Echolalic
	Echolalic	Does not initiate conversation
	Articulation WNL	Limited functions of language
	Responds more accurately when clinician uses gestures and speech	Does not consistently respond to verbal instructions
Noncommunicative	Separated easily	Stage VI on sensorimotor skills
	Attends preschool	Does not play interactively
	Cooperative	

■ REVIEW QUESTIONS

1. Which of the following groups of tests represent receptive tasks?
   a. Identification tasks, acting out, carrier phrase tasks
   b. Identification tasks, acting out, judgment tasks
   c. Identification tasks, judgment tasks, parallel sentence production tasks
   d. Identification tasks, acting out, delayed imitation

2. Which of the following statements about receptive language tasks is/are not correct?
   a. Judgment tasks are well suited and easy for children below 4 years of age.
   b. Identification can be achieved on the basis of recognition and superficial comprehension.
   c. Acting out may reveal knowledge of the real world rather than understanding of the linguistic features.
   d. All of the above are incorrect.
   e. None of the above are incorrect.

3. What type of validity is addressed by the question, "How well will Jim learn in the future?"
   a. Criterion-related diagnostic
   b. Construct
   c. Content
   d. Criterion-related predictive

4. The assessment domain which evaluates a child's ability to use foresight in simple problem solving is
   a. Object permanence
   b. Causality
   c. Schemes
   d. Means-end

5. Which of the following represent a set of developmental checklists?
   a. The REEL, the Uzgiris and Hunt, and the Symbolic Play Scale
   b. The REEL, the MacArthur, and the Preschool Language Scale
   c. The CDIS, the Uzgiris and Hunt, and the Peabody Picture Vocabulary Test
   d. All of the above contain at least one test that is not a developmental checklist.

6. Identification tasks are especially useful for assessing pragmatics.
   a. True
   b. False

7. Syntax should be assessed expressively and receptively since comprehension of form precedes production.
   a. True
   b. False

8. When assessing children who are largely at the single-word level, an analysis of presyntactic devices such as transitional elements and an analysis of lexical production should be done.
   a. True
   b. False

9. By definition, a standardized test is a valid test for all cultural groups.
   a. True
   b. False

10. During the constituent analysis phase of the diagnostic process, the clinician determines the meaning of the results and supports or rejects the hypothesis.
    a. True
    b. False

■ REFERENCES

Anastasi, A. (1968). *Psychological testing* (3rd ed.). New York: Macmillan.

Bernstein, D. K., & Tiegerman Farber, E. (2002). *Language and communication disorders in children* (4th ed.). Boston: Allyn and Bacon.

Bloom, L., & Lahey M. (1978). Language development and language disorders. New York: John Wiley and Sons.

Bzoch, K., & League, R. (1991). *The Receptive-Expressive Emergent Language Scale—2.* Los Angeles: Western Psychological Services.

Dunn, L. M., & Dunn, L. M. (1997). *The Peabody Picture Vocabulary Test-III.* Circle Pines, MN: American Guidance Services.

Dunst, C. (1980). *A clinical and educational manual for use with the Uzgiris and Hunt Scales of Infant Psychological Development.* Austin, TX: Pro-Ed.

Erickson, J. G. (1981). Communication assessment of the bilingual cultural child: An overview. In J. G. Erickson and D. R. Omark (Eds.), *Communication assessment of the bilingual bicultural child* (pp. 1–24). Austin, TX: Pro-Ed.

Fenson, L., Dale, P. S., Reznick, J. S., Thal, D., Bates, E., Hartung, J. P., Pethick, S., & Reilly, J. S. (1993). *MacArthur communicative development inventories: User's guide and technical manual.* San Diego: Singular Publishing Group.

Gardner, M. F. (1981). Expressive one-word picture vocabulary test. Novato, CA: Academic Therapy Publications.

Lombardino, L. J., & Kim, Y. T. (1986). *Symbolic play assessment for preschool children.* Unpublished manuscript.

Lombardino, L. J., Stapell, J. B., & Gerhardt, K. J. (1987, September-October). Evaluating communicative behaviors in infancy. *Journal of Pediatric Health Care, 1,* 5.

Lund, N., & Duchan, J. (1988). *Assessing children's language in naturalistic contexts* (2nd ed.). Englewood Cliffs, NJ: Prentice Hall.

Miller, J. F., Sedey, A. L., & Miolo, G. (1995, October). Validity of parent report measures of vocabulary development for children with Down syndrome. *Journal of Speech and Hearing Research, 38*(5), 1037–1044.

Nation, J. E., & Aram, D. M. (1984). *Diagnosis of speech and language disorders* (2nd ed.). San Diego: Singular Publishing Group.

Nelson, N. W. (1993). *Childhood language disorders in context: Infancy through adolescence.* New York: Merrill.

Owens, R. E. (1995). *Language disorders: A functional approach to assessment and intervention* (2nd ed.). Boston: Allyn and Bacon.

Penner, K., & Vinson, B. P. (1981). Facilitation of verb recognition by MR subjects through syntactic cuing. *Language, Speech, and Hearing Services in the Schools, 12,* 39–43.

Polakow, V. (1993). *Lives on the edge: Single mothers and their children in the other America.* Chicago: University of Chicago Press.

Reed, V. A. (1994). *An introduction to children with language disorders* (2nd ed.). New York: Merrill.

Shipley, K. G., & McAfee, J. G. (1998). *Assessment in Speech-Language Pathology: A Resource Manual* (2nd ed.). San Diego: Singular Publishing Group.

Sparrow, S. S., Balla, D. A., & Cicchetti, D. V. (1998). *Vineland social-emotional early childhood scales.* Circle Pines, MN: American Guidance Services.

Uzgiris, I., & Hunt, J. M. (1975). *Assessment in infancy: Ordinal scales of psychological development.* Urbana, IL: University of Illinois Press.

Uzgiris, I. C., & Hunt, J. M. (1978). *Assessment in infancy: Ordinal scales of psychological development.* Urbana: University of Illinois Press.

Wetherby, A. M., & Prizant, B. M. (1993). *Communication and Symbolic Behavior Scales.* Baltimore, MD: Brookes.

Wetherby, A. M., & Prizant, B. M. (2002). *Communication and Symbolic Behavior Scales-Developmental Profile.* Baltimore, MD: Brookes.

APPENDIX 3A

Assessment of Language Development

Name: _____ Age: _____ Date: _____

Examiner: _____

Instructions: Mark a plus (+) or a check if the child *does* exhibit the behavior, a minus (–) or a (0) if the child *does not* exhibit the behavior, and an *s* if the child exhibits the behavior *sometimes*. This form can be used during the informal observation and/or completed by a parent or knowledgeable caregiver. Because children develop at different rates, avoid using strict application of the age approximations. The time intervals are provided only as a general guideline for age appropriateness.

0–6 Months

_____ startle response to sound

_____ repeats the same sounds

_____ frequently coos, gurgles, and makes pleasure sounds

_____ uses a different cry to express different needs

_____ smiles when spoken to

_____ recognizes voices

_____ localizes sound by turning the head

_____ quieted by the human voice

_____ listens to speech

_____ uses the phonemes /b/, /p/, and /m/ in babbling

_____ imitates sounds

_____ uses sounds or gestures to indicate wants

_____ varies pitch and loudness

7–12 Months

_____ understands *no* and *hot*

_____ understands and responds to own name

_____ listens to and imitates more sounds

_____ recognizes words for common items (e.g., cup, shoe, juice)

_____ babbles using long and short groups of sounds

_____ uses a songlike intonation pattern when babbling

_____ uses a large variety of sounds in babbling

—— uses speech sounds rather than only crying to get attention

—— listens when spoken to

—— uses sound approximations

—— begins to change babbling to jargon

—— uses speech intentionally for the first time

—— production of one or more words

—— uses nouns almost exclusively

—— has an expressive vocabulary of one to three words

—— understands simple commands

13–18 Months

—— uses adult-like intonation patterns

—— uses echolalia and jargon

—— uses jargon to fill gaps in fluency

—— omits some initial consonants and almost all final consonants

—— produces mostly unintelligible speech

—— follows simple commands

—— has an expressive vocabulary of 3 to 20 or more words (mostly nouns)

—— produces two-word phrases

—— combines gestures and vocalizations

—— requests more of desired items

19–24 Months

—— uses words more frequently than jargon

—— has an expressive vocabulary of 50 to 100 or more words

—— has a receptive vocabulary of 300 or more words

—— starts to combine nouns and verbs

—— begins to use pronouns (*I* and *mine*)

—— maintains unstable voice control

—— uses appropriate intonation for questions

—— is approximately 25–50% intelligible to strangers

—— answers "what's that?" questions

—— enjoys listening to stories

—— knows five body parts

—— accurately names a few objects

—— follows two-part commands

2–3 Years

____ speech is 50–75% intelligible

____ understands *one* and *all*

____ verbalizes toilet needs (before, during, and after act)

____ requests items by name

____ responds to some yes/no questions

____ names everyday objects

____ points to pictures in a book when named

____ identifies several body parts

____ follows simple commands and answers simple questions

____ enjoys listening to short stories, songs, and rhymes

____ asks one- to two-word questions

____ uses three- to four-word phrases

____ uses some prepositions, articles, present progressive verbs, regular plurals, contractions, irregular past tense forms, and negation *no* or *not*

____ uses some regular past tense verbs, possessive morphemes, pronouns, and imperatives

____ uses words that are general in context

____ produces several forms of questions

____ understands *why, who, whose,* and *how many*

____ continues use of echolalia when difficulties in speech are encountered

____ has a receptive vocabulary of 500 to 900 words

____ has an expressive vocabulary of 50 to 250 or more words (rapid growth during this period)

____ exhibits multiple grammatical errors

____ understands most things said to him or her

____ frequently exhibits repetitions—especially starters, "I," and first syllables

____ speaks with a loud voice

____ increases range of pitch

____ uses vowels correctly

____ consistently uses initial consonants (although some are misarticulated)

____ frequently omits medial consonants

____ frequently omits or substitutes final consonants

____ uses approximately 27 phonemes

____ uses auxiliary *is* including the contracted form

3–4 Years

___ understands object functions

___ understands differences in meanings (stop-go, in-on, big-little)

___ follows two- and three-part commands

___ asks and answers simple questions (who, what, where, why)

___ frequently asks questions and often demands detail in responses

___ produces simple verbal analogies

___ uses language to express emotion

___ uses four to five words in sentences

___ repeats 6- to 13-syllable sentences accurately

___ identifies objects by name

___ manipulates adults and peers

___ may continue to use echolalia

___ uses up to six words in a sentence

___ uses nouns and verbs most frequently

___ is conscious of past and future

___ has a 1,200 to 2,000 or more word receptive vocabulary

___ has a 800 to 1,500 or more word expressive vocabulary

___ may repeat self often, exhibiting blocks, disturbed breathing, and facial grimaces during speech

___ increases speech rate

___ whispers

___ masters 50% of consonants and blends

___ speech is 80% intelligible

___ sentence grammar improves although some errors still persist

___ appropriately uses *is, are*, and *am* in sentences

___ tells two events in chronological order

___ engages in long conversations

___ uses some contractions, irregular plurals, future tense words, and conjunctions

___ consistently uses regular plurals, possessives, and simple past tense verbs

4 Years

___ imitatively counts to five

___ understands concept of numbers up to three

___ continues understanding of spatial concepts

___ recognizes one to three colors

___ has a receptive vocabulary of 2,800 or more words

___ counts to 10 by rote

___ listens to short simple stories

___ answers questions about function

___ uses grammatically correct sentences

___ has an expressive vocabulary of 900 to 2,000 or more words

___ uses sentence of four to eight words

___ answers complex two-part questions

___ asks for word definitions

___ speaks at a rate of approximately 186 words per minute

___ reduces total number of repetitions

___ enjoys rhythms, rhymes, and nonsense syllables

___ produces consonants with 90% accuracy

___ significantly reduces number of persistent sound omissions and substitutions

___ frequently omits medial consonants

___ speech is usually intelligible to strangers

___ talks about experiences at school, at friends' homes, and so on

___ accurately relays a long story

___ pays attention to a story and answers simple questions about it

___ uses some irregular plurals, possessive pronouns, future tense, reflexive pronouns, and comparative morphemes in sentences

5–6 Years

___ names six basic colors and three basic shapes

___ follows instructions given to a group

___ follows three-part commands

___ asks *how* questions

___ answers verbally to *hi* and *how are you?*

___ uses past tense and future tense appropriately

___ uses conjunctions

___ has a receptive vocabulary of 13,000 words

___ names opposites

___ sequentially names days of the week

___ counts to 30 by rote

___ continues to drastically increase vocabulary

___ reduces sentence length to four to six words

___ reverses sounds occasionally

___ exchanges information and asks questions

___ uses sentences with detail

___ uses grammatically complete sentences

___ accurately relays a story

___ sings entire songs and recites nursery rhymes

___ communicates easily with adults and other children

___ uses appropriate grammar in most cases

6–7 Years

___ names some letters, numbers, and currencies

___ sequences numbers

___ understands *left* and *right*

___ uses increasingly more complex sentences

___ engages in conversation

___ has a receptive vocabulary of approximately 20,000 words

___ uses a sentence length of approximately six words

___ understands most temporal concepts

___ recites the alphabet

___ counts to 100 by rote

___ uses most morphologic markers appropriately

___ uses passive voice appropriately

APPENDIX 3B

Sample Case History for Pediatric Language Cases

Identifying Information

Child's Legal Name: _____ Nickname: _____

Date of Birth: _____ Age: _____ Date History Form Completed: _____

Parents'/Legal Guardians' Names: _____

Address: _____
            Street   City/State   Zip Code

Mailing Address (if different): _____

Person Completing This Form: _____

Mother's Employer: _____ Job Title: _____

Mother's Daytime Phone #: _____ Evening Phone: _____

Father's Employer: _____ Job Title: _____

Father's Daytime Phone #: _____ Evening Phone: _____

Child's Social Security #: _____

Do you have Medicaid: Yes _____ No _____

If yes, please provide your 8-digit policy/care number: _____

Name of family doctor or referring physician: _____

Phone # of family doctor/referring physician: _____

Name of Insured Individual: _____

Name of Person Responsible for Payment: _____

Address/Phone (if different from above): _____

Referral Information

Who referred the child to this clinic:

☐ Pediatrician ☐ Relative ☐ Self/Parent

☐ Teacher ☐ Friend ☐ Other_____

Would you like the referring individual to receive a copy of the report? Yes _____ No _____

Address: _____
Street City/State Zip Code

Are there others who should receive a copy of the report? Yes _____ No _____

Name: _____

Address: _____
Street City/State Zip Code

Name: _____

Address: _____
Street City/State Zip Code

What is the reason for referral? (Check all that apply)

☐ Diagnosis ☐ School Placement

☐ Treatment ☐ Other _____

Present Communication Status

Please describe your child's speech: _____

_____

Have diagnostic or therapeutic services related to the speech problems previously been received?
Yes _____ No _____ If yes, by whom and when? _____

Results of previous diagnosis or therapy: _____

When did the problem first begin? _____

Has the problem: _____ remained the same

_____ gradually worsened

_____ worsened quickly?

Educational History

Name of current preschool/school: _____

Grade: _____ Primary Placement: _____ Regular Ed. Classroom

                                       _____ Self-Contained Classroom (full day)

                                       _____ Special Education (part day)

                                       _____ Other _____

Current Teacher's Name: _____

Describe your child's progress in school: _____

_____

In your opinion, does your child's speech/language problem have an effect on his/her school performance or school placement? _____ Yes _____ No If yes, please explain:

_____

Does your child receive speech-language therapy at school? _____ Yes _____ No

If yes, please indicate the following:

Name of Clinician: _____

Length and frequency of sessions: _____

Primary focus of therapy: _____

Family History

Mother's Name: _____ Age: _____ Highest Degree/Grade: _____

Father's Name: _____ Age: _____ Highest Degree/Grade: _____

Siblings: Name: _____ Age: _____ Highest Degree/Grade: _____

         Name: _____ Age: _____ Highest Degree/Grade: _____

         Name: _____ Age: _____ Highest Degree/Grade: _____

         Name: _____ Age: _____ Highest Degree/Grade: _____

Others in the Home: _____

              Name   Relationship

_____

              Name   Relationship

Pregnancy and Birth History

Did the mother have any illnesses or accidents during the pregnancy? _____ Yes _____ No

Did the mother receive/take any prescribed medications while pregnant? _____ Yes _____ No

If yes, what medications and for how long? _____

_____

Were the medications used during the _____ 1st trimester _____ 2nd trimester _____ 3rd trimester

Did the birth mother drink alcohol or use any illegal drugs while pregnant? _____ Yes _____ No

Were there any complications during the labor and/or delivery? _____ Yes _____ No

Was your baby's birth: _____ premature _____ term _____ late?

Did your baby have difficulty with any of the following in the first 48 hours following birth?

_____ breathing   _____ crying   _____ sleeping

_____ sucking   _____ responding to noise   _____ other

Comments on any of the above:

_____

_____

How long did your baby remain in the hospital following birth? _____

Developmental History

I have never been concerned about my child's developmental patterns. _____ Yes _____ No

I am concerned about my child's development because _____

_____

Please indicate the approximate ages at which each of the following occurred for the first time:

____ Cooing	____ Ask Questions	____ Feed Self/Hands
____ Babbling	____ Sit Unassisted	____ Feed Self/Utensils
____ Single words	____ Stand Unassisted	____ Toilet Trained
____ Combine words	____ Walk Unassisted	____ Dress Self

Is English your child's native language? ____ Yes ____ No

If not, what is your child's native language? _____

How many languages are spoken in the home? _____ Which languages? _____

_____

Medical History

General Health: ____ Excellent ____ Good ____ Fair ____ Poor

Please indicate any ongoing medical conditions: _____

Please indicate any regular medications: _____

Has your child ever been seen by any of the following specialists? Check all that apply:

____ ENT Physician	____ Psychologist	____ Nutritionist
____ Neurologist	____ Behavior Specialist	____ Orthodontist
____ Psychiatrist	____ Physical Therapist	____ Other
____ Physiatrist	____ Occupational Therapist	_____

Please list names/approximate dates/reasons for specialists:

Name: _____ Date: _____

Reason: _____

Name: _____ Date: _____

Reason: _____

Name: _____ Date: _____

Reason: _____

Please list previous surgeries/illnesses/injuries:

Problem	Dates	Comments

Please check all that apply and provide clarifying information under "Comment"

Illness	Comments	Yes	No
Allergies			
Recurrent colds/flu/sore throat			
Dizziness			
Dental problems			
Frequent laryngitis/hoarseness			
Epilepsy/seizure disorder			
Reading &/or spelling problems			
Other academic problems			
Attention Deficit Disorder (ADD)			
ADD with Hyperactivity			
Vision problems			
High fevers			
Kidney problems			
Swallowing/digestive disorders			
Respiratory difficulties			

Illness	Comments	Yes	No
Heart/circulatory problems			
Neurological disorders			
Cancer			
Endocrine/metabolic disorders			
Viruses (HIV, Herpes)			
Connective Tissue Disorders (Lupus, Arthritis, Scleroderma)			
Frequent &/or intense headaches			
Measles			
Mumps			
Chicken pox			
Meningitis			
Unusual fatigue/stress			
Mental illness			
Congenital disorders (list please)			

Audiological History

Please check the appropriate column:

	Yes	No
My child had 3+ ear infections between birth and 12 months of age.		
My child has had at least one ear infection that lasted more than 3 months.		
My child has been evaluated by an audiologist who determined that his/her hearing is within normal limits. Date of visit:		

	Yes	No
My child has failed a hearing screening in school. Date of screening:		
My child has passed a hearing screening in school. Date of screening:		
I suspect that my child has a hearing problem.		
My child has tubes in his/her ears. If yes, when:		
My child prefers one ear over the other. If yes, which ear?		
My child wears hearing aids. If yes, what type and for how long?		

Comments: _____

_____

_____

Speech and Language History

Please check the appropriate column:

	Yes	No
My child follows directions well.		
My child gives directions well.		
My child asks for help when needed.		
My child expresses himself/herself in a coherent manner that is understood by others.		
My child likes to have stories read to him/her. How long does he/she attend to the story?		
My child plays with age-appropriate toys appropriately.		

	Yes	No
My child has failed a speech screening in school. Date of screening:		
My child has passed a speech screening in school. Date of screening:		
My child communicates primarily through whining/crying.		
My child communicates primarily through gesturing/pointing.		
My child tries to communicate through verbalizing, but cannot be understood.		
My child primarily uses one-word utterances to communicate.		
My child primarily uses two-word phrases to communicate.		
My child primarily combines 3+ words to communicate.		
My child uses proper sentence structure for most of his/her utterances.		
My child's communication efforts are easily understood by familiar persons.		
My child's communication efforts are easily understood by unfamiliar persons.		
My child frequently drools.		
My child has difficulty chewing his/her food.		
I am concerned about my child's speech (how well what he/she says can be understood.)		
I am concerned about my child's language development (the content of what he/she says; how well he/she understands what others say).		

Overall, I would rate my child's speech intelligibility as:

_____ excellent _____ good _____ fair _____ poor _____ completely unintelligible

Comments:

_____

_____

_____

_____

APPENDIX 3C

Guidelines for Symbolic Play Scale Administration

This scale was developed from longitudinal and cross sectional data on the evolution and progression of play behaviors in normally developing children. The primary literature sources used for play levels, ordinal arrangement of play levels, and the corresponding ages were Bretherton (1984), Fenson (1984), McCune-Nicolich (1981), Watson & Fisher (1980), and Wolf, Rygh, & Altshuler (1984).

This scale is not a standardized assessment of play but rather it serves as an observational tool for use in approximating levels of nonverbal symbolic play development in language impaired preschool children. While there are not data to suggest that language-impaired children demonstrate differences in the developmental sequence of their play when compared to their normal developmental peers, studies have reported that language-impaired children are often delayed in their acquisition of play as observed in their restricted diversity of play schemes, shorter play schemes, and limited organization of play sequences (Lombardino, Stein, Kricos, & Wolf, 1986; Terrell et al., 1984).

SCALE ORGANIZATION

The scale is hierarchically organized for play levels spanning approximately 9 months to 5 years of age. Ages corresponding to each play behavior are only estimates and should be used by the therapist as developmental guidelines rather than as absolute indices. Age levels corresponding to the more advanced symbolic play behaviors (i.e., beyond the 3 year level) are based on very limited pool of empirical information as few studies have delineated ordinal levels of play at these higher stages of development.

RECOMMENDED PROCEDURES

No standard procedures have been developed for use with this scale; however, several procedures are recommended to help ensure (a) a representative sample of the child's play behaviors; (b) optimal level of play at which the child is capable of functioning; and (c) some degree of uniformity across test sessions and examiners.

Guidelines

1. Assess the child's play performance over a minimum of two 30–45 minute sessions. (If the child is verbal, this offers an excellent opportunity for collecting a language sample.)

2. Allow for approximately 10–15 minute preassessment warm-up period where the child is encouraged to play with a random set of toys in the presence of the parent and examiner (see list at end for recommended props). The parent and examiner should not actively participate in this play unless the child solicits their participation. The child should be permitted to direct the course of his play without restrictions (except in cases of disruptive behavior). If the child shows no initiative in playing with the toys, he can be prompted to do so or the child should be given the opportunity to choose a new set of toys.

3. Present the child with an organized set of toys to facilitate theme-related plays (e.g., cooking, grooming, doctoring). These toys or props will allow the child to represent familiar events or scripts in play. Scripts are ordered sequences of actions where temporal, causal, and spatial links are organized around a goal such as "making dinner," "bathing a baby," or "being examined by a doctor" (see list of recommended props for two scripts). These scripts are only examples of the types of organized play contexts that can be used.

There is empirical evidence to suggest that organized sets of toys facilitate more advanced action sequences in play (Largo & Howard, 1979; McCune-Nicolich & Fensen, 1985). Also, studies have shown that script contexts facilitate several aspects of language learning (Conti-Ramden & Friel-Patti, 1986; Snow, Perman, & Nathan, 1986; Harrison, Lombardino, & Farrar, 1989).

4. The child should be given the opportunity to play spontaneously with one theme-related set of toys (e.g., cooking set) at a time. The therapist can verbally prompt the child to enact a familiar script by suggesting, for example, that the child cook dinner for the baby. However, the child should not be coerced into following a script. Prompting is often not necessary because children will spontaneously enact a familiar routine.

While the child plays spontaneously, the examiner should note the child's highest level of spontaneous symbolic play. After approximately 15 to 20 minutes, the therapist should model[1] for the child levels of symbolic play that exceed those observed in the child's spontaneous play. For example, if the child produces multischemes spontaneously in a "dinner preparation" script but does not demonstrate object substitution and agent play behaviors, the examiner should model a "dinner preparation" script incorporating examples of object substitutions and agent play behaviors.

[1] Modeling is an important procedure in the assessment of sympolic play because research has shown that modeling is effective in eliciting levels of play that are within the child's action repertoire but not necessarily demonstrated in spontaneous play (Fenson, 1984). Additionally, children have been shown to simplify a modeled interaction when the model exceeds their level of conceptual development (Bretherton et al., 1984).

Following approximately 10 minutes of modeling, the therapist should encourage the child to reenact the play scripts for approximately 15 minutes while verbally prompting if necessary. It is at this time that the therapist should observe/record diversity of levels in the child's play schemes, diversity and length of play sequences, and optimal levels of play. Symbolic play sequences are defined as one or more schemes or action units uninterrupted by (1) social interaction; (2) object manipulation or exploratory behavior; (3) shift in focus of activity; and/or (4) unrelated or irrelevant activity. For example, *"child pretends to stir milk in a cup,* then *feeds the baby,* then *feeds mother"* is a symbolic gestural sequence comprised of three schemes.

Recording Data on Protocols

Developmental levels and other observations can be recorded on the scale assessment form during the evaluation session.[2] A summary form is provided as a quick reference for access to the child's most frequent (modal) and highest (optimal) levels of play. Additionally, the child's general developmental level in four major domains, cognitive domains, decentration (roles), decontextualization (objects), and integration (actions), can be recorded on the Three-Scheme Dimension summary form. This information can be used as one means for developing intervention objectives that target component actions of pretend play in addition to overall levels of play.

Interpreting Performance Information

The child's developmental play level should be examined relative to his chronological age (CA) if the child is not showing signs of having a generalized mental retardation. In cases where a child has mental retardation, performance levels should be examined relative to the child's mental age (MA). However, specific information regarding the child's cognitive status may not be available at the time of testing.

Clinical decisions for language intervention should be based on the child's: (a) highest level of symbolic play performance; (b) performance in the domains of objects, actions, and roles; (c) diversity of play schemes; and (d) structural complexity of play schemes. If the child is placed in treatment, scripted play formats should provide the contexts for facilitating both advanced nonverbal symbolic behavior and communication.

Note of Caution

Many contextual variables such as type of props (realistic vs. abstract), degree of modeling, complexity of modeled behavior, and immediate interests and preferences of the child can serve to enhance or depress play performance

---

[2] All child play behaviors occurring during random play, spontaneous organized play, and post-modeling play can be used to assess play performance.

(Bretherton et al., 1984). For example, the child may perform an object substitution spontaneously but reject a substitution modeled by the therapist. Bretherton et al. (1984) suggest that the therapist attempt to determine the child's range of symbolic play abilities in context of various types of play contexts. Such information could provide valuable directions for clinical intervention.

SOURCES FOR SCALE DEVELOPMENT

Bretherton, I. (1984). Representing the social world in symbolic play: Reality and fantasy. In I. Bretherton (Ed.), *Symbolic play: The development of social understanding*. Orlando, FL: Academic Press.

Bretherton, I., O'Connell, B., Shore, C., & Bates, E. (1984). The effect of contextual variation on symbolic play: Development from 20 to 28 months. In I. Bretherton (Ed.), *Symbolic play: The development of social understanding*. Orlando, FL: Academic Press.

Conti-Ramden, G., & Friel-Patti, S. (1986). Situational variability in mother-child conversations. In K. Nelson (Ed.), *Children's language* (Vol. 6). New York: Gardner Press.

Fenson, L. (1984). Developmental trends for action and speech in pretend play. In I. Bretherton (Ed.), *Symbolic play: The development of social understanding*. Orlando, FL: Academic Press.

Harrison, J., Lombardino, L., & Farrar, J. (1989). Language comprehension strategies used by young children in scripted-routines. Unpublished paper.

Largo, R. & Howard, J. (1979). Development progression in play behavior of children between nine and thirty months: Spontaneous play and imitation. *Development Medicine in Childhood Neurology, 21,* 229–316.

Lombardino, L., Stein, J., Kricos, P., & Wolf, M. (1986). Play diversity and structural relationships in the play and language of language-normal preschoolers: Preliminary data. *Journal of Communication Disorders, 19,* 475–489.

McCune-Nicolich, L. (1981). Toward symbolic functioning: Structure of early pretend games and potential parallels with language. *Child Development, 52,* 783–797.

McCune-Nicholich, L., & Fenson, L. (1984). Methodological issues in studying early pretend play. In T. D. Yawkey and A. D. Pellegrini (Eds.), *Child's Play: Developmental and Applied*. Hillsdale, NJ: Lawrence Erlbaum Associates, Inc.

Skarakis-Doyle, E. A. (1983, March). The development of symbolic play and language in language disordered children. Unpublished paper.

Snow, C., Perman, R., & Nathan, D. (1986). Why routines are different: Toward a multiple factors model of the relation between input and language acquisition. In K. Nelson (Ed.), *Children's language* (Vol. 6). New York: Gardner Press.

Terrell, B. Y., & Schwartz, R. G. (1983, November). Symbolic play: Is children's play determined by the objects used? Paper presented at the annual convention of the American Speech-Language-Hearing Association.

Watson, M., & Fisher, K. (1980). Development of social roles in elicited and spontaneous behavior during the preschool years. *Developmental Psychology, 16,* 483–494.

Wolf, D., Rygh, J., and Altshuler, J. (1984). Agency and experiences: Actions and states in play narratives. In I. Bretherton (Ed.), *Symbolic play: The development of social understanding*. Orlando, FL: Academic Press.

LIST OF PROPS

Props for Cooking Theme: Cooking Dinner Script

Baby doll	Regular spoon
Mother doll	Pretend food
Father doll	Pitcher
Bear	Block
Pots	Box
Bowls	Book
Large Wooden Spoon	Telephone

(Use imaginary items, e.g., salt, ice cream, refrigerator)

Props for Grooming Theme: Bathing Baby Script

Baby doll	Washcloth	Block
Mother doll	Shoe box on basin	Book
Father doll	Shampoo	Telephone
Bear	Comb/brush	Mirror

(Use imaginary items, e.g., hairdryer, towel)

Props for Random Play

Doll	Car	Tea set
Bear	Toy hammer	Blocks
Legos	Nesting cups	Telephone

APPENDIX 3D

Early Communication Checklist*†

Linda J. Lombardino, Ph.D., Jamie B. Stapell, M.A.,
Kenneth J. Gerhardt, Ph.D.

Child's Name _____ Date of Birth _____

Examiner _____ Test Date _____

Reactive Primitive Behaviors (1–3 months)
(Early perlocutionary)

____ Arouses from sleep by sudden noises

____ Startles to unexpected loud noises

____ Looks to/fixates on adult's face

____ Looks to/fixates on inanimate objects

____ Responds to adult's facial expressions and vocalizations (cooing sounds)

____ Smiles during face-to-face interactions

____ Responds differentially to familiar vs. unfamiliar, angry vs. happy, male vs. female voices

Purposeful Primitive Behaviors (4–7 months)
(Late perlocutionary)

____ Begins to make rudimentary head turns toward sound source

____ Searches for sound sources that are out-of-sight

____ Demonstrates a listening attitude

____ Reaches for an object held out to child or close by

____ Pushes away (or turns body away from) undesired object or event

____ Uses global body movements (vocal/gestural/eye contact) as a means to reinstate a desired activity

* Indicate whether behavior was directly observed (D) or reported by parent (P)

† Reprinted from *Journal of Pediatric Health Care, 1* (5), L. J. Lombardino, J. B. Stapell, and K. J. Gerhardt, Evaluating early communicative behaviors in infancy, pp. 240–246, © 1987, with permission from National Association of Pediatric Nurse Practitioners.

___ Responds to familiar phrases to reinstate a desired activity

___ Produces syllable repetitions

Transitional/Instrumental Communicative Behaviors (8–11 months)
(Transition from perlocutionary to illocutionary)

___ Turns to out-of-sight sound sources in the lateral plane

___ Enjoys shaking rattle or noise maker

___ Participates in social games such as pat-a-cake and peek-a-boo

___ Gives an object in response to adult's outstretched hand

___ Uses adult's hand to recreate a spectacle (does not look to adult's face as if to bid for help)

___ Reaches for objects at a distance (does not look back at adult)

___ Engages in "showing off" behaviors

___ Extends arms to be picked up

___ Waves "hi" or "bye" (with prompting from parent)

___ Responds to own name

___ Responds to "no," and a few single words

___ Uses ma-ma or da-da (void of any real meaning)

Intentional/Conventional Communicative Behaviors (11–14 months)
(Illocutionary)

___ Alerts to telephone ring

___ Looks to the television when certain programs or commercials come on

___ Initiates routine games

___ Spontaneously waves hi or bye

___ Spontaneously gives objects to adult

___ Spontaneously shows objects to adult

___ Spontaneously points to request objects from adult

___ Spontaneously points to request assistance

___ Shakes head "no" to indicate rejection

___ Uses a few words as performatives (proto-words)

___ Responds to a number of single words (names of family members, names of pets, labels for games or social routines, food-related items)

First Words (14–16 months)
(Locutionary)

___ Localizes to sounds in all planes (left, right, down, up, diagonal)

___ Responds to name when called from another room

___ Uses gestures, varying intonation patterns, and/or words to express a number of communicative functions

___ Draws attention to self

___ Draws attention to objects

___ Requests objects

___ Requests actions or social routines

___ Expresses dislikes or protests

___ Expresses pleasure or surprise

___ Greets

___ Answers

___ Uses a few words to refer to objects, events, actions, attributes, and locations

___ Responds to several words in addition to questions such as "Where's daddy?" "Where's your nose?"

APPENDIX 3E

Sampler of Frequently Used Tests to Assess Language of Preschoolers (Ages Birth–4:11)

Test	Author	Ages	Publisher
AGS Early Screening	Harrison et al.	2:0–6:11 years	AGS
Assessment for Persons Profoundly or Severely Impaired	Connard & Bradley-Johnson (1998)	Birth–8 months	Pro-Ed
Bankson Language Test	Bankson (1990)	3:0–6:11 years	Pro-Ed
Birth to Three Assess-Ment and Intervention System, 2nd ed.	Ammer & Bangs (2000)	Birth–3 years	Pro-Ed
Boehm-3 Preschool	Boehm (2001)	3:0–5:11 years	Psychological Corporation
Bracken Basic Concept Scale-revised	Bracken (1998)	2.6–7:11 years	Psychological Corporation
Bracken School Readiness Assessment	Bracken (2002)	2.6–7:11 years	Psychological Corporation
Carolina Picture Vocabulary Test for Deaf and Hearing Impaired Children	Layton & Holmes (1985)	4–11:6 years	Pro-Ed
Childhood Autism Rating Scale	Schopler, Reichler, & Renner	2 years and older	Psychological Corporation
Clinical Evaluation of Language Function-Preschool	Wiig, Secord, & Semel (1992)	3–6 years	Psychological Corporation
Comprehensive Assessment of Spoken Language	Carrow-Woolfolk	3:0–21 years	AGS
Communication and Symbolic Behavior Scales	Wetherby & Prizant (1993)	8–24 months	Brookes
Communication and Symbolic Behavior Scales-Developmental Profile	Wetherby & Prizant (2002)	6–24 months	Brookes
Comprehensive Receptive & Expressive Vocabulary Test, 2nd ed.	Wallace & Hammill (2003)	4:0–89:11 years	Psychological Corporation

Detroit Tests of Learning Aptitude-Primary, 2nd ed.	Hammill & Bryant	3:0–9:11 years	AGS
Developmental Activities Screening Inventory, 2nd ed.	Fewell & Langley (1984)	Birth–60 months	Pro-Ed
Developmental Assessment of Young Children	Voress & Maddox (1998)	Birth–5:11 years	Pro-Ed
Developmental Indicators for the Assessment of Learning (DIAL-3)	Mardell-Czudnowski & Goldenberg	3:0–6:11 years	AGS
Early Language Milestone Scale, 2nd ed.	Coplan (1993)	Birth–36 months	Pro-Ed
Evaluating Acquired Skills in Communication-Revised	Riley (1991)	3 months–8 years	Psychological Corporation
Expressive One-Word Picture Vocabulary Test	Brownell (2000)	2:0–18:11 years	Psychological Corporation
Expressive Vocabulary Test	Williams	2:6–90+ years	AGS
First STEp: Screening Test for Evaluating Preschoolers	Miller (1993)	2:9–6:2 years	Psychological Corporation
Fluharty Preschool Speech and Language Screening Test, 2nd ed.	Fluharty (2000)	3:0–6:11 years	Psychological Corporation
Joliet 3-Minute Pre-School Speech and Language Screen	Kinzler (1993)	2:6–4:6 years	Psychological Corporation
Kaufman Assessment	Kaufman & Kaufman	2:6–12:5 years	AGS
Miller Assessment for Preschoolers	Miller (1982)	2:9–5:8 years	Psychological Corporation
Kaufman Survey of Early Academic & Language Skills	Kaufman & Kaufman	3:0–6:11 years	AGS
Kindergarten Language Screening Test, 2nd ed.	Gauthier & Madison (1998)	3:6–6:11 years	Pro-Ed
MacArthur Communicative Development Inventories	Fenson et al. (2003)	8–30 months	Brookes
Mullen Scales of Early Learning	Mullen	Birth–68 months	AGS

OWLS: Listening Comprehension Scale & Oral Expression Scale	Carrow-Woolfolk	3:0–21:11 years	AGS
The Patterned Elicitation Syntax Test-Revised	Young & Perachio (1993)	3:0–7:5 years	Psychological Corporation
Peabody Picture Vocabulary Test-III	Dunn & Dunn	2:6–90+ years	AGS
Preschool Language Assessment Instrument, 2nd ed.	Blank, Rose, & Berlin (2003)	3:0–5:11 years	Pro-Ed
Preschool Language Scale, 4th ed.	Zimmerman, Steiner, & Pond (2002)	Birth–6:11 years	Psychological Corporation
Receptive-Expressive Emergent Language Scale, 3rd ed.	Bzoch, League & Brown	Infants & Toddlers	Pro-Ed
Receptive One-Word Picture Vocabulary Test	Brownell (2000)	2:0–18:11 years	Psychological Corporation
Rice-Wexler Test of Early Grammatical Impairment	Rice & Wexler (2001)	3:0–8 years	Psychological Corporation
Sequenced Inventory Of Communication Development-Revised	Hedrick, Prather, & Tobin	4 months–4 years	Pro-Ed
Structured Photo-Graphic Expressive Language Test, Pre-school	Werner & Kresheck (1983)	3:0–5 years	Psychological Corporation
Test for Auditory Comprehension of Language, 3rd ed.	Carrow-Woolfolk (1999)	3:0–9:11 years	Pro-Ed
Test of Early Reading Ability—Deaf or Hard of Hearing	Reid, Hresko, Hammill, & Wiltshire (1991)	3:0–13:11 years	Pro-Ed
Test for Examining Expressive Morphology	Shipley, Stone, & Sue (1983)	3:0–8 years	Psychological Corporation
Test of Early Language Development, 3rd ed.	Hresko, Reid, & Hammill (1999)	2:0–7:11 years	Pro-Ed
Test of Language Development-Primary, 3rd ed.	Newcomer & Hammill (1997)	4:0–8:11 years	Pro-Ed
Test of Word Finding, 2nd edition	German (2000)	4:0–12:11 years	Psychological Corporation

Test of Written Language, 3rd ed.	Hammill & Larsen (1998)	3:0–11 years	Psychological Corporation
The Token Test for Children	DiSimoni (1978)	3:0–12 years	Pro-Ed
Utah Test of Language Development, 4th edition	Mecham (2003)	3:0–9:11 years	Pro-Ed
Vineland Adaptive Behavior Scales	Sparrow, Balla, & Cicchetti	Birth–18:11 years	AGS
Wiig Criterion-Inventory of Language	Wiig (1990)	4:0–13 years	Psychological Referenced Corporation
The Wilson Syntax Screening Test	Wilson (2000)	Pre-K and K	Psychological Corporation

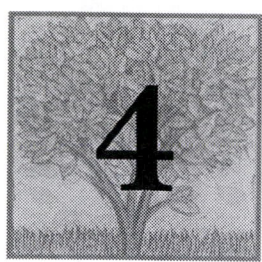

Treatment of Language Delays and Disorders in Preschool Children

■ LEARNING OBJECTIVES

After completion of this chapter, the reader will be able to

1. Differentiate between treatment principles, treatment procedures, and treatment goals and will be able to write a language goal for a preschooler with language deficits.

2. List characteristics of the perlocutionary stage, the illocutionary stage, and the locutionary stage with regard to pediatric language development.

3. Explain the functional model of intervention and differentiate between the more traditional model and the functional model.

4. Differentiate between the cycles approach to therapy and focused stimulation as explained by Cleave and Fey.

5. Describe at least four considerations when choosing therapy procedures for a child with a language-based delay or disorder.

6. Explain the evaluative planning process and discuss its role in the treatment sequence.

■ INTRODUCTION

One of the most important questions a clinician can ask when planning therapy is, "What are the reasons the child communicates?" MacDonald (1989) writes that children communicate for personal reasons, instrumental reasons, and social reasons. Personal reasons include talking for the child's own physical pleasure, and, in infants, babbling just to make sounds. Instrumental reasons include communication that occurs in order to get something to meet a need. Socially, communication is used to comment on the environment and create an exchange of information. As the child matures, the early sounds and gestures are replaced with more advanced symbols of language to produce an effective communicative exchange with another individual. But, MacDonald makes an important point that instrumental communication will not generalize to social use, but social communication will generalize to instrumental communication. Therefore, it is critical in therapy to emphasize the social uses of language in order to facilitate the communication process.

In this chapter, the reader will not find exact treatment procedures other than illustrative examples. Precise treatment procedures will always vary from client to client, so to provide the reader with procedures to use with a specific disorder would be of little value in the long run. However, to provide theoretical principles on which to base the decision-making process in treatment will give future clinicians the tools needed to deal with the range of language delays and disorders seen in preschool children.

■ THE ENVIRONMENT

A Historical Progression of Intervention

Historically, language stimulation activities were created in the context of behavioral paradigms. In the 1960s and 1970s, different techniques such as shaping, fading, modeling or imitation, and reinforcement procedures dominated the literature and provided many of the techniques that are still the foundation for many therapies. However, in the 1990s, the emphasis shifted away from behavioral procedures per se to focus on functional outcomes; that is to say, the goal is communication first, followed by expansion and generalization in the natural environment. Currently, the philosophy of "communication first" dominates many therapies owing to the possibility of fewer therapy sessions and a reliance on functional outcomes that results from the current emphasis in health care reform. It is important that therapy goals can easily be generalized to the child's natural setting. When a functional model of intervention is used, the child has the opportunity to develop an array of language structures, as well as communication skills. This learning is based on spontaneous conversations and social interactions with the child. It is beneficial to conduct the therapy in the child's natural contexts (home and preschool) to facilitate the generalization and maintenance of his or her language skills (Owens, 1999).

In addition to setting functional goals, a second concern when planning therapy is structuring the child's environment to facilitate the growth of his or her language and communication skills. An initial area of attention in this structuring is the concept of **sensory integration**—how much sensory input can the child tolerate? One way to measure this is to notice how distractible the child is and to monitor the visual and auditory stimulation present when the child is in therapy. Distractions that should be monitored include decorations and furnishings in the room, toys and other therapy materials, noise in the vicinity of the therapy room, and the clinician's attire (which should be conservative and businesslike, but comfortable).

Sensory integration. The organization and interpretation of input from the various sensory systems of the body.

The diagnostic and therapeutic materials available should be selected carefully to be safe, durable, and appropriate to the goals. When on a budget, it is wise to choose toys that can teach a variety of concepts, such as doll houses, play villages, cooking sets, and doctor kits. Regardless of the materials chosen, however, one of the biggest concerns of the clinician should be to keep the intervention procedures uncomplicated. Procedures should be designed to require minimal input from the clinician, to facilitate maximum responses from the child, and to ease the task of data collection. Schemes that involve role play with family members and other individuals with whom the child has contact are excellent therapy tools.

Another consideration in the historical progression of language intervention is the use of peer interactions to facilitate the development, maintenance, and generalization of language skills by children with language delays or disorders.

Until the passage of P. L. 94-142, the concept of least restrictive environment had received little attention in the education of children with handicaps. With subsequent expansion of the original legislation, the passing of P. L. 99-457 and the Individuals with Disabilities Education Act further mandated the inclusion principle as the model for school placement of children with handicapping conditions. As part of inclusion, it has become evident that time needs to be spent teaching the normally developing classmates about the handicaps exhibited by their classmates, as well as strategies the child with handicap(s) may use to communicate and become socially involved with their peers.

In addressing therapeutic intervention with children with specific language impairment (SLI), Hadley and Schuele (1998) "argue that it is particularly important for speech-language pathologists to target socially relevant language objectives with children with SLI because these children eventually must live up to standard societal expectations in social, educational, and vocational settings" (p. 25). Teaching pragmatic skills in a contrived setting based on one-on-one interactions between the clinician and child does not adequately address socialization demands with peer-groups beyond the therapy situation. Another problem that occurs in facilitating the development of social skills in children with SLI is the lack of emphasis on verbal skills needed for social competence in addition to (but separate from) nonverbal skills. Hadley and Schuele remind us that children with SLI have language impairments in the absence of motor, sensory, emotional, or intellectual problems. Thus, the speech-language pathologist may be the only special educator who provides intervention beyond the classroom placement. Also, children with SLI are at risk academically, so enhancing their peer interaction skills may have a side effect of making the child feel more positive about school and supporting their adjustment to the academic setting. It is important to identify children with SLI early so that intervention in all areas of language, including social interactions with peers, can be addressed to prepare the child for the social and academic demands he or she will face when beginning school.

Encouraging the Family to Facilitate Language Development

Schemes that reflect daily living situations encountered by the child should be the focus of preschool therapy. It is better to pick a few everyday situations to target in therapy and then encourage the family to generalize the concepts and techniques to other situations at home. Also, by using this approach, follow-through at home is more likely to occur because the suggestions made by the clinician can be used to facilitate language in the routine activities of the family, and anecdotal reports from the family (as opposed to specific data collection, which rarely gets done) are sufficient documentation.

One rule of thumb that can be used is to develop intervention strategies that can be done by the family in the car. Parents spend an inordinate amount of time driving family members hither and yon—and this is a great time to facilitate language development. The main instruction to the parent is that the adult's level of language should be equal to or slightly more complex than the child's level. This means the parent provides a reachable example for the child as he or she, the parents, and the clinician work toward the ultimate goal: effective communication at any time and any level.

Cleave and Fey (1997) conducted a study in which there were two groups of preschoolers, with one group receiving clinician-directed intervention only, and the other group receiving parent intervention only. All children in the study had expressive language deficits, particularly in the area of morphosyntactic development, but they "were judged to be normally responsive and able to plan an assertive role in conversation" (p. 23) with adults. Basic goals were defined as general goals of intervention based on the child's social-interactional skills. For each group, three basic goals of intervention were addressed:

1. To increase the frequency and consistency of the child's use of grammatical forms and operations that typically are used infrequently and inconsistently.

2. To foster the child's acquisition of new content-form interactions to perform available conversational acts.

3. To set the child's existing language-learning mechanisms in motion to promote the acquisition of general linguistic principles, and to foster broad, systematic changes in the child's grammar. (p. 23)

In treatment, the first basic goal was based on facilitating consistent use of the child's use of structures used inconsistently before therapy. The second goal focused on teaching the child new morphosyntactical constructions that were not previously in the child's repertoire. The final goal was developed to stimulate the child's existing language-learning processes in hopes of facilitating efficient learning of language beyond the clinical setting. Intermediate and specific goals were also developed for each child in the study. The list of specific goals for each child was quite large, and it was unreaslistic to expect that all the goals could be focused on in therapy. Thus, intermediate goals that encompassed a large number of specific goals were developed. It was hoped that this would lead to generalization of the skills learned when the intermediate goals were addressed. Within the context of the intermediate goals, four specific goals were selected for each child. A cyclical goal attack strategy, based on the cycles approach developed by Hodson and Paden (1991) for the treatment of phonological disorders, was incorporated into the treatment, along with focused stimulation procedures. In the cycles approach, the treatment focused on one goal per week for four consecutive weeks (e.g., goal 1 in week 1; goal 2 in week 2; goal 3 in week 3; goal 4 in week 4; goal 1 in week 5). Focused stimulation (Fey, 1986) was also used in the treatment protocol. In the focused stimulation procedures, the basis for intervention was natural conversation between the child and the adult. The child was bombarded with a chosen language form "in a variety of semantically and pragmatically appropriate contexts" (Cleave & Fey, 1997, p. 24). The adult would model the target behaviors, and the child would be encouraged to attempt the target.

As a result of their study, Cleave and Fey (1997) suggested that parents should be actively involved in the clinical process by combining the parent program with the clinic program. Although some parents may gain some knowledge about intervention by observing (as they did in the clinician-directed treatment), it is more beneficial to provide training for the parents to facilitate the learning of language beyond the clinical setting. Within the cycles approach and focused stimulation, sentence recasts helped the child meet the target by providing a model of correct productions that maintained the meaning of the child's utterance while simultaneously correcting or modifying the child's utterance (Cleave & Fey, 1997). All of these strategies enhanced the preschool child's mastery of grammatical structures and should be considered when planning an intervention program for preschoolers.

■ PRESYMBOLIC AND SYMBOLIC COMMUNICATION

Successful intervention with preschool children frequently hinges on the clinician's ability to determine if the child is at a presymbolic or a **symbolic level of communication** and on planning appropriate goals and activities based on the child's level.

Sensorimotor Skills as Foundations for Facilitating Language

Regardless of the approach a clinician chooses, it is critical that he or she look for basic **language parameters** that serve as precursors to effective communication skills. These parameters, as outlined in the *Ordinal Scales of Psychological Development* (Uzgiris & Hunt, 1975), include **means-end**, turn-taking, object permanence, use of gestures, requesting behaviors, **joint attention**, behavior regulation, play schemes, **causality**, and imitation skills. All of these skills help us to understand how the child relates to his or her environment, including objects and the people in it. The best success in therapy is when social contact, environmental exposures, and intact maturational systems are in place: these are needed for adequate development of language. As written by Dunst (1980),

> the description of the child's sensorimotor performance in *qualitative* terms represents the critical and most important step in the overall clinical-educational process. Procedures used to describe a child's performance in qualitative terms permit an assessment of the extent to

Symbolic level of communication. Communication in which the individual understands the relationships among words and objects and events (i.e., that the words represent the objects and events).

Language parameters. Aspects of language that form the basis of linguistic functioning.

Means-end. A language parameter in which the child has the ability to use foresight in simple problem solving (e.g., using a dowel to obtain an object that is out of reach).

Joint attention. The sharing of visual and auditory attention to the same stimulus.

Causality. The reactivation of a spectacle or event by bodily movement (e.g., turning the key to have a toy car reactivate).

which a child is delayed in development, whether or not a child's pattern of development is typical or atypical, a determination of a child's major strengths and weaknesses, and an identification of appropriate interventions designed to remediate or ameliorate any delays and/or deficits found. (p. vii)

Child-Centered Therapy

When beginning treatment, it is critical to remember that, regardless of the philosophical approach or the techniques chosen to accomplish the stated goals, the child is at the center of the treatment plan. Teachers and speech-language clinicians are usually highly directive individuals, meaning that they tend to give many directions that require specific responses. Although this may be satisfactory in some settings, therapy that is designed to generate maximum responses and facilitate generalization while keeping the child as the primary focus needs to be more experiential than directive. By nature, most preschoolers are exploratory creatures. However, some children have handicaps that limit their ability to explore their environments and, in turn, restrict the development of language.

Learned helplessness. A state of nonaction that a child learns because his or her needs are constantly anticipated by his or her caregivers so that there is little or no need for the child to communicate or initiate communication.

In addition, many children with disabilities experience **learned helplessness** because their caregivers or clinicians, or both, anticipate their needs and fulfill them before the child has to communicate them using idiosyncratic or conventional means of expression. Whenever a child's needs are met before he or she expresses them overtly, the child may lose motivation to communicate. However, this can be a problem at the opposite end of the spectrum as well. In some cases, children desperately try to communicate their needs but, due to the idiosyncratic nature of their communication signals, their attempts may not be understood. In these cases, as a child is misinterpreted over time, he or she may give up attempting to initiate communication through conventional methods. The goal is to help this child avoid being frustrated by getting him or her to use more conventional signals to communicate needs and to engage in social exchanges for a range of communicative functions.

For example, a child with many autistic behaviors had a communication system that consisted of a gesture for "eat" and arm movements to signal the clinician to restart a spectacle such as a battery operated toy. In this case, the adults in his environment imitated these movements and always paired giving food for the gestural request to eat and always restarted the toy and paired the child's arm movements with the word "more." By doing so, the clinicians validated the child's two primary attempts at communication. In this case, social contact and environmental manipulation were used to increase the child's communicative attempts, despite his underdeveloped communication signals. Eventually, meaning was assigned to other movements the child made; and within six months, he had a communicative repertoire of approximately 10 gestures that were used in effective communication exchanges. In his case, his social-emotional development was enhanced through appropriate early intervention.

Interactive Environmental Frameworks

Morris (1982) developed a chart that demonstrates the interactive frameworks that affect speech and language development in children with disabilities (Figure 4–1). The critical message of this framework is that assessment and therapy must be child-centered and based on the clinician's knowledge of normal development.

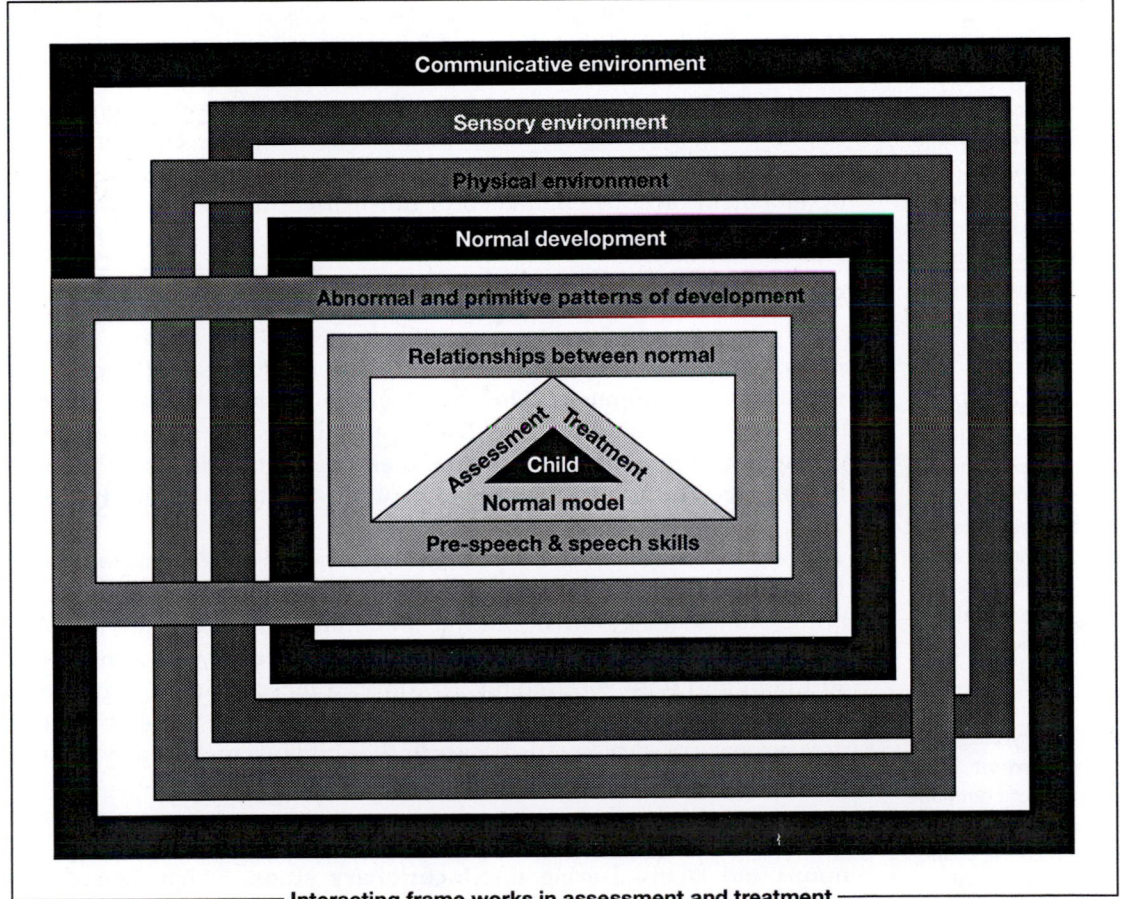

FIGURE 4–1. Interactive frameworks to facilitate communication. (From *The Normal Acquisition of Oral Feeding Skills: Implications for Assessment and Treatment*, by S. E. Morris, 1982, Central Islip, NY. © 1982 by Therapeutic Media, Inc.)

As noted previously, the child is at the center of the figure, representing the fact that assessment and treatment are based on the child's abilities and deficits. The next box stresses the relationships among normal prespeech and speech skills. Thus, when studying the sensorimotor stages and social stages of the child's development, a clear correlation is observed among prespeech activities such as gestures, babbling, and jargon and a child's development of normal speech and language patterns.

The third box stresses the importance of looking at abnormal and primitive patterns of development. By doing so, the clinician is able to determine if the child has a delay or a disorder, particularly when considered in the context of the next box, which represents normal development. The outer three boxes emphasize the fact that there must be an analysis and manipulation of the physical, sensory, and communicative environments of the child in order to facilitate growth of speech and language skills. It is particularly important to recognize the fact that the outer box (communicative environment) and the fourth box (normal development) are represented by solid lines, with one break where abnormal and primitive patterns of development interrupt the flow of normal development in the communicative environment. This alerts the clinician to the fact that any abnormal or primitive patterns of development must be eliminated or normalized in order to have complete development of the communicative environment.

Social Stages of Development

Bates, Camaioni, and Volterra (1975) described three social stages of communication development. The first stage, the **perlocutionary stage**, lasts from birth to 8 months of age. During this time period, children are nonverbal, but communicative; however, their communication is unintentional. In this stage, the adult assigns meaning to the behaviors of the child.

The second stage is the **illocutionary stage**, which develops around 10 months of age. In this stage, the infant is still nonverbal (he or she does not use any specific words), but the communication efforts are intentional. The infant may use eye gaze, conventional gestures (e.g., waving good-bye and pointing), and vocalizations to convey a message in an organized and coordinated manner. During this stage the use of jargon is noted as the child uses protowords. Protowords are words the child invents that may or may not sound like standard English words.

During the third stage, the child starts to use real words, which are primarily nouns and labels. During this **locutionary stage**, which begins around 12 months of age, the child uses intentional linguistic communication. Around 18 months of age, the child combines words and develops an expressive vocabulary of 50 words. However, receptive language (i.e., what the child understands) exceeds expressive language.

Perlocutionary stage of development. The social stage of communication development, during which the child is interactive but uses nonverbal and unintentional communication.

Illocutionary stage of development. The social stage of communication development, in which the child is interactive and communication efforts are intentional, although some of the communication may still be nonverbal.

Locutionary stage of development. The social stage of communication development, during which the child develops intentional, linguistic communication and speech consists primarily of nouns and labels.

Although the Bates model does not explain language acquisition, it does provide a focus on language use that is based on the social interactions between the child and his or her caregiver. It also provides a basis from which to judge if a child may be developing a delay in expressive language. If a child is not using single words by 18 months and is not combining words by 30 months, there is reason to suspect that he or she may have a language deficit.

Again, it is critical to identify children with language deficits early in their development in order to facilitate socially appropriate and effective communication before they become frustrated communicators. In early childhood, the listener provides interpretation of a child's vocalizations and verbalizations to determine the intent of the communicative effort. Halle, Brady, and Drasgow (2004) note that preschoolers with disabilities often have a limited repertoire of communication and social skills. The authors point out that a preverbal preschooler who is engaged in an activity but has limited communication skills may begin to cry, with that crying having several possible implications. For example, the child could be bored, frustrated, finished with the activity, requesting another task, lonely, and/or needing attention. It is up to the listener to interpret the cry and respond appropriately. Incorrect interpretation leads to a communication breakdown, and the need for the child to initiate a communication repair strategy to meet his/her needs. "Hence, it is important to carefully consider variables affecting communication breakdowns as well as strategies that may be effective in facilitating communication success following a breakdown" (pp. 43–44).

Halle et al. (2004) identify three types of communication breakdowns: (1) requests for clarification, (2) nonacknowledgments, and (3) topic shifts. Brady (2003) has some preliminary data that indicate that when faced with a communication breakdown, beginning communicators are more likely to respond positively to requests for clarification (e.g., the listener asking "What?" or "Do you mean . . . ?") than they will to nonacknowledgments and topic shifts. Nonacknowledgements refers to the listener's lack of response to the child's attempt at communication and does not adequately communicate to the child that he or she needs to use a repair strategy in order to get a response. Whether the lack of acknowledgment is intentional or not, the child's communication effort is not reinforced, which may lead to frustration, lack of motivation to communicate, and fewer attempts to communicate in the future.

Topic shifts may be an attempt to distract the child from his or her original effort to communicate. Once again, this is a communication breakdown because the child does not achieve his or her communicative goal or intent. Sometimes a topic shift occurs because the listener chooses not to honor the child's request and wishes to distract the child. If the distraction is equally desirable to the child (e.g., the parent offers a cup of juice when the child requested milk), then the child will not be motivated to implement a repair strategy. In other instances, it is possible that the child does not desire the intended outcome enough to make the effort to engage in a repair strategy.

Generally speaking, there are two types of repair: repetition and modifications. When using repetition, the initiating communicator simply repeats verbatim the original signal. Modifications can consist of additions (adding information to the original signal), reductions (omitting information in the original comunication), and substitutions which provide information in place of any of the original signal (Halle et al., 2004; Brady & Halle, 2002; Wetherby, Alexander, & Prizant (1998). Halle and colleagues (2004) have listed five factors that determine the response efficiency of the child's communication:

1. Response effort

2. Immediacy of obtaining the desired outcome

3. Consistency of obtaining the desired outcome

4. Quality or magnitude of outcome

5. History of punishment. ("any likelihood that reduces the likelihood of the response" (p. 46) such as screaming or throwing materials)

All of these factors together help determine what repair strategies the child will attempt as well as affecting his or her motivation to continue a communicative exchange. Clearly, the environment plays a significant role in the use of repair strategies and in maintaining a child's desire to communicate.

■ THERAPEUTIC PRINCIPLES AND PROCEDURES

Therapeutic Principles

With the development of a scientific approach to assessment and treatment of communication disorders, it has become abundantly clear that learning is not a random process. Rather, learning to be an effective communicator is the result of an organized, data-based program designed to capitalize on strengths to improve deficits. Succinctly put, a therapy program is formulated to delineate the principles and procedures that will be used to achieve the therapy objectives.

Principles. Summary statements of experimental evidence that provide the rules from which treatment procedures are developed.

Principles form the basis of a therapy program. Principles are conceptual in nature and are relatively broad-based compared to procedures. They are summary statements of experimental evidence that provide the rules from which the treatment procedures are developed (Hegde, 1995). For example, a principle could be how the clinician approaches therapy. A clinician may choose to do either within-discipline therapy, interdisciplinary therapy, or transdisciplinary therapy. Which principle is selected depends on the clinician's philosophy about the need to interact with other professionals treating a client. In the within discipline therapy, the clinician does not interact with other professionals (physical therapy, occupational therapy, social work, nursing) who are working with the client. In the interdisciplinary approach, the clinician works within his or her own discipline but participates in regular (usually weekly) meetings with other professionals for the purpose of sharing information about the client's progress in the varying programs of intervention. The transdisciplinary approach takes the interdisciplinary approach a step farther in that the clinicians all learn the various therapy programs a patient is undergoing and incorporate information and procedures from all programs into each therapeutic discipline. Table 4–1 provides

TABLE 4–1. Model of a transdisciplinary goal.

Physical Therapy Goal: The child will exhibit a protective righting response while on the ball in 8 of 10 attempts.

Physical Therapy Procedures:

1. Place child on stomach on large ball.

2. While holding onto the child's feet, roll the child forward.

3. Have assistant assist the child in extending his or her arms and placing the palms on the floor as if breaking a fall.

4. Roll the child back toward the clinician and repeat the procedure.

Language Therapy Goal: In 8 of 10 trials, the child will choose the correct item from an array of three when asked to select an item based on a description of its function.

Language Therapy Procedures:

1. An array of three items, each with a different function (eat, play, dress, write) will be placed in front of the child.

2. When the function of one of the items is described, the child will select the intended object and give it to the clinician.

Occupational Therapy Goal: The child will use a pincer grasp when picking up objects on 90% of all trials.

Occupational Therapy Procedures:

1. The child will imitate a model of bringing the tips of the index finger and thumb together.

2. The child will pick up a small object using a pincer grasp.

Transdisciplinary Procedures:

1. While on the ball, the child will demonstrate a protective righting response as he or she is rolled forward.

2. As the child extends arms and hands, he or she will select the designated object using a pincer grasp.

an example of combining therapy goals from speech-language pathology, occupational therapy, and physical therapy.

Therapy Procedures

Procedures. Concrete, measurable, and objective clinical activities based on the experimental evidence, which form the foundation for therapy outlined in the principles.

In contrast to principles, **procedures** are concrete, measurable, and objective. It is also important that they be replicable, which means that another clinician could implement the plan with similar results as the original clinician obtained. Procedures can be thought of as clinical activities based on the experimental evidence, which forms the foundation outlined in the principles (Hegde, 1995). Another difference between procedures and principles is that principles are generic, whereas procedures are written specific to the client, the disorder, or both (Hegde, 1995).

When choosing which treatment procedures to use, the clinician should keep in mind the six questions outlined in Table 4–2. The first question addresses the issue of whether or not the technique has been evaluated in a controlled setting. One of the major concerns of the profession relates to the need to have experimental evidence on the abilities of the procedures to create a positive, functional outcome. To gather the data, more structured clinical research is required to evaluate experimentally the procedures used in speech-language therapy. Tied closely to this first question is the second question, which addresses the issue of whether or not the evaluation of the procedures was favorable. In other words, has the evidence from controlled research settings in therapy yielded a positive outcome for the patients?

A third critical question relates to the replicability issue: Can the procedures be used by different clinicians in different settings with results similar to those obtained in the experimental evaluation? A procedure that works only under highly controlled circumstances, which cannot be readily replicated in other settings, should not be considered part of a clinician's repertoire of therapy procedures.

TABLE 4–2. Questions to answer in the selection of treatment procedures.

Has the technique been evaluated experimentally?

Have the results been favorable?

Has the technique been replicated across settings, clinicians, and clients?

Is the procedure appropriate for my client?

Can the environment be manipulated to implement the procedure?

Is my client improving?

In some cases, as the fourth question shows, the procedures may be replicable, but they may not necessarily be appropriate for the client. For example, if a piece of equipment is required to use the procedure and the clinician does not have that equipment available, it is not a procedure that can be duplicated in that circumstance with that particular client. Another example is the teaching of eye contact to children of Native American descent. Native American culture teaches children that it is disrespectful to have eye contact with elders. However, a clinician may identify this as a goal for a Native American child. Procedures to teach eye contact are well documented, yet they would be inappropriate as a goal for many Native American children.

The fifth question relates to the clinical environment in which the procedure is being used. Procedures that require a child's total attention would not be appropriate procedures to use in most hospital units for children owing to the presence of other stimulations inherent in that environment. Some activities require more space than others and thus would be impractical to implement in a small therapy room.

Of all the questions, the sixth question is without doubt the most important. A client may fail to progress for many reasons, but one of the easiest to rule out is the choice of incorrect procedures. A common mistake made by beginning (and some experienced) clinicians is to choose a procedure that is too difficult for a child. This often occurs because the clinician has not carefully analyzed the task at hand. Task analysis is a critical clinical tool that must be mastered in order to choose correct procedures. In a task analysis, the clinician works through a task step by step, ensuring that the child has the skills necessary to master the procedure. For example, many sequencing activities require an intact short-term memory. Thus, if a child is unable to remember a simple sequence, he or she cannot be expected to succeed on a task that requires remembering one step before another.

Regardless of the principles and procedures selected by the clinician, the overall goal in therapy is to increase the number of options available to the client to help him or her reach his maximum potential. For a 3-year-old preschooler who does not talk, therapy should not focus solely on getting the child to talk. Rather, therapy should concentrate on teaching the child to communicate in some manner, as by gestures, sounds, sign language, or a communication board. Speech should be modeled in all communication exchanges, but it should not be the sole focus of therapy. Otherwise, it is possible the child will become extremely frustrated and shut down on all communicative attempts. It is important to remember that all children learn to communicate by exploring the use of a variety of systems—cognitive, sensory, and motor—before adapting to the most common form—speech. Clinicians do not help the child by demanding only one form of communication. Children learn speech and language by exploring their environment through a myriad of sensory and motor experiences. Thus, for children functioning below the level of age of 24 months, it is critical to guide a child through a variety of sensorimotor experiences to facilitate the neurological maturation needed for effective communication.

Going With the Flow

Another common mistake made by beginning clinicians is not tempering the demand for therapeutic compliance with some flexibility as opportunities present themselves in the clinical setting. A clinician was observed teaching a 3-year-old child the concept of *over* and *under*. The activity required the child to sit in a chair at the table and to identify *over* and *under* on a series of illustrations. After doing about 10 cards, the child slid out of his seat and took refuge under the table. The clinician was so determined to complete the task with the illustrations that she completely missed the opportunity to use the fact that the child was under the table to reiterate and demonstrate the concept being taught! Children are playful creatures who present many opportunities to teach a variety of concepts. It is critical for clinicians not to miss these incidental learning opportunities by adhering to a rigid lesson plan.

The Clinician-Client Interaction

Rapport

Rapport. A harmonious connection between two individuals based on mutual respect and a level of trust.

In order to set appropriate goals, or target behaviors, time must spent on developing the clinician-client interaction. A crucial element is **rapport** which is described by Hegde (1995) as "a harmonious connection." Rapport consists of mutual respect and a level of trust between the client and the clinician. It is frequently established through small talk, in which the clinician spends time learning about the client as a person. In the process of taking a case history, the clinician should interject questions that will help him or her understand the child as a person, not as a diagnostic case. These questions should include such information as the child's favorite toys, special activities that the child enjoys, whether he or she enjoys books, and other such questions. Above all, the parents of a preschool child need to trust the clinician who is responsible for telling them if their child has a problem and what can be done about the problem. If a level of respect and trust has not been established, most likely the client will not return to the clinician for intervention.

Another critical element in establishing rapport is the clinician's enthusiasm. No client wants to spend a therapy session with a clinician who is not enthusiastic about his or her work. If clinicians think back over their educational careers, certain teachers stand out as favorite teachers who taught the student in a meaningful and effective manner. Most of these teachers would be described as being enthusiastic about their task. As speech-language pathologists, we deal with many different types of children and families, but the

TABLE 4–3. Elements of rapport (RAPPORT)

Respect: to hold in mutual regard the roles the child, the family, and the clinician play in addressing the communication deficit

Admiration: to hold in esteem the families' efforts to facilitate language and communication in their child

Participation: to develop a therapy program that empowers the child and the family to be active participants in the diagnostic and therapeutic processes

Professional Interaction: to maintain a professional, yet personal, level of interaction with the child and family

Opportunity: to go with the flow and take advantage of situations that present themselves in accordance with the therapy procedures and goals

Restraint: to be less directive and more accommodating of the child's language and communication efforts, thereby encouraging active participation in therapy

Timing: to be cognizant of a family's readiness to receive and accept the fact that their child may have a communication deficit

basic skills with regard to establishing a rapport with the child and his or her family remain the same.

Actually, the word rapport can be described using an acronym, as outlined in Table 4–3.

Analyzing the Client's Temperament

When dealing with the preschool population, clinicians must understand the biological foundations for the behaviors the child exhibits and appreciate how they influence the provision of treatment for a communication deficit. Table 4–4 delineates nine areas that should be considered when analyzing a client's temperament in preparation for therapy.

Activity Level. It is normal for preschoolers to move about and fidget as part of their attempts to explore their world and determine where they fit into the broad picture of life. Beginning clinicians should spend time in a preschool setting to learn about the wide ranges of activity that occur in the process of normal growth and development. This understanding will keep many children from having their normal activity levels diagnosed as hyperactivity. Children need to move around, and therapy should be structured to accommodate that need.

Rhythmicity. The body has a normal heart rate of about 60 beats a minute, or 1 per second. Children who have not developed a normal body rhythm, as explained in the discussion of babies suffering the effects of drug and

TABLE 4–4. Nine areas of assessment when determining a client's temperament.

Category	Description
Activity level	The degree to which the child moves around
Rhythmicity	The child's regularity with regard to sleep patterns, eating, and bowel and bladder functions
Approach or withdrawal	The reaction of the child to any new stimulus, including people, food, places
Adaptability	The child's ability to adapt to a new situation even if the initial response was withdrawal
Intensity of reaction	The child's tendency to scream or whimper when hungry, shriek with laughter or smile when amused
Threshold of responsiveness	The degree of sensitivity to environmental stimuli and to changes in the environment
Quality of mood	The child's overall disposition, whether pleasant and friendly or grumpy and unfriendly
Distractibility	The ease with which the child can be interrupted in an ongoing activity
Attention span and persistence	The length of time a child pursues an activity or persists despite interruptions

Source: Adapted from *Applied Behavior Analysis for Researchers*, by P. A. Alberto and A. C. Troutman, 1986, Columbus, OH: Merrill. Copyright 1986. Merrill Publishing Company.

alcohol abuse, need special consideration in developing this rhythm. If an infant is having difficulty coordinating sucking and swallowing, simply patting the baby at a rate of one pat per second can provide external control which, through consistent and persistent application, will lead to the establishment of an internal rhythm. This is important because, if a child is trying physiologically to determine a normal rhythm, he or she has little energy left to learn the use and power of communication and language.

Approach or Withdrawal. Some children are easily separated from their parents; others are not. To fully participate in therapy activities, a child must learn to separate physically and emotionally from his or her parents. In this category of functioning, the clinician also should analyze carefully how a child reacts to the introduction of new environments and new stimuli. If a clinician is in a facility with several different therapy rooms, he or she may find that a child will react negatively to being seen in a therapy room other than the one in which therapy is typically received. Other children may need a gradation in presentation of stimuli because they are physiologically incapable of handling multiple stimulations. Generally, approach is considered to be a positive response and withdrawal a negative one (Leith, 1984).

Intensity of Reaction. Along with observing approach or withdrawal of the child, the clinician needs to determine the child's threshold of responsiveness. Is the child reticent in the presence of strangers, or in the presence of known adults making specific demands for responses? Is the child overly responsive, which may interfere with his or her attention span on a given task? It is important to be able to "read" the child to determine if he or she is anxious or relaxed about the tasks. The quality of the child's mood will be greatly affected by his or her level of reaction to novel and familiar settings and stimuli. Children who are underresponsive or overly responsive may have difficulty exhibiting the persistence and attention span needed to complete a task. All humans, including children, have a level of responsiveness beyond which they cannot be pushed without negative ramifications. The child's temperament needs to be evaluated carefully so the clinician can obtain maximum responses in the therapy setting.

Adaptability. Adaptability is defined as an individual's ability to adjust to new or changing circumstances (Guralnik, 1968). By carefully studying the child's approach and withdrawal systems and the intensity of his or her reactions, the clinician can determine how adaptable a child is. The child's adaptability will rely in part on the clinician's ability to motivate the child. Motivation is affected by receiving the cooperation of significant others, carefully grading the environmental support and reinforcers for the communication attempts, and using the proper contingencies in a variety of settings.

Motivation. Success in therapy will not occur if the clinician is unable to motivate the child. Motivation is affected by receiving the cooperation of significant others, carefully grading the environmental support and reinforcers for communication attempts, and using the proper contingencies in a variety of settings.

Cause and Effect. A good clinician always thinks in terms of cause-and-effect relationships. Every behavior has a cause, and every behavior has an effect. The question that begs an answer in therapy is how do the causes create the desired or undesired effects. For example, if a child has a low sensory threshold, the clinician needs to present stimuli carefully to encourage desired responses. If the child reacts by withdrawing from the stimulus, the cause of this withdrawing needs to be analyzed carefully. Is it a matter of offering too much stimulation in too short a period of time? Is the stimulus too complex for the child to tolerate? Does the stimulus demand a reaction from different physiological levels that the child has not fully integrated? Addressing these questions adequately can lead to a better understanding of the causes of the child's responses and lead to more effective therapy planning.

Quality of Mood. Quality of mood is closely related to approach and withdrawal. Is the child excited about attending therapy? Is the child friendly (positive approach) or unfriendly (negative approach or withdrawal)? Is the child grumpy or "in a bad mood"? All of us have days when we would rather be doing something else, but with maturity comes the ability to alter our mood to the situation at hand. When a child is "not in the mood" to participate in the therapy activities, it may be necessary for the clinician to alter the lesson plan to facilitate the child's participation. This is part of the "going with the flow" approach mentioned previously.

Distractibility, Attention Span, and Persistence. All of us are distractible under certain conditions, but how well we learn is affected by our ability to attend to and participate in the activities that should be dominating us at any given time. A child with attention deficit disorder will have difficulty prioritizing events in the environment in such as way that he can stay attuned to the important stimuli and minimize his attention to the distracters. For example, a child sitting in a classroom may have difficulty paying attention to the teacher if there is noise on the playground outside the classroom window. The distractible child will give more energy and focus to the extraneous noise than he will to the primary stimulation being provided by the teacher. More information on this topic can be found in Chapter 8.

■ THE TREATMENT SEQUENCE

The Evaluative-Planning Process

The treatment sequence consists of two major portions: the evaluative-planning process and the clinical process. The evaluative planning process includes the evaluation of the client and the determination of behavioral change goals. The clinical process, or what is more commonly referred to as **therapy**, consists of establishing and habituating the new skills, then generalizing the skills to the client's natural environment (Leith, 1984).

Therapy. The process of establishing and habituating new skills, then generalizing the skills to the client's natural environment.

Evaluate the Client

It cannot be stressed enough that evaluation is the first step of the therapeutic process. It is through a careful analysis of the evaluation results that the clinician makes decisions about the goals, procedures, and principles for the therapy. During the evaluative planning process, four issues need to be addressed (Table 4–5). Describing the nature of the problem includes identifying whether the child is exhibiting a delay, a disorder, or a difference with regard to language and communicative functioning. Within each category, the current level of functioning the child exhibits should be described. In infants and toddlers this is frequently done in terms of the stages of social-communication and sensorimotor development (see additional information in Chapter 3). For the preschool child (age 3 to 4 years old), the child's communication skills are described relative to stages of normal development in expressive and receptive language acquisition.

Table 4–5. Four purposes of the evaluative-planning process.

1. To describe the nature of the problem

2. To define the severity of the problem

3. To determine the etiology (cause), if possible

4. To make recommendations

Source: Adapted from *Handbook of Clinical Methods in Communication Disorders*, by W. R. Leith, 1984. San Diego: Singular Publishing Group.

Defining the severity of the problem is a second critical purpose in the evaluative planning process. The clinician first offers a description of the child's abilities and deficits. In defining the severity of the problem, the clinician applies objective measures to determine how much of a delay is present or how severe a disorder the child exhibits when compared with a normative sample. In other words, the description is based on observation, and judgments on the severity can be based on normative samples.

A third purpose of the evaluative-planning process is to identify the etiology, if possible. As discussed thus far, etiologic information is sometimes required to determine if a child is expected to progress or regress, and possibly it is needed to place a child into treatment. Procedural and fiscal needs often dictate the identification of the etiology; thus whenever possible, this information should be obtained.

The final purpose of the evaluative-planning process is to make recommendations with regard to treatment. This step entails recommending whether or not therapy should be initiated and defining specific areas of concentration for the therapy program if needed.

Determine Behavioral Change Goals

As already explained, goals are based on the results of the evaluation. One of the questions that needs to be answered in determining goals is: What does the child need to be able to communicate successfully in his or her environment? The answer to this question should help determine the mode or method of communication the child will use. Will he or she be taught to rely on speech, or will he or she use an augmentative or alternative communication strategy? In light of the answer to this question, a second important question is: What skills is the child currently demonstrating? If the child has an effective gestural system, it may be beneficial to increase the use of gestures while encouraging the child to vocalize with each gesture. Over time, it would be hoped that the vocalizations could be shaped into appropriate words.

A third question in determining goals is: How do you facilitate the child's use of the newly learned skill in his or her natural environment? This is the step in which the support of the child's caregivers is critical. No child is going to develop into an effective language user in one hour of therapy per week. The natural environment must be structured to facilitate language exploration and use.

The choice of goals will be affected by many of the same questions that were answered during the testing portion of the process. One of those determinants of a goal is whether the child is exhibiting a language delay, a language disorder, or a language difference. If the child has a language delay, the focus will be on determining where the child is, developmentally, with regard to language competence and language performance, and then moving on from that point through a normal progression of language acquisition. If the child is displaying a language disorder, the focus will shift to getting rid of the abnormal behaviors and replacing them with language behaviors that would normally be observed in developing children. Finally, if the child has a language difference, therapy will concentrate on structuring the environment in such a way as to facilitate the development of both languages and to teach the child to code switch. **Code switching** is the transferring of a person's use of a language or dialect to the setting at hand.

Code switching. The ability of an individual to switch dialects or languages depending on the communicative situation.

Other factors that will affect the choice of goals are the severity of the delay or disorder and the presence of organic factors in the etiology. Obviously, the more severe a disorder, the greater the challenge for the clinician. If the child's insurance or Medicaid coverage requires limitations in the number of visits that can be made, this is an additional area of concern. If the child has severe limitations in language, enlisting the support of his or her significant others will be critical to structure the environment so that language learning and use are facilitated on a daily basis. Of course, structuring the environment is important regardless of the level of the severity of the communication and/or language deficit, but as the severity increases, the need for environmental structuring also increases. In addition, certain etiological factors may present obstacles the clinician cannot change that could affect progress. In these cases, it is important to work with interdisciplinary teams and the families to facilitate progress and provide opportunities that the child can use despite any etiological factors. For example, if a child has severe oral-motor problems, the likelihood of using speech as a primary communication mode is lessened. The use of an augmentative system may be of paramount importance to help the child be an effective communicator. The timing of the introduction of an augmentative system and the development of a system a child can use in light of other disabling conditions are crucial.

Determination of the child's cognitive level is important. This may be more complex than it appears because the lack of ability to use language effectively can be misinterpreted as a cognitive problem instead of a language problem.

Thorough and careful analysis of a child's psycho-educational abilities is critical in determining the long-term goals for a child with multiple deficits.

Set up an Environment to Facilitate Language. In actuality, the child will be learning in three different environments. First, incidental teaching occurs in his or her daily living. Incidental teaching is done by the caregivers and the clinician as the child presents opportunities to reinforce a language concept. A second environment is the formal therapy setting in which the clinician plays the primary role in facilitating the child's growth in receptive and expressive language skills. The third teaching strategy based on environment is stimulation in contrived settings, which is followed through by the clinician and the caregivers in formal and informal circumstances.

In all cases, regardless of whether the child has a language delay, disorder, or difference, and regardless of the severity, synergy must occur between therapy and everyday contexts in the child's family and educational settings. As expressed by Owens (1995), "Language facilitators should be trained to recognize the communicative intentions of child's behaviors, to implement the training program, and to assess functionality and practicality of intervention methods, materials, and adaptations" (p. 119). Success hinges on the ability of everyone in the child's natural environment to recognize opportunities to stimulate language and to structure the environment to facilitate language learning opportunities.

Efforts to Modify the Environmental Factors of Poverty

Many poor children come from disorganized, nonregulated worlds, and when put into an overly structured school system, they fail (Polakow, 1993). During his presidential administration, Lyndon Baines Johnson declared a war on poverty as part of his vision of a "Great Society." In 1965, The Equal Opportunity America program funded the Head Start program in hopes that the provision of cognitive enrichment programs would lead to higher IQs and fewer special education placements for elementary school-age children. The Head Start program differed from other similar programs because it was holistic in its approach, consisting of four components: education, health, nutrition, and social services (parent education) (Polakow, 1993). Another major difference between this initiative and others with similar goals was that the programs were justified "in terms of avoidance of future economic costs, rather than on positive humanitarian grounds" (Polakow, 1993, p. 101). That is to say, the justification was that, through participation in Head Start, children were less likely to need expensive special education placements once they attained school age. In addition, when children are ready to start school by age 5 years, they are more likely to have successful experiences, which helps ensure that, as they progress through the educational system, fewer will drop out.

The Clinical Process

Skill. A sequence of responses that are learned through the coordination of various sensory and motor systems and are eventually organized into complex response chains.

Throughout the clinical process, the clinician is assisting the client in developing new skills. A **skill** is defined as a sequence of responses. The responses are learned through the coordination of various sensory and motor systems that are eventually organized into complex response chains (Hegde, 1995).

Effective therapy will occur only if the clinician and the child understand the relationship between the stimulus presented by the clinician, the response of the child, and the consequence (positive or negative reinforcement) offered by the clinician. The child has to understand that, when a stimulus is presented, he or she is expected to integrate his or her own knowledge to respond appropriately.

Development of New Skills

In teaching a new skill, a logical sequence must be followed. In actuality, a skill is taught in three different stages: the cognitive stage, the fixation stage, and the autonomous stage. Development of New Skills (Hegde, 1995).

The Cognitive Stage. The cognitive stage is also referred to as the acquisition stage because it is the stage at which the child acquires the new skills. Therapy begins as the clinician introduces the goals and procedures to the client. During this stage, the clinician provides information using several different techniques, and the client demonstrates the behavior in response to the techniques and stimuli presented by the clinician. During this stage, the clinician should be aware of the prompting hierarchy outlined in Figure 4–2.

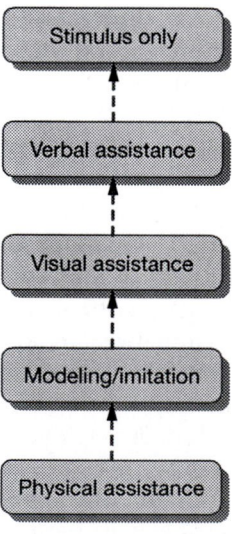

FIGURE 4–2. The prompting hierarchy.

At the beginning of the therapy, the clinician may find it necessary to offer physical assistance by actually guiding the child through the expected responses. For example, a clinician may offer an array of three items (stimuli), such as a toy truck, a spoon, and a shirt, and then ask the child to choose the item he or she uses to eat. If the child does not point to the desired item, the clinician could offer verbal assistance by offering a verbal prompt such as, "I eat soup with a spoon. Show me spoon." If the child does not respond correctly, the clinician could offer visual assistance such as moving the spoon a little closer to the child than the foil items, or pretending to use a spoon to eat. Lack of an appropriate response after visual assistance could indicate the need for modeling the desired response. If the child is physically capable of reaching for the spoon but doesn't, the clinician may model the behavior by pointing to the spoon and having the child imitate the response. If the child still points to the wrong item, the clinician could gently guide the child through the act of pointing to or selecting the spoon. It is important that the clinician move through the prompting hierarchy as quickly as possible so that the child does not come to rely on the clinician's assistance to make the correct response.

The Fixation Stage. Otherwise known as the proficiency stage, the purpose of the fixation stage is to stabilize the new skills in the clinical setting. During this stage, the clinician fades out the consequences with the assumption that the use of the new skills will provide its own reinforcement. The client works at habituating the new behavior by practicing and perfecting the skill in a controlled clinical setting. The goal is for the client to continue the performance of the new skills after the contingencies have been withdrawn. This is one of the most difficult stages of therapy.

Clinical activities during the fixation stage include varying the stimuli presented to elicit the response, varying the conditions under which the response occurs, and varying the presenter of the stimulus. This is a good time to bring in the caregivers and have them assume the role of the clinician so that the next stage of therapy, the autonomous stage, will be facilitated.

The Autonomous Stage. Also known as the maintenance stage, the autonomous stage is the phase of therapy in which the goal is getting the new behavior to occur in the client's everyday settings. The client generalizes the skill to make it functional in all settings.

Specific Therapy Procedures Based on a Behavioral Paradigm

Physical Assistance. During the cognitive stage of therapy, the clinician can utilize a variety of therapy procedures borrowed from the psychology literature for addressing the creation of new skills. With children, frequently the first step is to have the clinician physically guide the child through making the correct choice from a myriad of stimuli (see Figure 4–2).

Modeling. The demonstration of a desired behavior to elicit an imitative response.

Modeling and Imitation. A second type of intervention is **modeling** and imitation. In this approach, the clinician demonstrates a desired behavior in order to prompt an imitative response. Imitation is a powerful teaching tool and forms the foundation for the development of many different skills in normal development.

However, many children with cognitive disabilities do not have the ability to imitate, which negates this method as a teaching tool. In cases in which the child does not imitate, physical assistance will be needed to teach the skill of imitation. Another problem is that some behaviors are difficult to model, although this is more problematic in speech therapy than in language therapy. Research principles support modeling and imitation and indicate that "subjects reinforced for imitating various responses will eventually also imitate unreinforced responses" (Alberto & Troutman, 1986, p. 279).

Shaping. The differential reinforcement of successive approximations to a specified target to create a new behavior.

Shaping. A third technique, **shaping**, is rarely used in its purest form. Shaping is the differential reinforcement of successive approximations to a specified target to create a new behavior.

In its pure form, no model is offered, and the clinician does not tell a client why he or she is being reinforced. When used without other techniques, shaping is a very slow process. To use shaping effectively, the clinician must define the target precisely and grade the steps carefully. If the steps are too small, the therapy is inefficient; if steps are too large, reinforcement is not sufficient to keep the child on task. Similarly, it is important to choose the correct place to start in teaching the sequence of behaviors. Each task should be analyzed carefully or broken into small steps. The starting point should be determined systematically by assessing the child's performance on each small step, with therapy beginning at the step in which the child fails. It is also important for the clinician to know when to progress. If the progression is too slow, the child may plateau; that is, he or she will not continue to progress through the sequence of tasks. If, on the other hand, the progression is too fast, the behaviors may extinguish, or disappear, before the entire sequence can be learned. Shaping could be used if a child does not demonstrate any vocalizations and the clinician wants the child to go from being nonvocal to being able to vocalize appropriately. Initially, each sound the child makes would be reinforced. As the child increases the frequency of vocalizations, the clinician could begin to focus on the quality of the vocalizations and reinforce differentially only those sounds which approximate a specific phoneme.

Prompt. A supplementary antecedent that is added to the original stimulus to increase the probability of a correct response.

Prompting With Verbal Assistance. Offering verbal instruction as a **prompt** is another effective therapy technique. A prompt is also referred to as a supplementary antecedent because it is added to the original stimuli in the hope that it will increase the probability that the child will perform the desired response in reaction to the stimulus. Returning to the example in which the child is shown the toy truck, the spoon, and the shirt, if the child did not correctly select the spoon when asked to show the clinician what the child uses to eat, the clinician could provide a prompt by sounding out the first phoneme, /s/, to stimulate the child to choose the correct item. The clinician should always use the weakest prompt possible and should be sure that the prompt focuses the client's attention on the stimulus, not on the additional prompt.

Chaining. Chaining is a therapy technique used to teach a skill that consists of many different components. Specifically, chaining is a sequence of behaviors, all of which must be done to be rewarded. There are three types of chaining: forward chaining, backward chaining, and total task presentation. In **forward chaining**, each step is taught in sequence, and the child is rewarded for completing each step as it is learned. Forward chaining is used more frequently than the other types of chaining in language and cognition tasks. **Backward chaining** is used to teach many self-help skills. In backward chaining, the final step of the sequence is taught first, followed by each step as the sequence regresses back to the original step. In **total-task presentation**, the child is required to perform all steps in the correct sequence to obtain a reward. This would be used after the chain is learned using either backward or forward chaining.

Total-task presentation can be used when the child can do each individual component but does not sequence properly. Thus, it is not the learning of the discrete steps that is rewarded, but rather the proper sequencing of the steps.

Fading. During the fixation stage, fading is a critical technique. **Fading** is the gradual removal of prompts and reinforcers so that the client responds independently to the stimulus. The key words in the definition of fading are "gradual removal." If the prompts and reinforcers are removed too quickly, the child will lose the response and it will be necessary to go back to the cognitive stage to relearn the skill. Another aspect of fading is bringing an already learned behavior under the control of a different stimulus. Going back to the truck-spoon-shirt example again, the clinician would substitute a different spoon to be sure the response, "spoon," is learned and generalized and is not specific to the one stimulus. Thus, in fading the antecedent stimulus may change, but the desired response remains the same (Alberto & Troutman, 1986).

■ TREATMENT SUGGESTIONS BASED ON ETIOLOGY

Therapy Approaches for Preschool Children Who Are Cognitively Challenged

The motor and/or hearing disabilities combined with cognitive, speech and/or language deficits make a neurodevelopmental approach to therapy the most realistic and promising. In a neurodevelopmental approach, all

Forward chaining. A series of sequenced behaviors in which the first steps of the sequence are taught first; the typical chaining approach used in teaching academic skills.

Backward chaining. A series of sequenced behaviors, in which the last steps of the sequence are taught first, working backward to the beginning of the chain; frequently used to teach self-help skills.

Total-task presentation. A series of sequenced behaviors, all of which must be done completely and in sequence in order to master the skill and be reinforced.

Fading. The gradual withdrawal of prompts used to facilitate a response.

aspects of the child's development are addressed, with the child achieving improved function in all modalities simultaneously. Emphasis should be placed on assisting the child through the normal stages of sensorimotor, cognitive, speech, and language development, with the use of environmental stimulation and experiential learning to facilitate the language growth.

Most children need to be at Piagetian sensorimotor stage late IV or early V before they are able to use symbols such as words and pictures to represent concepts. It is possible to use some augmentative communication systems without any presymbolic training, but these systems are limited to one icon representing one message. For example, the speech-language pathologist in a self-contained classroom for children with multiple disabilities in the severe to profound mental disability group placed black and white photographs of essential self-help items around the classroom. The teacher, classroom aides, and clinicians all provided assistance in pointing to a picture prior to the child's using the item. For example, if a child was thirsty, the teacher had the child point to a picture of a cup before receiving a cup of water. Although these children were not likely to combine photos to make early word combinations or to function at the symbolic level, they did learn to point to the picture to receive the item with prompting. Another way to encourage communication is to put something the child desires out of reach and then observe the child as he or she problem solves how to get the desired item. For example, the boy in Figure 4–3 is reaching for the cookies that are slightly out of his reach as part of a "temptation" exercise designed to have him request assistance.

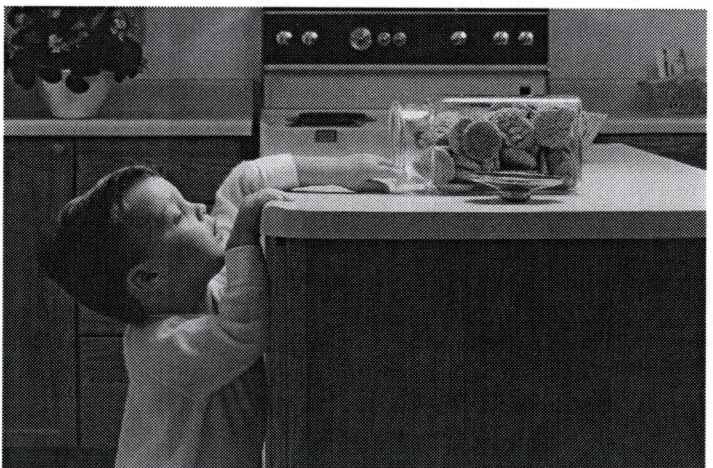

FIGURE 4–3. Temptation exercises are an excellent way to elicit communication from children who have delayed expressive language.

The use of generative language in augmentative communication requires that a child be at the symbolic level of functioning. It is critical that the clinician use an integrated model that includes presymbolic skills and communication-first approaches and then move to symbolic play schemes, followed by teaching words and symbols as a communication mode.

For children with mental disabilities, repetition is a key factor in achieving success in therapy. Therapy is an ongoing process that should be integrated into all daily activities. Early patterns of teaching should provide good models of communication. The adults in the child's environment must act as though they expect an answer; they should not anticipate every need. Otherwise, the child learns to be helpless instead of learning to take the initiative in communication efforts. The environment needs to be structured to facilitate learning through a variety of sensory systems, but at the cognitive level of the child.

Speech and Language for Hearing-Impaired Individuals

Speech and language can be taught to persons who are hearing impaired using a variety of methods of communication. Manualists support the use of sign language, including finger-spelling. American Sign Language was developed within the deaf community and is one of the most widely used signing systems. Cued speech is a supplementary system that uses a series of signals to facilitate the comprehension of spoken language. Typically, oralists do not support the use of supplementary signing systems. However, to return to one of the basic philosophies of this book, no clinician should be a purist in terms of being a manualist or oralist. Rather, whichever system works best for the child who has the hearing loss is the system that should be used. Some children may benefit from a combination of systems (total communication), and this should be analyzed carefully before assigning one communication system arbitrarily on the basis of the clinician's biases.

Interventions for Babies Exposed Prenatally to Drugs

In addition to patting the baby at a rate of one beat per second, caregivers can use other external structuring and soothing techniques for children who are suffering the effects of maternal drug use. Swaddling the baby will help reduce the self-disrupting movements the child makes as part of his or her own distress system. Developing a consistent sucking pattern will facilitate the use of a pacifier, which can also provide some soothing to the baby. The development of consistent, well-structured, predictable environments is absolutely critical, and this needs to be done primarily by providing support, structure, and guidance to the mother during high-stress tasks and situations. Finally, teaching the mother to keep a behavioral log to identify triggers and early warning signs can help provide a focus for intervention to facilitate the relationship between the baby, the mother, and the baby's general environment (Griffith, 1992).

TABLE 4–6. Questions for a behavioral log for drug-exposed babies.

1. What is the infant's usual threshold for overstimulation?
2. What are his or her distress signals?
3. Where is the baby at this time?
4. How much stress does this activity cause?
5. What interventions were attempted?
6. What interventions worked?

Source: Adapted from "Prenatal Exposure to Cocaine and Other Drugs: Developmental and Educational Prognoses," by D. R. Griffith, 1992, September, *Phi Beta Kappan*, pp. 30–34.

In the behavioral log, questions that identify the point at which the baby becomes overstimulated should be used as guidance to provide the information needed to make environmental modifications (Table 4–6). These questions are critical in that they lead the parent through a problem-solving mode to assist the parent in helping the child. The key to helping these babies is to keep them below their threshold of tolerance. Once the level of tolerance is determined, intervention can begin. However, it is critical to respect the threshold level, because once the baby is overstimulated, it is too late. Gradually, with structured transitions, the level of tolerance can increase, and the baby's neurological systems will become increasingly organized. This physiological organization is what could, eventually, separate children who will do well in school from those who will struggle academically and socially.

■ SUMMARY

At this point, it should be clear that learning is not a random process. It is a well-orchestrated sequencing of tasks through which the language skills needed to be an effective communicator are produced. Learning is based on principles, procedures, and programs.

A therapy program encompasses fundamental principles and best practices into a comprehensive plan of action. A quality program also identifies specific activities that may be implemented to help the client achieve his or her therapy goals, including treatment variables that are used to stimulate, change, and eliminate behaviors in the therapy setting.

Regardless of the procedures selected for a child's therapy, it is critical to remember to treat the child and not the label or disability. Even though labels are sometimes necessary for financial or placement reasons, the clinician must remember to react to the child and to assess and treat the child, not the label. Also, the clinician needs to make sure the child's various systems—sensory, motor, neurological, and anatomical—are intact. This is important because a clinician should not attempt remediation of behaviors that are not responsive to behavioral interventions.

CASE STUDY

History

T is a 2-year, 5-month-old girl whose father contacted the University of Florida Speech and Hearing Clinic in Gainesville, Florida because he was concerned about her language and speech development. T's history is positive for spastic cerebral palsy, and she has not received any speech or language therapy. The family lives on a farm about 30 miles from the clinic, but both parents work in Gainesville. There are no other children in the family. While her parents are at work, T stays at home with her maternal grandparents.

Evaluation

Her speech and language were informally assessed using the Assessment of Language Development (see Appendix 3A) and judged to be in the 13- to 18-month-age range. The Early Communication Checklist (Lombardino, Stapell, & Gerhardt, 1987) (Appendix 3B) was also used, with T scoring in the 14- to 16-month range. Overall, she exhibited approximately a 12-month delay receptively and expressively.

	Strengths	Weaknesses
Communicative	Excellent eye contact	Delayed receptive language
	Engages adults in play	Delayed expressive language
	Uses jargon and pointing to communicate	Oral motor weakness
		Lack of means-end and causality
		Limited symbolic play skills
Noncommunicative	Supportive family	Spastic cerebral palsy
	Attends therapy regularly	Limited language experiences beyond the home setting
	Great personality!	

Long-Term Therapy Goals

1. T will be age appropriate in her receptive language skills.

2. T will be age appropriate in her expressive language skills.

3. T will enhance her oral-motor skills through a series of oral-motor exercises.

Language Short-Term Therapy Goals

1. T will spontaneously use 20 words to refer to objects, events, and attributes of objects/toys presented by the clinician.

2. T will problem solve in situations set up to tempt her by putting a toy or food item out of her reach. T will get the item or request help on four out of five trials for three consecutive sessions.

3. T will engage in interactive play in schemes set up by the clinician. Interactive play schemes will be set up using a doctoring kit and a baby doll, a kitchen set, a play garage, a dollhouse, and a toy farm.

4. T will produce multischemes spontaneously such as "cooking" a meal in the play kitchen, feeding it to a doll, and putting the doll to bed. T will complete two multischeme tasks per session.

5. T will request help on 100% of the tasks that she is unable to complete independently.

6. In a tea party setting, T will request food and drink (that were used to facilitate her oral motor goals).

Oral-Motor Short-Term Therapy Goals

1. With 90% accuracy on 10 trials, T will imitate tongue and lip movements made by the clinician.

2. With 90% success on 10 trials, T will pucker her lips and drink through a straw.

3. With 90% accuracy on 10 trials, T will lick a lollipop held by the clinician at the corners of T's mouth and at midline above the lips and below the lips.

4. T will resist having the clinician pull a life saver tied to a string out of T's mouth when the life saver is held beween her lips and teeth.

5. T will use lateral and rotary chewing movements on a piece of caramel wrapped in gauze and held in T's mouth by the clinician, transferring the caramel from right to left and back a minimum of 10 times in one minute.

6. T will bite through a sandwich cookie when it is held between her front incisors five times.

Results

T met all goals and was dismissed from therapy after eight months. Her receptive language and play skills were age appropriate, and she was combining words. For example, she said "Daddy bye-bye" when her father went to get a drink of water, and "baby broke" when the arm fell off a plastic doll with which she was playing. In addition, she was addressing her clinicians by name. T was augmenting her speech with gestures and simple signs when she was not understood. She showed an example of generalization when she had a rhizotomy (a surgical procedure to release some of the spasticity in her legs). Living on a farm, T had received mild injuries and pain when she had been bitten by animals. This was the only pain she knew, and after her surgery she reached back toward her incision and said, "Bepbep (what she called the clinician), bite hurts." The family is to be commended for their interactive support in the therapy sessions and for following up with the goals and procedures at home. Their involvement certainly contributed to the rapid progress T made in therapy.

▨ REVIEW QUESTIONS

1. The treatment stage in which the client practices, perfects, and stabilizes the new behavior is the
   a. Cognitive stage
   b. Autonomous stage
   c. Fixation stage
   d. Director's stage

2. Observable, measurable, replicable items that are based on information gleaned from careful study of the available research are
   a. Principles
   b. Procedures
   c. Theorems
   d. Of no use in therapy

3. Which of the following represent the prompting hierarchy?
   a. Stimulus → physical assist → verbal assist → visual assist → imitation/ modeling
   b. Stimulus → imitation/modeling → physical assist → visual assist → verbal assist
   c. Stimulus → verbal assist → physical assist → visual assist → imitation/ modeling
   d. Stimulus → verbal assist → visual assist → imitation/modeling → physical assist

4. The stage of communication development in which the child's efforts are nonverbal but intentional is the _____ stage.

   a. Perlocutionary
   b. Illocutionary
   c. Locutionary
   d. Stationary

5. An interactive framework for assessment and treatment of a child with multiple handicaps is best implemented in a transdisciplinary or inter-disciplinary setting.

   a. True
   b. False

6. IDEA funds can be used to pay for therapy for school-aged children who have a language difference.

   a. True
   b. False

7. Divergent stimuli are those that produce one or only a few possible answers.

   a. True
   b. False

8. Sensorimotor integration is the sequence of responses that are derived through the coordination of sensory and motor systems of the body.

   a. True
   b. False

9. The use of schemes and scripts to simulate real-life settings in therapy is an excellent approach to therapy for preschool children and eventually facilitates the everyday use of skills learned in therapy.

   a. True
   b. False

10. Knowledge of the child's communicative environment is at the center of the assessment and treatment model proposed by Suzanne Morris.

    a. True
    b. False

■ REFERENCES

Alberto, P. A., & Troutman, A. C. (1986). *Applied behavior analysis for teachers* (2nd ed.). Columbus, OH: Merrill Publishing Company.

Alberto, P. A., & Troutman, A. C. (1990). *Applied behavior analysis for teachers* (3rd ed.). Columbus, OH: Merrill Publishing Company.

Bates, E., Camaioni, L., & Volterra, V. (1975). The acquisition of performatives prior to speech. *Merrill-Palmer Quarterly, 21*, 205–226.

Brady, N. (2003, March). *Communication repair strategies by young children with developmental disabilities.* Paper presented at the 36th annual Gatlinburg Conference on Research and Theory in Intellectual and Developmental Disabilities. Annapolis, MD.

Brady, N., & Halle, J. (2002). Breakdowns and repairs in conversations between beginning AAC users and their partners. In J. Reichle, D. Beukelman, & J. Light (Eds.), *Exemplary practices for beginning communicators: Implications for AAC* (pp. 323–352). Baltimore, MD: Paul H. Brookes.

Cleave, P. L., & Fey, M. E. (1997, February). Two approaches to the facilitation of grammar in children with language impairments: Rationale and description. *American Journal of Speech-Language Pathology, 6,* (1), 22–32.

Dunst, C. (1980). *A clinical and educational manual for use with the Uzgiris and Hunt scales of infant psychological development.* Austin, TX: Pro-Ed.

Fey, M. E. (1986). *Language intervention with young children.* San Diego: College-Hill Press.

Griffith, D. R. (1992, September). Prenatal exposure to cocaine and other drugs: Developmental and educational prognoses. *Phi Delta Kappan,* 30–34.

Guralnik, D. B. (Ed.). (1968). *Webster's new world dictionary of the American language.* New York: World Publishing Company.

Hadley, P. A., & Schuele, C. M. (1998, November). Facilitating peer interaction: Socially relevant objectives for preschool language intervention. *American Journal of Speech-Language Pathology, 7,* (4), 25–36.

Halle, J., Brady, N. C., & Drasgow, E. (2004, February). Enhancing socially adaptive communicative repairs of beginning communicators with disabilities. *American Journal of Speech-Language Pathology, 13,* (1), 43–54.

Hegde, M. N. (1995). *Clinical methods and practicum in speech-language pathology.* San Diego: Singular Publishing Group.

Hodson, B. W., & Paden, E. P. (1991). *Targeting intelligible speech* (2nd ed.). Austin, TX: Pro-Ed.

Lambardino, L. J., Stapell, J. B., & Gerhardt, K. J. (1987, September-October). Evaluating communicative behaviors in infancy. *Journal of Pediatric Health Care, 1,* 5.

Leith, W. R. (1984). *Handbook of clinical methods in communication disorders.* San Diego: Singular Publishing Group.

MacDonald, J. (1989). *Becoming partners with children: From play to conversation.* San Antonio, TX: Special Press.

Morris, S. E. (1982). *The normal acquisition of oral feeding skills: Implications for assessment and treatment.* Central Islip, NY: Therapeutic Media.

Owens, R. E. (1995). *Language disorders: A functional approach to assessment and intervention* (2nd ed.). Boston: Allyn and Bacon.

Owens, R. E. (1999). *Language disorders: A functional approach to assessment and intervention* (3rd ed.). Boston: Allyn and Bacon.

Polakow, V. (1993). *Lives on the edge: Single mothers and their children in the other America.* Chicago: University of Chicago Press.

Uzgiris, I. C., & Hunt, J. M. (1975). *Assessment in infancy: Ordinal scales of psychological development.* Urbana: University of Illinois Press.

Wetherby, A. M., Alexander, D. G., & Prizant, B. M. (1998). The ontogeny and role of repair strategies. In A. M. Wetherby, S. F. Warren, & J. Reichle (Vol. Eds.), *Communication and language intervention series:* Vol. 7, *Transition in prelinguistic communication* (pp. 135–161). Baltimore, MD: Paul H. Brookes.

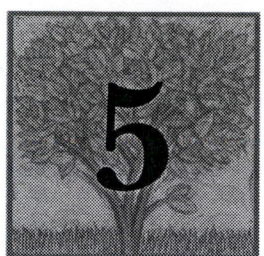

Persistence of Language Deficits Throughout the Lifespan

■ **LEARNING OBJECTIVES**

After completion of this chapter, the reader will be able to

1. Identify predictors of a child's need for special services in adolescence.

2. List Damico and Oller's seven pragmatic referral criteria for elementary education teachers.

3. Differentiate characteristics of language development in the early and later childhood years as noted by Nippold.

4. Identify residual language problems experienced by school-age children with a history of language deficits.

5. Describe the pragmatic and form components of language in children with mental handicaps.

6. Describe the impact of language deficits on the development of academic, language, and psychological skills in children with any of the following disorders: Down syndrome, fetal alcohol syndrome, fragile X syndrome, and velo-cardio-facial syndrome.

■ **INTRODUCTION**

Becoming school age and then entering the preadolescence and adolescence years are times of tremendous change and growth in the physical, social, academic, and personal segments of a child's life. Rosenkoetter (1995) listed some of the changes that accompany the transition from preschool to kindergarten:

1. The adult/child ratio is reduced.

2. There is an increased number of children in educational and social groups.

3. The child may be riding a school bus or participating in a carpool instead of being driven to school by the parents.

4. The family's involvement may differ between preschool and kindergarten.

5. There are increased expectations for academic performance placed on the child.

6. There is a different and more structured curricular content in kindergarten.

7. The manner of teacher instruction differs, with increased expectations for knowledge of classroom rules and routines.

Children who have a language delay or disorder will frequently find these school-year transitions more difficult than normally developing children would. The transition to school creates additional demands on a child's language that are introduced by teachers and peers in the classroom setting. Children who have a language-based disorder or delay are certainly at risk of failure when they enter the academic segment of their lives. Many of the children who have transition difficulties will qualify for school-based intervention, with therapy directed at reducing the impact of the language deficit on the child's academic and social progress. The involvement of the school-based speech-language pathologist in identifying children who have language deficits and in facilitating the school-year transitions is critical in establishing language competencies that play a role in the curricular transitions as the child progresses through school. Nelson (1994) writes the following:

> To succeed in the new communicative context of the early grades, children must learn to process language that is more complex and decontextualized than at home. They must recognize on their own when repairs are needed and how to make them. They must also learn new rules of communicative interaction that involve expectations for making formal requests to take communicative turns (e.g., by raising their hands) and for keeping their turns short, to the point, and responsive to topics raised by the teacher rather than initiating turns of their own. (p. 120)

Effects of Speech and Language Deficits on Social and Academic Achievement

There have been many studies showing that speech and language deficits manifested during the preschool years have residual effects on social and academic achievement in the school years. In a 1980 study, Aram and Nation conducted a chart review of children seen at the Cleveland Hearing and Speech Center in 1973–1974 who were diagnosed with developmental speech and language disorders. A follow-up study was done four to five years after diagnosis, relying on teacher and parent ratings and the teachers' reports of the children's status based on academic achievement as measured by standardized tests. Approximately 40% of the children who were originally seen for developmental speech and language problems continued to have difficulties with language or articulation and reading and spelling. In a similar study done by King, Jones, and Lasky (1982), 50 adolescents who had been seen as preschoolers at the Kent State University Speech and Hearing Clinic were assessed by parent report. Forty-two percent of the 50 adolescents still had communication problems.

There are obvious problems with retrospective studies. For one thing, the investigators must rely on whatever information was available in the child's record of his or her preschool development. Secondly, there was no control over who was in the study because severity of the problem could not always be determined retrospectively. Children with serious motor problems and children with mild articulation problems were all included. A third problem is the subjectivity of relying on reports from parents and teachers for the follow-up study.

Longitudinal Study by Aram, Ekelman, and Nation

Aram, Ekelman, and Nation (1984) did a 10-year follow-up study of children who had been diagnosed with a language disorder and enrolled in ongoing therapy at the Cleveland Hearing and Speech Center as preschoolers. The children ranged in age from 3:5 to 6:11. Each of the 47 children was given an extensive battery of language tests in 1971. The tests measured "comprehension, formulation, and repetition of certain semantic, syntactic, and phonological features" (p. 233). Also, each child was assessed for nonverbal intelligence using the Arthur Adaptation of the Leiter International Performance Scale (1952). If the child failed a hearing screening, had craniofacial or neurological deficits, or had begun first grade, he or she was excluded from the study. In 1981, the researchers located 20 (16 boys and 4 girls) of the original 47 children and retested. They ranged in age from 13:3 to 16:10, and the mean age was 14:10. The 1981 retesting included measures of intelligence, speech and language, academic achievement, and social adjustment. In addition, the parents of each adolescent completed a parent questionnaire (the Child Behavior Checklist by Achenbach, 1981) addressing behavior problems and social competence.

The results from the follow-up testing are summarized by the study's authors as follows:

> 60% of the Verbal IQs, 80% of the Performance IQs, and 70% of the Full Scale IQs fall within or above the low average range. Yet, with few exceptions, most subjects continue to present deficiencies in language abilities, have required special academic attention, are less socially competent, and present more behavioral problems than their peers. Thus, it would appear that for most of this group, the language disorders recognized in the preschool years are only the beginning of long-standing language, academic, and often behavioral problems.

Five of the adolescents had not been in special education and had not repeated a grade. These students had the highest IQs, the best performance on diadochokinetic tasks, and the best language abilities. The other 20 had special education services that ranged from tutoring to placement in a class for educably mentally handicapped children. These children had the lowest IQs, the most problems with **diadochokinetic tasks** (tasks requiring rapid and repetitive movements of the articulators), and the poorest language

Diadochokinetic tasks.
Tasks requiring rapid, repetitive movements of the articulators; frequently elicited by having the child repeat pʌtʌkʌ as quickly as possible.

performance. "Those with mid-range IQs and language skills required either tutoring, grade repetition, or self-contained LD class placement" (p. 240). The reader is referred to this study (Aram et al., 1984) for a complete explanation of the test procedures used, and a more extensive discussion of the results.

■ LANGUAGE DEVELOPMENT IN SCHOOL-AGE CHILDREN

There are numerous factors that can be used to predict a child's need for special services at different developmental stages. For example, parental traits such as the education level of the mother "are better predictors of disabilities in adolescence than children's own behavior" (Nelson, 1998, p. 289) during the early years (birth to 3). However, from ages 4 to 7, child-centered skills (i.e., cognitive abilities and speech/language/communication skills) as measured by standardized tests are better predictors of a child's need for special services in adolescence (Kochanek, Kabacoff, & Lipsitt, 1990). Furthermore, teachers are the main source of referral for children in the school years. Thus, the speech-language pathologist should spend time educating the teachers about receptive and expressive language problems that can negatively impact a child's social and academic achievement. Damico and Oller (1980) noted seven pragmatic referral criteria for elementary education teachers. These criteria are outlined in Table 5–1.

TABLE 5–1. Pragmatically oriented referral criteria for elementary education teachers. Suggested by Damico and Oller (1980).

- *Linguistic nonfluency.* Disruption of speech production by a disproportionately high number of repetitions, unusual pauses, and excessive use of hesitation forms.

- *Revisions.* Breakup of speech production by numerous false starts or self-interruptions; multiple revisions are made as if the child keeps coming to a dead end in a maze.

- *Delays before responding.* Pauses of inordinate length following communication attempts initiated by others.

- *Nonspecific vocabulary.* The use of expressions such as *this, that, then, he,* or *over there* without making the referents clear to the listener; also, the overuse of all-purpose words such as *thing, stuff, these,* and *those.*

- *Inappropriate responses.* The child's utterances appear to indicate that the child is operating on an independent discourse agenda—not attending to the prompts or probes of the adult or others.

- *Poor topic maintenance.* Rapid and inappropriate changes in the topic without providing transitional clues to the listener.

- *Need for repetition.* Requests for multiple repetitions of an utterance without any indication of improvement in comprehension.

Source: From *Language, Speech, and Hearing Services in Schools,* 1980, Vol. 11, p. 88, by J. S. Damico and J. W. Oller, Jr. Copyright 1980 by American Speech-Language-Hearing Association. Reprinted with permission.

Another frequent predictor for the need of special services is the age at which a child began to talk. Girolametto et al., (2001) studied 21 children at age 5 who had previously been diagnosed as late talkers. The children had all previously received intervention that included a parent program implemented when the children were 2 to 3 years of age and direct intervention for approximately 50% of the children who did not show adequate language growth in the parent program. At age 5 the children were tested on their language, with the results being compared to those of normally developing peers. Following intervention, 86% of the language-impaired children matched the control group in the areas of expressive grammar and vocabulary but had weaknesses in some higher-level standardized tests designed to measure the child's ability to meaningfully engage in teacher-child discourse, his or her use of pragmatic cues for resolving ambiguous sentences, and other narrative tasks. This and other studies have found that by the time the late talkers attain school age, most of them score within normal limits on norm-referenced expressive language tests. However, many of the children who achieve these normal scores "continue to have difficulties with higher level linguistic tasks that clearly distinguish them from their peers and that could place them at risk for learning and academic difficulties during the early school years" (p. 359). Girolametto and his colleagues cite several studies in which the assessment of children's narrative skills found that the late talkers had similar mean length of utterances and content when compared to children with normally developing **expressive language** which is the ability to convey a message through conventional means using words and symbols, but they used "significantly fewer cohesive ties and were less mature" (p. 359).

Rescorla, Hadicke-Wiley, and Escarce (1993) assessed the language of 6-year-old children who had been late talkers and found that the children scored lower than their peers on word definition tasks, verbal reasoning tasks, and auditory short-term memory tasks. When they retested the late talkers at ages 7 and 8, the children had difficulty on sentence formulation tasks. At age 8, they also demonstrated problems in auditory processing, verbal memory, and fluency in word retrieval. Certainly, all these residual problems can affect the child's ability to succeed in school.

Even when children's early language problems appear to resolve (as documented by tests of basic communication skills), they often show evidence of difficulties when more abstract and decontextualized language is assessed, or when multiple language skills must be coordinated as when engaged in narrative retelling tasks.

The adolescent years are particularly daunting in the changes that occur not only related to academics, but also related to physical, social, emotional, and vocational growth. Some of these changes are highlighted in Table 5–2.

When considering the impact of language development on the various features of language, it is evident that children continue to acquire skills in

Expressive language. The ability to convey a message through conventional means using words and symbols; the content of what is expressed.

TABLE 5–2. Characteristics of stages and tasks of normal adolescence.

Task	Stage of Adolescence		
	Early (10–14)	Middle (14–16)	Late (16–20)
Acceptance of the Physical Changes of Puberty	• Physical changes occur rapidly but with wide person-to-person variability • Self-consciousness, insecurity, and worry about being different from peers	• Pubertal changes almost complete for girls; boys still undergoing physical changes • Girls more confident; boys more awkward	• Adult appearance, comfortable with physical changes. • Physical strength continues to increase, especially for males.
Attainment of Independence	• Changes of puberty distinguish early adolescents from children, but do not provide independence. • Ambivalence (childhood dependence unattractive, but unprepared for the independence of adulthood) leads to vacillation between parents and peers for support	• Ability to work, drive, date; appear more mature; dependence lessens and peer bonds increase. • Conflict with authority, limit testing, experimental and risk-taking behaviors at a maximum	• Independence a realistic social expectation. • Continuing education, becoming employed, getting married—all possibilities that often lead to ambivalence about independence
Emergence of a Stable Identity	• Am I OK? Am I normal? • How do I fit into my peer group? • Paradoxical loss of identity in becoming a member of a peer group.	• Who am I? • How am I different from other people? • What makes me special or unique?	• Who am I in relation to other people? • What is my role with respect to education, work, sexuality, community, religion, and family?
Development of Cognitive Patterns	• Concrete operational thought: present more real than future, concrete more real than abstract. • Egocentrism. • Personal fable. • Imaginary audience.	• Emerging formal operations: abstractions, hypotheses, and thinking about future personal interests and emerging identity.	• Formal operations: thinking about the future, things as they should be, options, consequences can be considered.

Source: From *Communication Solutions for Older Students* (p. 36), by V. L Larson and N. McKinley, 2003, Eau Claire, WI, Thinking Publications © 2003 by Thinking Publications. Reprinted with permission.

each feature throughout childhood, but the most prevalent growth is in the areas of pragmatics and semantics. One reason for this is the expansion of the child's world beyond the home as the child enters the structured academic experience. He or she is interacting with more people in a variety of contexts that exceeds the interactions focused primarily on the family and narrow preschool group. In addition, the **metalinguistic skills** and **metapragmatic skills** show rapid growth during this transition time.

The Development of Metalinguistic Skills

The development of metalinguistic skills is most marked at 4 to 8 years of age, but the development continues to mature well into adolescence. Metalinguistic skills constitute a language awareness that enables the child to "think and talk about language" as something more than simply being a tool that enables communication (Bernstein, 1997). The development of metalinguistic skills is particularly important because some researchers believe that they appear to be critical in the child's ability to attain literacy skills (van Kleek, 1994). Other areas of change as the child progresses from childhood to adolescence include the development of **metacognition** skills, the ability to develop alternative ways to solve a problem or resolve a situation, the ability to form hypotheses and task analyze them in a constructive manner, and the capacity to make personal decisions (Larson & McKinley, 1995).

The growth accompanying the change from preschool to kindergarten, as well as from elementary school to middle school and middle school to high school, requires an increased responsibility for problem solving and making personal decisions (Larson & McKinley, 1995), both of which are frequently problematic for children who have a language delay and/or disorder that extends beyond the preschool years.

Miller (1989) listed developmental tasks, some of which begin in childhood and extend into the preadolescent and adolescent years:

- The development of a self-identity

- Adjusting to physical and psychological changes in the body

- The development of **abstract thought processes** about the physical and social world, "thinking beyond the here and now," and forming opinions based on fact

- The acquisition of interpersonal skills to foster the development of peer relationships

- The development of a new relationships with family members as the child increases his or her independence and lessens the emotional dependence on family

Metalinguistic skills. Skills that allow an individual to think about language in a critical manner and to make judgments with regard to the accuracy and appropriate use of language skills and functions.

Metapragmatic skills. Conscious and intentional awareness of ways in which to use language effectively in different contexts.

Metacognition. The ability to develop alternative ways to solve a problem or resolve a situation, the ability to form hypotheses and task analyze them in a constructive manner, and the capacity to make personal decisions.

Abstract thought processes. Thinking beyond the limits of a fact and developing opinions and expansion on a given piece of information.

- The development of a personal system of values that impact problem solving and the development of relationships

- The ability to consider the future and set goals

Another prominent change is the fact that children move from having primarily an auditory mode of learning language to also having a visual mode of learning language as they begin to read and write in the early grades in school (Bernstein, 1997).

Later Stages of Language Development

The academic, social, and vocational demands of language as the child progresses through the school years are astounding! Nelson's (1998) later stages of language development include children from third grade through adulthood; they are divided into the preadolescent age group (8 to 12 years of age) and the adolescence/transition to the adulthood stage (12 to 21 years of age). During the later stages of development, children make gradual changes in their language acquisition as opposed to the rapid changes in the early and middle age periods. Nippold (1988) conducted research aimed at differentiating between the early (ages 0 to 9) and later (ages 9 to 19) stages of language development. One factor stressed by Nippold is that up to age 8, emphasis is on the acquisition of spoken language skills, whereas at age 9 and later, the emphasis is on written language skills. As children get older, they learn language from both auditory and visual input, whereas younger children learn primarily from auditory input (the speech of others). Other differences include the growth of metacognitive and metalinguistic abilities in later childhood and adolescence, as well as the processing of more abstract notions.

Syntactic Growth

Embedded sentences. Compound sentences in which a minimum of two independent clauses are combined to form one sentence.

Syntactic growth during the school years includes expansion of noun and verb phrases, the use of **embedded sentences** (also known as compound sentences consisting of at least two independent clauses) using words such as *unless, therefore,* and *although* (even though interpretation of these words does not occur until approximately age 7 years); the comprehension of gerunds (around age 6 years); and the use of derivational morphemes (-er, -man, -ist) that change verbs into nouns around 6½ years of age. Other areas of syntactic and morphological growth include the comprehension of irregular noun-verb agreement (by the end of second grade), and the use of reflexive pronouns (Menyuk, 1969; Carrow, 1973; Bernstein, 1997).

Growth of Lexicon in School-Age Children

Lexicon. A composite list of the words and signs that comprise an individual's vocabulary.

There is a significant increase in **lexicon**, or vocabulary, in school-age children, both in terms of learning new words and being able to more clearly define them. Growth in these areas extends throughout the school years.

There is a dramatic increase in the use of words denoting temporal, spatial, logical, and familial relationships between the ages of 7 to 11 years, as well as an increase in the use of words with multiple meanings (Bernstein, 1997; Menyuk, 1971; Owens, 1996). Bernstein (1997) writes that there is a high correlation between lexicon, "general linguistic competence, and academic aptitude" (p. 131). Throughout the school years, children increase their abilities to comprehend and use **nonliteral language** (abstract and symbolic) that includes metaphors, idioms, humor, and proverbs.

Nonliteral language. Language that is abstract and symbolic.

An example of growth of humor is evident as children of different ages attempt to share the "Why did the chicken cross the road" joke during a conversation at dinnertime:

7-year-old: "Why did the chicken cross the road?"

Father: "I don't know! Why did the chicken cross the road?"

7-year-old: "To get to the other side."

Family: Robust laughter.

4-year-old: "Why did chicken cross the road?"

Mother: "I don't know! Why did the chicken cross the road?

4-year-old: "Cross the road."

Family: Laughter, with the 4-year-old's laughter being the most raucous.

18-month-old: "Chicken" and laughter.

Family: Light-hearted laughter to indicate enjoyment of the attempt.

Clearly, the 4-year-old was beginning to implement the ability to analyze language using **metalinguistic devices** to convey humor in that she understood the concept of a riddle but still needed development in order to understand the punch line! The 18-month-old clued in on one word that had possibly made everyone else laugh and uttered it in order to provoke a reaction.

Metalinguistic devices. The ability to think about and analyze language, including the ability to understand humor, multiple meanings, inferences, and figurative language.

Another area of significant growth through the school years is pragmatics as children "learn how to become good conversational partners, how to make indirect requests, and how to process the language of the classroom" (Bernstein, 1997, p. 133). The development of social, emotional, and cognitive skills as the child progresses through school results in an expansion of the child's pragmatic capabilities. White (1975) noted communicative skills demonstrated by school-age children.

1. They can obtain and maintain adults' attention in a socially acceptable manner.

2. They can assume the roles of leader and follower among their peers.

3. They can use other individuals as a resource for help in obtaining desired information.

4. They can express appropriately emotions such as affection, hostility, and anger.

5. They can show pride in themselves and their accomplishments.

6. They can actively engage in role play.

7. They can compete with their peers in storytelling activities.

Similar growth occurs in the use of narratives, conversation, indirect requests, and topic maintenance. Children age 5 use direct requests, but by age 7 they begin to make indirect requests, an ability that grows in complexity as the child advances in age (Bernstein, 1997).

As one can see, there are many changes that children, preadolescents, and adolescents experience, and certainly all of these changes and areas of growth have the potential to be negatively impacted by the presence of a language delay or disorder. This chapter will explore these effects.

■ SPECIFIC LANGUAGE IMPAIRMENT

Children with specific language impairment (SLI) face numerous academic and social challenges in the school transition years due to the well-documented existence of problems with peer relationships. However, it should be noted that not all children with SLI will have problems with social competence (Fujiki, Brinton, & Clarke, 2002). The degree of variability of social skills in children with SLI begs for further study. Gertner, Rice, and Hadley (1994) found that many preschool children diagnosed with SLI were considered by their peers as not being a preferred playmate. In addition, Rice, Sell, and Hadley (1991) found that children with SLI preferred adults as their conversational partners instead of their peers. In another study, Fujiki et al. (2001) studied the social behaviors of children on the school playground as opposed to the structured format of the academic classroom. They found that language-impaired children were typically more withdrawn and spent significantly less time interacting with peers than did children who did not have a language impairment. The root of these social difficulties in part can be traced back to the poor language abilities characteristic of children with SLI.

Emotional regulation. The ability to control one's emotions and express them appropriately based on the myriad components of a setting.

Fujiki and colleagues (2002) proposed that one variable affecting social development in a child with SLI is **emotional regulation**. They suggest that children's language impairments can influence their ability to regulate, or control, their emotions. These children are frequently teased because they laugh and cry more easily than their peers, with the laughter often being out of proportion when compared to that of their classmates. They may become more frustrated when unable to do a task that is accomplished more readily by their peers. Additional factors that influence emotional regulation include the child's temperament, socialization practices, and cognitive functioning. Children who do not have deficits in these areas may account for those who have SLI but do not have significant social difficulties.

Participation in Collaborative Activities

Difficulties with social interaction certainly place a child at risk in the classroom given the emphasis on group projects and other **collaborative activities**.

Children with SLI usually find such activities difficult. Indeed, in research on language-impaired children's participation in group activities, Brinton, Fujiki, and Higbee (1998) found that these children participated significantly less often than their nonlanguage-impaired peers, both verbally and nonverbally. This led to the conclusions that (1) language-impaired children who have difficulty in group work situations do not use nonverbal methods to compensate for verbal deficits, and (2) that the success of children with SLI becoming actively involved in cooperative learning groups may depend largely on their level of social functioning. Brinton and colleagues (2000) did a pilot study to look at the functioning of children with language impairments in cooperative learning groups. Their findings verified those of Brinton et al. (1998), particularly that the social functioning of a child with SLI significantly impacted their ability to integrate into a cooperative work group. However, they also found that some of the children did have more success in these small groups when compared to their performance in a full classroom activity, possibly because these groups are usually made up of children with different ability levels. This sets ups a **scaffolding system** in which the higher functioning children provide models for those who do not function as well.

Literacy Skills and Phonological Processing in Children with SLI

A critical factor in the development of literacy skills is early exposure to books as depicted in Figure 5–1.

In a longitudinal study by Stothard et al. (1998), there was a difference in literacy skills and phonological processing with the language-impaired children (resolved) performing worse than the controls. Those children whose language impairment had not resolved by age 5:6 and those who had general

Collaborative activities. Those activities that involve the joint participation and cooperation of the members of a group.

Scaffolding system. A "stair-step" approach to problem solving in a group consisting of students at varying levels of ability in which a high functioning child provides a model for a lower functioning child.

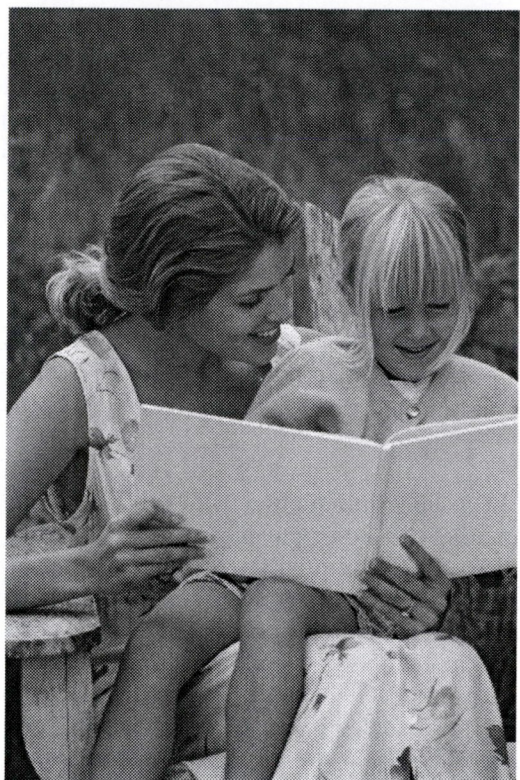

FIGURE 5–1. Exposing a child to books and reading with him or her at an early age is a crucial factor in developing literacy.

delay all exhibited "significant impairments in all aspects of spoken and written language functioning" (p. 407). Stothard and colleagues did a longitudinal follow-up study of 71 adolescents who had been diagnosed as having a speech-language impairment as preschoolers, and who were in an original study by Bishop and Edmundson (1987). When the children were 4 years of age, they were divided into two groups. The general delay group had a measured nonverbal IQ that was 2 standard deviations below the mean. The SLI group had normal nonverbal intelligence. When the children were 5:6, the children in the SLI group were divided into those whose language problems had resolved, and those whose SLI persisted. The general delay group was also followed. When the children with SLI were 15 to 16 years of age, they were given a test battery consisting of tests of spoken language and literacy skills, and their performance was compared to those of age-matched normal-language children. It is interesting to note that on tests of language comprehension and vocabulary, there was no difference between the children in the control group and those whose language impairments had resolved by age 5:6. In addition, it should be noted that the children whose language impairment did not resolve also had deficits on nonverbal tasks on the Weschler Intelligence Scale for Children-III. In fact, 47% of those children scored one deviation below the mean on nonverbal composite scores, and 20% fell more than two standard deviations below the mean. Also, with time, the children with general delay and those with unresolved SLI increasingly fell behind their peer groups in vocabulary. Based on these results, it is clear that 15-year-old-children who had a long-standing history of general delay or unresolved specific language impairments had significant deficits in verbal and nonverbal language that could negatively impact academic success. Approximately 50% of the 15-year-old adolescents were receiving special education services, and the majority had academic problems. Even those children whose language impairments had resolved by age 5:6 exhibited "residual, but mild, processing impairments that place them at risk of later failure (e.g., in literacy skills)" (p. 417). The children in the resolved group were not diagnosed as dyslexic, and even though their "reading skills were significantly poorer than those of controls, they were not generally outside of the normal range as predicted by IQ" (p. 417).

Johnson and her colleagues (1999) did a longitudinal study in which they followed children for a 14-year period. The 142 children in their study were originally diagnosed at age 5 as having language impairments and were retested at 12 and 18 to 20 years of age. Twenty-seven and one-half percent of the 142 children had speech impairments only, 43.6% had language impairments only, and 28.9% had impairments in speech and language. There were also 142 controls selected from among the children who passed the initial screening. The results of the study indicated the following:

1. Those children diagnosed at age 5 with speech impairment had only "subtle, residual speech problems as young adults but showed no long-term deficits in language, cognitive, and academic performance" (p. 755) when compared to age-level nonimpaired peers.

2. Children who were diagnosed as age 5 with language impairment "showed clear long-term deficits in language, cognitive, and academic domains relative to peers without early language difficulty" (p. 755).

In all these studies, it is evident that even those children whose problems appeared to be resolved in the early academic years demonstrated deficits in middle school and high school that had an impact on their social and academic success. Thus, children with SLI need to be followed by a team of specialists throughout school. This team should consist of the child's teachers, a guidance counselor, a psychologist, and a speech-language pathologist, at least. This is particularly important as the child enters the late elementary grades and middle school and high school, because this is a critical time not only in academic demands, but also in the growth of importance of peer relationships.

■ FETAL ALCOHOL SYNDROME/FETAL ALCOHOL EFFECTS

In addition to the facial and physical characteristics, central nervous system dysfunction is always present in fetal alcohol syndrome (FAS) and is very common in children with fetal alcohol effects (FAE). With regard to mental functioning, a child with fetal alcohol syndrome typically functions in the mildly to moderately impaired range of intelligence. Language deficits and delays are common, including echolalia and **perseveration**. In addition, their expressive language frequently exceeds their receptive language abilities. However, they may exhibit difficulties with word order and word meanings (Owens, 2004).

Perseveration. "Getting stuck," usually involuntarily, on a motor, verbal, or nonverbal activity.

Academic problems are characteristic of FAS/FAE. These are the result of conceptual deficits (such as time and space), difficulties with comprehension of spoken and written materials, deficits in basic problem solving, and visual and spatial memory deficits (Ratner & Harris, 1994).

Behavioral problems, including attention deficit disorder, are also common. In the classroom, these children can be somewhat disruptive. Subtle learning problems due to cognitive deficits are often exhibited by children with fetal alcohol effects, including poor attention skills, poor judgment, and memory deficits (Owens, 2004). The poor development of interpersonal skills also affects children with FAS/FAE. For example, they typically have problems with the reciprocal nature of a conversation. In addition, they have difficulty understanding the expectations and rules associated with social language interactions and generally have poor communication "because it lacks substance, cohesion, meaning, and relevance" (Larson & McKinley, 1995, p. 9). The picture is further complicated by the frequent presence of impulsivity and hyperactivity, tremors, restlessness, and temper tantrums. Adolescents with FAS/FAE often have sexual difficulties. They may be depressed (possibly due to social isolation from their peers), and they frequently drop out of school (Ratner & Harris, 1994).

The above characteristics compound the problems of adolescents trying to demonstrate the growth presented in the introduction to this chapter. In addition, the same problems typically carry over into adulthood, and children and adults with either of these disorders are frequently considered to be underachievers. Their impulsiveness, poor judgment, and attentional deficits create problems for those who are either in school or who are employed (Ratner & Harris, 1994).

■ CHILDREN PRENATALLY EXPOSED TO COCAINE AND/OR OTHER DRUGS

Polydrug exposed. The use of multiple drugs, including alcohol, by a pregnant mother.

In Chapter 2, a baby who is cocaine or **polydrug exposed** is typically disorganized with regard to his/her central nervous system. It is known that many individuals who use cocaine often use other drugs concurrently. Thus, it is often difficult to determine the exact effects on a fetus of a particular drug used by the mom during pregnancy.

As the baby gets older, he or she will have difficulty adjusting to new environments with much the same type of difficulty as in the initial months of life (see Chapter 2). At a time when he or she should be learning basic cognitive processes through developmental tasks, the infant may have trouble learning through environmental stimulation, particularly in learning those skills that lead to the ability to master complex tasks at the later stages of development. Finally, it is possible that babies who are not able to organize themselves in a disorganized environment will also have difficulty shifting tasks and handling change as they get older. When drug-exposed children attain school age, their language is typified by their word retrieval problems and poor pragmatics (Rivers & Hedrick, 1992). Weak pragmatic skills can be further confounded by frequent changes in living arrangements and care settings as is common.

■ CHILDREN WITH COGNITIVE DISABILITIES

As stressed in Chapter 2, children with cognitive disabilities display a wide array of deficits. By definition (American Association on Mental Retardation, 2002), the deficits must be manifested prior to age 18, and include deficits in at least two of the following adaptive skill areas:

communication	community use	leisure
self-care	self-direction	work
home living	health and safety	
social skills	functional academics	

Children with cognitive handicaps usually follow the same path of acquisition in the various features of language as do normally developing children, but at a slower rate. In approximately 50% of the children with cognitive handicaps, there is no gap between their language abilities and their cognitive skills. Many school districts use this as criteria for placement in school-based speech/language therapy (Miller & Chapman, 1984). A sample criterion would be that a child must demonstrate a gap of 12 months between his or her language and cognitive skills in order to be enrolled in therapy.

With regard to the features of language, the delays indicate that the child with a cognitive handicap will acquire the features in the same sequence as those who do not have a cognitive handicap, but with a delay in terms of onset times. Owens (2004) studied the pragmatic skills of children with cognitive disabilities and found that, in the preschool years, children with cognitive handicaps used gestures to express intent at approximately the same rate as nondisabled children. However, asking for clarification and asking other questions were problematic for children with cognitive handicaps (Owens, 2004; Mundy, Seibert, and Hogan, 1985). Generally, the early expressive language skills of preschool children with cognitive disabilities is on par with their cognitive abilities. They do, however, tend to be less assertive when engaged in conversations (Bedrosian & Prutting, 1978).

In 1973, Brown found that when the mean length of utterance (MLU) is below 3, "children with MR display few differences in the sequence of learning grammatical rules when compared with mental-age mates" (Paul, 2001, p. 119).

However, the syntactic and morphological features of their language are reflective of a child with a cognitive handicap, and they do not develop forms of language as fully as those of nonhandicapped children. Specifically, their sentences lack complexity and are shorter than those of their age-level peers. While the sequence of the acquisition of morphemes is similar to that of nonhandicapped age peers, the rate in which syntax and morphology are learned is slower (Paul, 2001).

When one analyzes the content of the language of children with cognitive handicaps, he or she finds that these children tend to use more concrete words such as nouns and verbs than adjectives and adverbs (Owens, 2004). Again, in the early stages, the child's sequence of acquisition of words tends to follow that of their age-level peers, with delays becoming more evident as the child advances in age. Layton (2001) found that it appears that semantics develop more easily than syntax in the language of children with cognitive handicaps, particularly in children with Down syndrome.

Severe to Profound Cognitive Disabilities

Children with profound cognitive disabilities will have difficulty mastering the basic skills needed for academic success. Their curriculum should focus on the development of fundamental skills such as self-help skills, basic communication, and motor development. Instruction for these children should also include efforts to teach functional reading and math skills needed to participate safely in the environment. These children will typically need complete care and supervision, even into adulthood.

Children who fall into the category of severe cognitive disabilities will have significant difficulties when they reach school age. As a rule, these children do not develop functional academic skills. They may learn to talk and communicate at a rudimentary level, frequently being limited to single words and basic communication via an alternative/augmentative communication device.

Education of these children will often focus on the development of early cognitive skills such as mean-end, causality, imitation, and symbolic play schemes. This is in keeping with Piaget's theories with regard to the interaction between innate cognitive precursors to language and the development of language through organization of a child's world and environmental opportunities. Education of these children will require systematic, focused, repetitive training. For example, photos of key objects in the child's environment should be posted in the appropriate areas of the classroom or therapy room. The child should be encouraged (and assisted if necessary) to point to the appropriate picture when the object is being used. When the child is given a cup of water to drink, he or she should point to a picture of the cup. In addition, the development of **sensorimotor** skills that require the integration of feedback from the sensory system and the resultant motor behaviors should be a curricular focus as these may help lay a foundation for the development of early cognitive and language skills.

Sensorimotor. Skills involving the integration of sensory feedback and motor behaviors.

Mild to Moderate Cognitive Disabilities

As stated in Chapter 2, preschoolers with IQs of 50 to 70 (American Association on Mental Retardation, 2002) fall in the mild range of cognitive disabilities and will typically have delayed social and communication skills. Actually, mild cognitive disabilities may not even be noticed until the child begins school or later. However, their academic skills usually do not progress beyond the sixth grade level at which time they will need special education and may be labeled as educable mentally disabled. As adults, they may have some social and vocational independence but will need guidance in times of social and economic stress.

Children with moderate cognitive disabilities (IQ in the 40 to 54 range) will usually not progress beyond the fourth grade level in regard to their academic growth. As adults, they "may be able to work independently at unskilled or semiskilled occupations but often need supervision and guidance under conditions of even mild social or economic stress" (Nelson, 1993, p. 99)

■ DOWN SYNDROME

Children with Down syndrome have intelligence quotients that range from mildly impaired to profoundly handicapped. Regardless of the level of functioning, as the child with Down syndrome advances in age, the gaps between his or her language skills and those of his peers at the same mental age widen. This is particularly true in the areas of morphology and syntax. Chapman and colleagues (1998) found that children with Down syndrome tend to omit morphemes and grammatical function words more than their mental-age peers. Thus, it would make sense that therapy with children who have

TABLE 5–3. When children with Down syndrome use –ed to form the past tense.

Age	Never	Sometimes	Often
2	100%		
3	93%	7%	
4	78%	19%	3%
5	77%	18%	5%

Source: From *Early Communication Skills for Children with Down Syndrome,* by L. Kumin, p. 111. © 2003 by Woodbine House.

TABLE 5–4. When children with Down syndrome use –ing.

Age	Never	Sometimes	Often
2	96.3%	3.7%	
3	73%	13%	13%
4	61%	27%	12%
5	52%	36%	22%

Source: From *Early Communication Skills for Children with Down Syndrome,* by L. Kumin, p. 111. © 2003 by Woodbine House.

mental handicaps, and particularly those with Down syndrome, would have syntax and morphology as major foci of therapy. Chapman and colleagues stated that adolescents with Down syndrome can improve these areas of expressive language, thereby increasing the length and complexity of their sentences. Kumin, Councill, and Goodman (1998) conducted a study to determine when children with Down syndrome start talking about events in the past and in the future, as well as when they use –ed and –ing word endings. Their findings are summarized in Tables 5–3 and 5–4.

In 1979, Gillham documented that, in children with Down syndrome, the average age at which the first word is spoken is 18 months. Typical mean length of utterance in children with Down syndrome at age 4 years is 1.5 words, 3.5 words at 6 years of age, and 5+ words at 15 years (Kumin, 2003). In the early years, their lexicon consists primarily of concrete, referential words that denote objects or things experienced by the child. Grammatical classification words such as "or" and "however" are typically not used until age 5 at the earliest, and use of words with grammatical meanings does not usually develop until approximately age 6 (Kumin, Councill, & Goodman, 1998). It should be noted that when children with Down syndrome are compared to their chronological-age peers, they have a smaller vocabulary. But, when compared to mental-age peers, they may have a larger vocabulary. This may be explained, in part, by the fact that when compared to mental-age peers the child with Down syndrome will most likely be older chronologically and will have had more life experiences (Rondal, 1978; Miller, 1988; Kumin, 2003). This is important clinically in that these children need to be taught to organize their vocabulary into concepts, thus forming a basic organization to their language that enables them to generalize their vocabulary.

Children with Down syndrome usually have language deficits that are greater than would be predicted when looking at their nonverbal cognitive skills (Chapman, 1995). Using a test of nonverbal intelligence, Buckley (1993, 1995a) tested 12 teenagers who had Down syndrome. The mean age of the teenagers was 14:11. On the Ravens Progressive Matrices Test (Raven, 1995), which tests nonverbal reasoning skills, they scored a mean age of 7:0. On a picture vocabulary comprehension test, the mean age for the group was 5:6, and on a grammar comprehension test, the average score was 5:0 years.

Reading levels in children with Down syndrome frequently exceed their language and cognitive levels. Several studies have been done to evaluate reading skills in children with Down syndrome. Buckley and her colleagues (1995b) did a study in which a group of cognitively matched children with Down syndrome were divided into two subgroups. One subgroup was taught to read, and the other was not. When the study concluded, they found that the language and memory skills of those children who were taught to read were more advanced than those in the nonreader group. In addition, the speech, language, and educational achievements by the readers were more advanced by the time the children reached age 10 to 11. These findings support the importance of introducing a literacy component into the educational and therapeutic plans for students who have Down syndrome.

In another study on reading ability in children with Down syndrome, Kay-Raining Bird, Cleave, and McConnell (2000) followed 12 children with Down syndrome over a 4.5 year period, looking at the impact of three literacy skills (language, cognition, and phonological awareness) on reading acquisition. The purpose of the study was to determine the roles of word recognition and decoding abilities in the reading of children with Down syndrome. Two predictors of literacy development in the Down syndrome population are cognitive ability (Sloper et al., 1990) and expressive-receptive language skills (Carr, 1995). Children who have better cognitive and language skills typically do better in the academic setting.

Sloper and colleagues (1990) studied 123 children with Down syndrome aged 6 to 14 years. They investigated child, parental/family, and school variables and their effects on academic achievement. Their findings were that mental age was the most predictive variable. Other predictors included "older ages, mainstream placements, female gender, and fathers' feelings of control over the outcomes of their children" (Kay-Raining Bird et al., 2000, p. 320).

Carr (1995) did a longitudinal study in which she followed 54 children with Down syndrome. When the individuals were 11 and 21 years of age, she assessed their language, cognition, and academic achievement. She assessed reading using the Neale Analysis of Reading Ability (Neale, 1958), and found that two-fifths of her sample could be scored, even though some additional subjects had letter recognition skills. Carr's findings supported the findings of Sloper and colleagues in that IQ is a significant predictor of reading success, and that there are "significant correlations between reading and both vocabulary comprehension and production skills" (Kay-Raining Bird et al., 2000, p. 320).

In a study by Fowler, Doherty, and Boynton (1995), 33 young adults with Down syndrome were divided into four subgroups based on their reading performance. The assessment consisted of three subtexts of the Woodcock Reading Master Test-Revised: Word Identification, Word Attack, and Passage Comprehension (Woodcock, 1987), and the Auditory Analysis Test (AAT) (Rosner & Simon, 1971). Kay-Raining Bird and colleagues, summarized Fowler's findings as follows:

1. As measured by the Word Attack subtest, decoding skills lagged behind Word Identification abilities except in the most skilled readers.

2. The poorest performances were on the Passage Comprehension subtest.

3. Even taking out the variable of cognitive status, the children's performance on the AAT was generally poor; however, the performance was variable across participants and it significantly correlated with their performance on the Word Attack and the Word Identification reading.

4. Those individuals who scored beyond the first grade level on Word Attack Skills on the WRMT-R also scored at least a 10 on phonological awareness on the AAT.

5. Based on #4, phonological awareness is a necessary component of decoding, but alone is not sufficient for decoding ability to develop.

6. Other measures correlating significantly with reading ability in the subjects with Down syndrome (again, after cognition was partialled out) were word retrieval, auditory memory, and visual memory.

Other studies have supported these findings and shed additional light on the role of phonological awareness in reading, both in normally developing populations and Down syndrome populations (Kay-Raining Bird & McConnell, 1994; Kay-Raining Bird et al., 1998).

The implications of these studies for therapy with children with Down syndrome are that it appears that it may be beneficial to incorporate preliteracy and literacy skills commensurate with their cognitive age into the therapeutic curriculum of children with Down syndrome.

■ FRAGILE X SYNDROME

The incidence of fragile X syndrome is much higher in boys than in girls. When girls are affected, they are typically not as severely impaired as are their male counterparts. The IQ of individuals who have fragile X syndrome can range from low normal to severe, but typically they exhibit moderate levels of mental handicaps. Girls tend to function in the mild range, more characteristic of learning disabilities than mental retardation (Paul, 2001).

The physical characteristics are discussed in Chapter 2, but there are also cognitive and language deficits that can hinder the academic and social growth of children with fragile X syndrome. As in children with autism, many of these characteristics are typical of those seen in individuals with attention deficit disorder/hyperactivity. Specifically, a boy with fragile X syndrome may be hyperactive, have a short attention span, be impulsive, and have poor interactive skills (Paul, 2001). Boys may also exhibit some signs of autism such as repetitive hand flapping, lack of eye contact, hypersensitivities, and **tactile defensiveness**, which means that they usually have a negative reaction to being touched. They also frequently have fine motor control deficits. (Spiridigliozzi et al., 2001).

Tactile defensiveness. A pronounced dislike of being touched, usually accompanied by a negative emotional reaction.

With regard to cognitive skills, Paul (2001) writes that the individuals with fragile X syndrome do better on tasks that require "simultaneous processing" than on those that require "sequential processing." For example, identifying the missing part of an object when shown an incomplete picture of that object is an easier task than reproducing a series of words in the same order as presented. Strengths which can foster academic progress include good long-term memory and visual memory. They are good at repetition and verbal imitation that can also contribute to academic success when provided with a good model (Spiridigliozzi et al., 2001).

However, they also have several weaknesses than can hinder academic, social, and vocational growth. Spiridigliozzi and colleagues (2001) found that calculation, abstract reasoning, and problem solving are problematic for children with fragile X syndrome. Initiating and completing tasks are also problematic, but they do respond to prompts to help in these areas. They also found that IQ in this population declines over time because their rate of development slows down as they get older (when compared to normally developing peers). Because of the decline as the boys get older, efficient and effective early intervention is critical.

The extent to which these children have speech and language deficits is tied, to some degree, to the level of retardation that is present. Thus, one could expect to see some of the same behaviors and characteristics that are described in the section on cognitive handicaps. In addition, children with fragile X syndrome demonstrate delays in expressive language. Receptive language and semantics are relatively unaffected when compared to the level of expressive language. They use numerous phonological processes for an extended amount of time when compared to their age-level peers. Their speech is also characterized by a rapid rate and reduced intelligibility, particularly as sentences increase in length (Scharfenaker, 1990). In addition, they demonstrate word-finding difficulties (which impacts their abilities to answer direct questions), have delayed syntax, and exhibit pragmatic deficits including lack of clarifying gestures, poor turn-taking, and poor maintenance of a topic (Schopmeyer & Lowe, 1992).

■ AUTISM AND PERVASIVE DEVELOPMENTAL DISABILITIES

Mutism. Not speaking; may be selective, meaning a child does not talk in certain settings, or elective, meaning there is no organic or physical disability that prevents the child from talking.

As delineated in Chapter 2, the criteria for the diagnosis of autism includes language deficits as well as qualitative impairments in social interaction and communication. Many children with autism go through a period of **mutism**, or silence, in the early years. However, when the child does begin to speak, he typically has excellent articulation.

In fact, this is one marker to differentiate between children with autism and children with cognitive retardation; children with cognitive retardation do not demonstrate the articulatory acumen that children with autism do. Hurford (1991) writes that if a functional language system has not developed by age 5 years, there is little likelihood of its developing. DeMyer and colleagues (1973) found that approximately 65 percent of children with autism who were mute at age 5 remained mute several years later in their development. As the child with autism progresses through the developmental period, there appear to be periods of rapid growth and development as opposed to the slow consistent development exhibited by normally developing children.

Paul (2001) and Lord and Paul (1997) indicate that that the majority (maybe as high as 80%) of individuals with autism test out as being mentally deficient on cognitive tests by the time they are school age, and that approximately 40% do not develop expressive language by the time they are 5 years of age (school age). For individuals who do not develop a system of expressive language, the prognosis as adults in guarded. However, for the 15 to 20% of individuals with autism who are cognitively within normal limits (based on intelligence testing), the outlook is more positive.

Paul (2001) writes the following:

> A few of these individuals seem to "outgrow" their autism by mid-childhood, but most remain autistic or at least very odd as adults. They may be able to live on their own; they can learn functional job skills, and some can graduate from college in fields such as mathematics or

computer science. But even these very bright autistic individuals continue to have difficulty with human relationships, social judgment, and appropriate use of language. (p. 108)

Other researchers indicate that for more than 95% of the individuals who are diagnosed as autistic, the disorder is a lifelong disorder (Volkmar et al., 1997; Grandin, 1997).

Social deficits are at the core of the diagnosis of autism. Schopler and Mesibov (1986) have found that when children with autism reach adolescence, they appear to demonstrate an increased awareness and interest in other people. They state that their problems seem to be a "lack of social skills rather than a lack of social interest" (p. 5). Thus, implications for treatment would suggest that the clinician target pragmatic skills in therapy. Children and adults with autism also may demonstrate splinter skills representing unusual abilities such as being able to memorize the phone directory (Nelson, 1998). Young children with autism are usually unresponsive to others, and they engage in solitary activity during the early years. As Schopler and Mesibov found, as the children get older, they show interest in interacting with others socially but find such interaction difficult. Volkmar and colleagues (1997) found that older children with autism have difficulty establishing a shared frame of reference with their social partner, frequently speaking tangentially without providing background information needed for the listener to understand the conversation. They are also somewhat impulsive in their language, failing to adhere to accepted social norms. For example, they may blurt out, "That is an ugly dress." Volkmar and colleagues also found that these children use **stereotypical phrases** as the norm for social interaction, and fail to recognize and use nonverbal cues when interacting with others.

Stereotypical phrases. Fixed, nonvarying utterances that are often heard produced by others and used in excess by children with social interaction deficits.

Asperger's Syndrome

Asperger's syndrome is a label used to identify children who are at the higher end of the autism spectrum. These children will usually have difficulty making friends in school, in some part because they have difficulty comprehending nonverbal communication behaviors, and they lack spontaneity in their communication endeavors. Organization of information is also problematic which can significantly impact their academic success. Thus, this should be a major focus of therapy for children with Asperger's syndrome.

Children who have Asperger's syndrome often demonstrate splinter skills at a high level such as proficiency in music or mathematics, but at the same time have difficulty with organizational skills and the generalization of skills learned in one setting to a novel setting. An illustration of this is that the child may be able to comprehend complex mathematical or scientific principles but fail to bring his or her homework home at the end of the school day due to lack of organizational skills. In addition, these children may have temper tantrums, but not as a manipulative effort; rather, the tantrums are usually in response to fear, stress, and/or frustration.

The classroom for children with autism or Asperger's syndrome should stick to a regular schedule as much as possible because these children typically have difficulty with transition to new activities and schedules. The classroom should not be overstimulating in terms of noise and visual distractions. In fact, the child with Asperger's syndrome will share many of the characteristics of children with **attention deficit disorder** (with or without hyperactivity).

Attention deficit disorder. The presence of behavior that typically includes inattention, hyperactivity, and impulsivity that exceed that expected by children at a given age.

Remaining seated for an extended period of time and being able to focus on the task at hand are quite taxing for children who fall on the autism spectrum. He or she may have auditory processing problems, leading to failure to comprehend instructions provided by teachers and therapists, so the students will benefit from having directions broken down into small steps and using visual cues when possible.

Comprehension may lag behind expression in children with Asperger's syndrome. This certainly interferes with the progression of his or her academic skills once in school. Likewise, poor organization skills and possible auditory processing deficits may impact his or her ability to achieve academic success. Children who fall on the autism spectrum often have **dysgraphia**, or difficulty writing, making it difficult to listen to the teacher and take notes simultaneously. It will be helpful to the student to have the teacher make copies of his or her notes for the child, or to assign a fellow student as his or her notetaker in the class.

Dysgraphia. Impaired ability to write, usually due to brain damage.

The development of friendships with other students is a big problem for children with Asperger's syndrome. As mentioned earlier, they often lack comprehension of basic social skills, and this interferes with the ability to establish and maintain friendships. It may be helpful for the family members, the teacher, and other professionals who interact with the child to lead a classroom discussion with the students in the child's class in order to explain the nature of the disorder and solicit their help in forming relationships with the student.

With regard to a prognosis for children with autism, Paul (1987) suggests their language skills and their performance on intelligence tests are two markers. Those children who fall within or close to the normal range of intelligence quotients are more successful in achieving independence in adulthood. Also, the development of speech by age 5 is indicative of a more promising prognosis. Those children who have a relatively normal developmental history followed by a regression have a poorer prognosis than children who do not regress (Watson & Ozonoff, 2001). Some children with autism who have a normal to high IQ may attend college, live independently, and become employed. However, they remain socially handicapped, having difficulty with pragmatics, empathy, and other social skills (Schroeder, LeBlanc, & Mayo, 1996; Paul, 2001).

■ VELO-CARDIO-FACIAL SYNDROME

Learning disabilities are characteristic in children with velo-cardio-facial syndrome (VCF), a genetic syndrome. In fact, 99% of individuals with VCF will experience learning disabilities. Golding-Kushner, Weller, and Shprintzen (1985) found that, regardless of age, children with VCF had perceptual motor weaknesses. Intellectual functioning and language skills were essentially normal by the time the child turned age 6. However, as they grew older, the children with VCF demonstrated poor abstract reasoning skills when compared to normally developing children, partially due to the fact that they remain at a relatively concrete level of cognitive functioning. Thus, the academic, language, and psychological skills were negatively impacted. This impact would be expected given that as the child advances in school, there are increased linguistic and cognitive demands. Complicating the speech, language, and academic problems is the fact that children who have VCF characteristically will have recurrent bouts of fluid accumulation and infection otherwise known as otitis media with effusion (Faires, Topping, & Cranford, 1993; Gravel & Wallace, 1996).

As children with VCF get older, the ability to form appropriate social interactions may be negatively affected by stress. Papolos and colleagues (1996) have documented that approximately 70% of the cases they assessed presented with some form of bipolar affective disorders such as dysthymia and psychotic manic depression (Shprintzen, 1997). In addition, a study by Goldberg and colleagues (1993) found a wide variety of psychiatric disorders including attention deficit disorder with hyperactivity, generalized anxiety disorder, obsessive compulsive disorder, severe personality disorder, and paranoid disorder. All these factors vary in terms of their occurrence, but nearly all children with VCF will have "some degree of cognitive impairment and social communication deficits" (Carneol, Marks, & Weik, 1999, p. 28). These impairments may be relatively subtle, and the lack of proper diagnosis may prevent the child from receiving appropriate services in the public schools.

■ ATTENTION DEFICIT DISORDER WITH OR WITHOUT HYPERACTIVITY

Children and adolescents who have attention deficit disorder (ADD) will need guidance in understanding how they process information, and how they should participate in social and academic settings. **Impulsivity** is a major

Impulsivity. The performance of actions done without thinking or premeditation.

component of attention deficit disorder with hyperactivity (ADHD), and these students should work closely with an adult (teacher, counselor, parent, etc.) who can help them understand the nature of their impulsivity and how it interferes with learning and social interactions.

Co-morbidity. The coexistence of one or more disorders.

They should receive instruction in problem solving, working with others, and understanding themselves as participants in academic situations (Tattershall, 2002). Rutter, Tizard, and Whitmore (1970) did a study to document **co-morbidity** of psychiatric, neurological, and learning disorders. They found that 25% of the children who had reading problems also had either ADD, ADHD, or oppositional disorders.

Students who have ADD without hyperactivity will need some of the same direction as is provided for students with ADHD, particularly in the areas of problem solving and understanding themselves and the nature of ADD. They should receive counseling about how to self-monitor their attention, and what to do when attentional problems interfere with their social and academic progress. Teachers, counselors, and parents should be sure the adolescent understands the nature of ADD and its impact on learning.

Adolescents with ADD/ADHD are likely to have problems with pragmatics. They need instruction in the rules that govern how to be a communication partner. Tattershall (2002) suggests that the adolescents collect and report anecdotes about communication exchanges in which they believed they were successful, and in which they felt unsuccessful. Sharing these anecdotes with an adult can help the student analyze the strengths and weaknesses in social conversations and academic settings. Likewise, they can observe communication exchanges among their peers, analyze them (including role play), and adopt strategies that were effective in the conversations. Larson and McKinley (1987) make the point that language therapy for adolescents (with or without ADD/ADHD) should focus primarily on pragmatics, with semantics, syntax, and phonology being addressed under the umbrella of pragmatics. Teenagers need to learn survival language and be able to relate to their peers in order to succeed socially and academically.

■ SUMMARY

The development of language has been studied heavily in the preschool population. However, it is only in the last 10 years or so that much attention has been paid to the continuing development of language in school-age children. Care should be taken to analyze the language of a child based on semantics, syntax, morphology, phonology, and pragmatics. Children who have demonstrated a delay or disorder in one or more areas of language as a preschooler should be tested and enrolled in therapy as soon as possible in order to minimize the impact of the delay or disorder on social and academic functioning. There is substantial evidence for the need to incorporate preliteracy skills into the education of all preschool children, and particularly of those preschoolers who have language delays or disorders. Literacy intervention will probably be needed when the child begins and progresses through the academic curriculum.

Evidence exists in some of the recent research that indicates that even preschool-age children whose language deficits appear to have been resolved by the time they enter first grade may have some residual effects that are not noticed until the academic demands increase. Typically, there is a substantial increase in academic demands when the child enters third grade and begins to face the demands of reading textbooks for comprehension. Dealing with problem solving, abstract concepts, and increased linguistic complexity can tax a child's linguistic system, particularly if there have been previous problems. Thus, it is probably a good idea to monitor the language skills of all third graders who have a history of language delays or disorders in case there are residual elements that could impact the child's academic and social success.

CASE STUDY

Instead of the usual case study, I am including a story written by Preston Lewis who has an 18-year-old brother who is cognitively challenged with an IQ in the 30 to 40 range. The name of the story is "A Case for Teaching Functional Skills" and I believe it captures the need to have therapy goals that are aimed at helping individuals with life-long impairments to get the most benefit out of life.

A Case for Teaching Functional Skills*

By Preston Lewis

It is not uncommon to find instances of curricular content for students with moderate to severe handicaps based primarily on information from the administration of norm-referenced evaluation instruments. A dilemma often results when an attempt is made to translate test items failed at particular levels or mental ages into actual tasks to be taught. Not only were these evaluation tools never intended to be used in this manner, but the result is that students end up spending a majority of their school years being taught skills that are totally artificial or extremely age inappropriate. Given the time it takes students with moderate to severe handicaps to acquire and maintain even functional skills, there is no time or justification for devoting instruction to teaching items that are selected from a developmentally based hierarchy of supposed "prerequisite" selected skills. A scenario of the outcome for one such student is portrayed below.

My Other Brother Daryl

18 years old. TMH (30 to 40 IQ). Been in school 12 years. Never been served in any other setting than elementary school. He has had a number of years of "individual instruction." He has learned to do a lot of things!

Daryl can now do lots of things he couldn't do before!

He can put 100 pegs in a board in less than 10 minutes while in his seat with 95% accuracy. But, he can't put quarters in vending machines.

Upon command, he can "touch nose, shoulder, food, hair, ear." He's still working on wrist, ankle, hips. But, he can't blow his nose when needed.

He can now do a 12-piece Big Bird puzzle with 100% accuracy and color an Easter Bunny and stay in the lines! But, he prefers music, but was never taught how to use a radio or record player.

He can now fold primary paper in halves and even quarters. But he can't fold his clothes.

He can sort blocks by color, up to 10 different colors! But, he can't sort clothes (whites from colors) for washing.

He can roll Play Dough and make wonderful clay snakes. But, he can't roll bread dough and cut out biscuits.

He can string beads in alternating colors and match it to a pattern on a DLM card. But, he can't lace his shoes.

He can sing his ABCs and tell me names of all the letters of the alphabet when presented on a card in uppercase with 80% accuracy. But, he can't tell the men's room from the ladies' room when we go to McDonald's.

He can be told it's a cloudy/rainy day and take a black felt cloud and put it on the day of the week on an enlarged calendar (with assistance). But, he still goes out in the rain without a raincoat or hat.

He can identify with 100% accuracy 100 different Peabody Picture Cards by pointing! But, he can't order a hamburger by pointing to a picture or gesturing.

He can walk a balance beam forwards, sideways, and backwards! But, he can't walk up the steps or bleachers unassisted in the gym to go to a basketball game.

He can count to 100 by rote memory. But, he doesn't know how many dollars to pay the waitress for a $2.59 McDonald's coupon special.

He can put the cube in the box, beside the box, and behind the box. But, he can't find the trash bin in McDonald's and empty his trash into it.

He can sit in a circle with appropriate behavior and sing songs and play "Duck, Duck, Goose." But, nobody else in his neighborhood his age seems to want to do that.

I guess he's just not ready yet.

*Reprinted with permission from *TASH Newsletter,* December 1987.

■ REVIEW QUESTIONS

1. There have been many studies showing that speech and language deficits manifested during the preschool years have residual effects on social and academic achievement in the school years.

   a. True
   b. False

2. Parental education is a better predictor of a child's language behaviors in adolescence than are the child's language abilities during the birth-to-3 years.

   a. True
   b. False

3. The development of metalinguistic skills is most marked at 3 to 6 years of age.

   a. True
   b. False

4. Skills that reflect the child's ability to develop alternative ways to solve a problem or resolve a situation, the ability to form hypotheses and task analyze them in a constructive manner, and the capacity to make personal decisions are _____ skills.

   a. Metalinguistic skills
   b. Metanarrative skills
   c. Metacognitive skills
   d. Metapragmatic skills

5. Academic problems of children with fetal alcohol syndrome/fetal alcohol effects include which of the following?

   a. Conceptual deficits such as time and space
   b. Difficulties with comprehension of spoken and written materials
   c. Deficits in basic problem solving
   d. Deficits in visual and spatial memory
   e. All of the above
   f. None of the above

6. In approximately 70% of children who are cognitively challenged, there is no gap between their language abilities and their cognitive abilities.

   a. True
   b. False

7. Academically, children with moderate cognitive challenges plateau in their academic skills around grade 6.

   a. True
   b. False

8. It is useless to introduce a literacy component into the educational and therapeutic plans for students with Down syndrome because learning to read is too big a challenge.

   a. True
   b. False

9. Typically, girls with fragile X syndrome are more severely affected in terms of their cognitive and language functioning than are boys.

   a. True
   b. False

10. It is rare that a child with velo-cardio-facial syndrome will exhibit a learning disability.

    a. True
    b. False

■ REFERENCES

Achenbach, T. M. (1979). The child behavior profile: An empirically based system for assessing children's behavioral problems and competencies. *International Journal of Mental Health, 7,* 24–42.

Achenbach, T. M. (1981). *Child behavior checklist.* Burlington, VT: University of Vermont.

American Association on Mental Retardation (AAMR) (2002). *Definition of mental retardation.* www.aamr.org/Policies/faq_mental_retardation.shtml.

Aram, D. M., Ekelman, B. L., & Nation, J. E. (1984, June). Preschoolers with language disorders: 10 years later. *Journal of Speech and Hearing Research, 27,* 232–244.

Aram, D. M., & Nation, J. E. (1980). Preschool language disorders and subsequent language and academic difficulties. *Journal of Communication Disorders, 13,* 159–170.

Arthur, G. (1952). *The Arthur adaptation of the Leiter international performance scale.* Washington, DC: Psychological Service Center Press.

Bedrosian, J. & Prutting, C. (1978). Communicative performance of mentally retarded adults in four conversational settings. *Journal of Speech and Hearing Research, 21,* 79–95.

Bernstein, D. K. (1997). Language development: The school-age years. In D. K. Bernstein and E. Tiegerman-Farber (Eds.), *Language and communication disorders in children* (pp. 127–151). Allyn and Bacon.

Bernstein, D. K., & Tiegerman-Farber, E. (1997). *Language and communication disorders in children.* Boston: Allyn and Bacon.

Bishop, D. V. M., & Edmundson, A. (1987). Language-impaired 4-year-olds: Distinguishing transient from persistent impairment. *Journal of Speech and Hearing Disorders, 52,* 156–173.

Brinton, B., Fujiki, M., & Higbee, L. (1998). Participation in cooperative learning activities by children with specific language impairment. *Journal of Speech, Language, and Hearing Research, 41,* 1193–1206.

Brinton, B., Fujiki, M., Montague, E. C., & Hanton, J. L. (2000). Children with language impairment in cooperative work groups: A pilot study. *Language, Speech, and Hearing Services in Schools, 31,* 252–264.

Brown, R. (1973). *A first language: The early stages.* Cambridge, MA: Harvard University Press.

Buckley, S. (1993). Language development in children with Down's syndrome: Reasons for optimism. *Down Syndrome Research and Practice, 1,* 3–9.

Buckley, S. (1995a). Improving the expressive language skills of teenagers with Down syndrome. *Down Syndrome Research and Practice, 3*(3), 110–115.

Buckley, S. (1995b). Teaching children with Down syndrome to read and write. In L. Nadel & D. Rosenthal (Eds.), *Down syndrome: Living and learning in the community* (pp. 158–169). New York: Wiley-Liss.

Carneol, S. O., Marks, S. M., & Weik, L. (February, 1999). The speech-language pathologist: Key role in the diagnosis of velocardiofacial syndrome. *American Journal of Speech-Language Pathology, 8,* 23–32.

Carr, J. (1995). *Down's syndrome: Children growing up.* New York: Cambridge University Press.

Carrow, E. (1973). *Test of auditory comprehension of language.* Austin, TX: Urban Research Group.

Chapman, R. S. (1995). Language development in children and adolescents with Down syndrome. In Fletcher, B., & MacWhinney, B. (Eds.), *Handbook of child language* (pp. 641–663). Oxford: Blackwell Publishers.

Chapman, R., Seung, H., Schwartz, S., & Kay-Raining Bird, E. (1998). Language skills of children and adolescents with Down syndrome. II: Production deficits. *Journal of Speech, Language, and Hearing Research, 41*(4), 861–873.

Damico, J., & Oller, J. W., Jr. (1980). Pragmatic versus morphological/syntactic criteria for language referrals. *Language, Speech, and Hearing Services in the Schools, 19,* 51–66.

DeMyer, M., Barton, S., DeMeyer, E., Norton, J., Allen J., & Steele, R. (1973). Prognosis in autism: A follow-up study. *Journal of Autism and Childhood Schizophrenia, 3,* 199–216.

Faires, W., Topping, G., & Cranford, J. L. (1993). The long term effects of chronic ottitis media with effusion on language and auditory sequential memory. *Journal of Medical Speech-Language Pathology, 1,* 163–169.

Fowler, A., Doherty, B., & Boynton, L. (1995). The basis of reading skill in young adults with Down syndrome. In L. Nadel & D. Rosenthal (Eds.), *Down syndrome: Living and learning in the community.* New York: John Wiley & Sons.

Fujiki, M., Brinton, B., & Clarke, D. (April, 2002). Emotional regulation in children with specific language impairment. *Language, Speech, and Hearing Services in Schools, 33,* 102–111.

Fujiki, M., Brinton, B., Isaacson, T., & Summers, C. (April, 2001). Social behaviors of children with language impairment on the playground: A pilot study. *Language, Speech, and Hearing Services in Schools, 32,* 101–113.

Gertner, B. L., Rice, M. L., & Hadley, P. A. (1994). Influence of communicative competence on peer preferences in a preschool classroom. *Journal of Speech and Hearing Research, 37,* 913–923.

Gillham, B. (1979). *The first words language programme: A basic language programme for mentally handicapped children.* London: George Allen & Unwin.

Girolametto, L., Wiigs, M., Smyth, R., Weitzman, E., & Pearce, P. S. (November, 2001). Children with a history of expressive vocabulary delay: Outcomes at 5 years of age. *American Journal of Speech-Language Pathology, 10*(4), 358–369.

Goldberg, R., Motzking, B., Marion, R., Scambler, R. J., & Shprintzen, R. J. (1993). Velo-cardio-facial syndrome: A review of 120 patients. *American Journal of Medical Genetics, 45,* 313–319.

Golding-Kushner, K., Weller, G., & Shprintzen, R. J. (1985). Velo-cardio-facial syndrome: Language and psychological profiles. *Journal of Craniofacial Genetics Developmental Biology, 5,* 259–266.

Grandin, T. (1997). A personal perspective on autism. In D. Cohen and F. Volkmar (Eds.), *Handbook of autism and pervasive developmental disorders* (pp. 1032–1042). New York: John Wiley and Sons.

Gravel, J. S., & Wallace, I. F. (1996). Early otitis media, auditory abilities, and educational risk. *American Journal of Speech-Language Pathology, 4*(3), 89–94.

Hurford, J. (1991). The evolution of the critical period for language acquisition. *Cognition, 40,* 159–201.

Johnson, C. J., Beitchman, J. H., Young, A., Escobar, M., Atkinson, L., Wilson, B., Brownlie, E. G., Douglas, L., Taback, N., Lan, I., & Want, M. (1999). Fourteen-year follow-up of children with and without speech/language impairments: Speech/language stability and outcomes. *Journal of Speech, Language, and Hearing Research, 42*(3), 744–760.

Kay-Raining Bird, E., Cleave, P. L., & McConnell, L. (November, 2000). Reading and phonological awareness in children with Down syndrome: A longitudinal study. *American Journal of Speech-Language Pathology, 9,* 319–330.

Kay-Raining Bird, E., Cleave, P. L., McFarlane, H., & Hackett, A. (1998, July). Written language abilities in children with Down syndrome. Poster presented at the XVth biennial meetings of ISSBD, Bern, Switzerland.

Kay-Raining Bird, E., & McConnell, L. (1994, November). Language and literacy relationships in children with Down syndrome. Poster presented at the Annual American Speech-Language-Hearing Association Convention, New Orleans, LA.

King, R. R., Jones, C., & Laskey, E. (1982). In retrospect: A fifteen year follow-up report of speech-language disordered children. *Language, Speech, and Hearing Services in Schools, 13,* 24–32.

Kochanek, T. T., Kabacoff, R. I., & Lipsitt, L. P. (1990). Early identification of developmentally disabled and at-risk preschool children. *Exceptional Children, 56,* 528–538.

Kumin, L. (2003). *Early communication skills for children with Down syndrome: A guide for parents and professionals.* Bethesda, MD: Woodbine House.

Kumin, L., Councill, C., & Goodman, M. (1998). Expressive vocabulary development in children with Down syndrome. *Down Syndrome Quarterly, 3,* 1–7.

Larson, V. L., & McKinley, N. (1987). *Communication assessment and intervention strategies for adolescents.* Eau Claire, WI: Thinking Publications.

Larson, V. L., & McKinley, N. (1995). *Language disorders in older students: Preadolescents and adolescents.* Eau Claire, WI: Thinking Publications.

Layton, T. (2001). Young children with Down syndrome. In T. Layton, E. Crais, and L. Watson (Eds.). *Handbook of early language impairment in children: Nature* (pp. 302–360). Albany, NY: Delmar Publishers.

Lord, C., & Paul, R. (1997). Language and communication in autism. In D. Cohen and F. Volkmar (Eds.), *Handbook of autism and pervasive developmental disorders* (2nd ed.) (pp. 195–225). New York: John Wiley and Sons.

Menyuk, P. (1969). *Sentences children use.* Cambridge, MA: MIT Press.

Menyuk, P. (1971). *The acquisition and development of language.* Englewood Cliffs, NJ: Prentice Hall.

Miller, J. F. (1988). Individual differences in vocabulary acquisition in children with Down syndrome. *Progress in Clinical and Biological Research, 393,* 93–103.

Miller, J., & Chapman, R. (1984). Disorders of communication: Investigating the development of mentally retarded children. *American Journal of Mental Deficiency, 88,* 536–545.

Miller, P. (1989). Theories of adolescent development. In J. Worell and F. Danner (Eds.), *The adolescent as decision-maker: Applications to development and education* (pp. 13–49). San Diego: Academic Press.

Mundy, P., Seibert, J., & Hogan, A. (1985). Communication skills in mentally retarded children. In M. Sigman (Ed.), *Children with emotional disorders and developmental disabilities: Assessment and treatment* (pp. 45–70). Orlando, FL: Grune and Stratton.

Neale, M. D. (1958). *Neale analysis of reading ability manual.* London: Macmillan.

Nelson, N. W. (1993). *Childhood language disorders in context.* New York: Merrill Publishing Company.

Nelson, N. W. (1994). Curriculum-based language assessment and intervention across the grades. In G. P Wallach and K. G. Butler (Eds.), *Language learning disabilities in school-age children and adolescents: Some principles and applications* (pp. 104–131). New York: Merrill/Macmillan Publishing Company.

Nelson, N. W. (1998). *Childhood language disorders in context: Infancy through Adolescence* (2nd ed.). Boston: Allyn and Bacon.

Nippold, M. A. (1988). The literate lexicon. In M. A. Nippold (Ed.), *Later language development: Ages nine through nineteen* (pp. 29–47). Austin, TX: Pro-Ed.

Owens, R. (1996). *Language development: An introduction* (3rd ed.). Columbus, OH: Merrill/Macmillan.

Owens, R. (2004). *Language disorders: A functional approach to assessment and intervention* (4th ed.). Boston: Allyn and Bacon.

Papolos, D. F., Faedda, G. L., Veit, S., Goldberg, R., Morrow, B., Kucherlapati, R., & Shprintzen, R. J. (1996). Bipolar spectrum disorders in patients diagnosed with velo-cardio-facial syndrome: Does a hemizygous deletion of chromosome 22q11 result in bipolar affective disorder? *American Journal of Psychiatry, 153,* 1541–1547.

Paul, R. (1987). Communication. In D. J. Cohen and A. M. Donnellan (Eds.), *Handbook of autism and pervasive developmental disorders* (pp. 61–84). New York: John Wiley and Sons.

Paul, R. (2001). *Language disorders from infancy through adolescence: Assessment and intervention.* St. Louis, MO: Mosby.

Ratner, V., & Harris, L. (1994). *Understanding language disorders: The impact on learning.* Eau Claire, WI: Thinking Publications.

Raven, J. C. (1995). Raven's Progressive Matrices Test. San Antonio, TX: PsychCorp/Harcourt Assessment, Inc.

Rescorla, L., Hadicke-Wiley, M., & Escarce, E. (1993). Epidemiological investigation of expressive language delay at age two. *First Language, 13,* 5–22.

Rice, M. L., Sell, M. A., & Hadley, P. A. (1991). Social interactions of speech- and language-impaired children. *Journal of Speech and Hearing Research, 34,* 1299–1307.

Rivers, K. L., & Hedrick, D. (1992). Langauge and behavioral concerns for drug-exposed infants and toddlers. *Infant-Toddler Intervention: The Transdisciplinary Journal, 2*(1), 63–71.

Rondal, J. A. (1978). Maternal speech to normal and Down's syndrome children matched for mean length of utterance. In C. E. Myers (Ed.), *Quality of life in severely and profoundly mentally retarded people: Research foundations for improvement.* Washington, DC: American Association on Mental Deficiency.

Rosenkoetter, S. E. (1995) *It's a big step.* Topeka, KS: Bridging Early Services Task Force, Coordinating Council on Early Childhood Developmental Services.

Rosner, J., & Simon, D. P. (1971)., The auditory analysis test: An initial report. *Journal of Learning Disabilities, 4,* 384–392.

Rutter, M., Tizard, J., & Whitmore, K. (Eds.). (1970). *Education, health, and behavior.* London: Longmans Green.

Scharfenaker, S. (1990). The fragile X syndrome. *ASHA, 32,* 45–47.

Schopler, E., & Mesibov, G. B. (Eds.) (1986). *Communication problems in autism.* New York: Plenum Press.

Schopmeyer, E., & Lowe, F. (1992). *The fragile X child.* San Diego: Singular Publishing Group.

Schroeder, S., LeBlanc, J., & Mayo, L. (1996). Brief report: A life-span perspective on the development of individuals with autism. *Journal of Autism and Developmental Disorders, 26,* 251–256.

Shprintzen, R. (1997). *Genetics, syndromes, and communication disorders.* San Diego: Singular Publishing Group.

Sloper, P., Cunningham, C., Turner, S., & Knussen, Cl. (1990). Factors related to the academic attainments of children with Down syndrome. *British Journal of Educational Psychology, 60,* 284–298.

Spiridigliozzi, G., Lachiewicz, A., Mirrett, S., & McConkie-Rosell, A. (2001). Fragile X syndrome in young children. In T. Layton, E. Crais, and L. Watson, *Handbook of early language impairment in children: Nature* (pp. 258–301). Albany, NY: Delmar Publishers.

Stothard, S. E., Snowling, M. J., Bishop, D. V. M., Chipchase, B. B., & Kaplan, C. A. (1998). Language-impaired preschoolers: A follow-up into adolescence. *Journal of Speech, Language, and Hearing Research, 41*(2), 407–418.

Tattershall, S. (2002). *Adolescents with language and learning needs: A shoulder to shoulder collaboration.* Albany, NY: Singular/Thomson Learning.

van Kleek, A. (1994). Metalinguistic development. In G. P. Wallach and K. G. Butler (Eds.), *Language learning disabilities in school-age children and adolescents: Some principles and applications.* New York: Merrill/Macmillan Publishing Company.

Volkmar, F., Carter, A., Grossman, J., & Klin, A. (1997). Social development in autism. In D. Cohen and F. Volkmar (Eds.), *Handbook of autism and pervasive developmental disorders* (pp. 173–194). New York: John Wiley and Sons.

Wallach, G. P. & Butler, K. G. (1994). *Language learning disabilities in school-age children and adolescents: Some principles and applications.* New York: Merrill/Macmillan Publishing Company.

Watson, L. R., & Ozonoff, S. (2001). In T. Layton, E. Crais, and L. Watson (Eds.), *Handbook of early language impairment in children: Nature* (pp. 177–257). Albany, NY: Delmar.

White, B. (1975). Critical influences in the origins of competence. *Merrill-Palmer Quarterly, 22,* 243–266.

Woodcock, R. W. (1987). *Woodcock reading mastery tests-revised.* Circle Pines, MN: American Guidance Service.

II

LANGUAGE DISORDERS IN SCHOOL-AGE CHILDREN

Chapters 6 through 11 are dedicated to the study of language disorders in school-age children. It is not unusual for language delays in the preschool population to persist as language disorders in the school-age years.

Many preschoolers who are diagnosed as having specific language impairment are considered learning disabled in elementary school. Even those who improve their expressive language will still have problems with subtle language skills and with complex and advanced language skills. They may also have trouble with socialization. In addition, it is not uncommon to see children with specific language impairment or with attention deficit disorder (with or without hyperactivity).

Kamhi and Catts (1989) noted that reading requires the same factors as does language, but the weighting of the factors is different. Two of these factors are biology and environment. Human biology is designed so that the auditory system is adapted and refined to process speech at a subconscious level. The visual system is not as well adapted, so additional "attentional resources" are needed. The second factor is environment. Almost all environments use spoken language, but it is not necessarily the same as written language. We are "biologically endowed" and socialized to use oral language. Some cultures do not value written language, so they do not provide formal reading instruction. The impact of this is an underlying theme to Chapters 6 through 11.

In Chapter 6, language-based learning disabilities are reviewed. So-called "red flags" and "soft signs" that could serve as precursors to reading and spelling disorders are delineated in the hope that readers will learn possible warning signs of language-based learning disabilities. If these warning signs are observed in the preschool population, they prompt early intervention in the preschool years to avoid more catastrophic learning disabilities in the school years. In Chapter 7, the impact of language deficits on spelling and reading disorders is discussed. In Chapter 8, issues related to attention deficit disorder (ADD) and attention deficit disorder with hyperactivity (ADHD) are delineated. The impact of these two disorders on learning is reviewed. Chapter 9 focuses on traumatic brain injury (TBI). Although the focus of this chapter is on TBI in the school-aged population, much of what is true in this population is also found in traumatic brain injury in adults. Thus, the reader can extrapolate the information contained in this chapter to address TBI in adults. Chapter 10 focuses on general assessment issues in the school-age population, and Chapter 11 addresses treatment considerations.

Just as it was important to understand language delays, disorders, and differences to bridge the age gap between preschool and school-age children, so is it important to understand the impact of language-based learning disabilities in the adult population.

■ REFERENCE

Kamhi, A. B., & Catts, H. W. (1989). *Reading disabilities: A developmental language perspective.* Austin, TX: Pro-Ed.

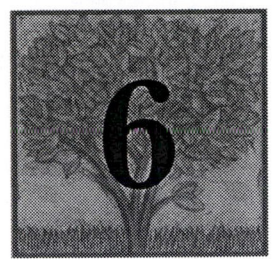

Language-Based Learning Disabilities in the School-Age Population

▥ **LEARNING OBJECTIVES**

After completion of this chapter, the reader will be able to

1. Explain why speech-language pathologists should be part of the team that treats children with language-based learning disabilities, particularly with reading and spelling problems

2. Describe some of the problems an educational team (including the SLP) faces in diagnosing learning disabilities in school-age children, particularly those 10 years of age and older

3. List and briefly discuss red flags for the development of a language-based learning disability.

4. Compare and contrast categories of language-learning disabilities based on the historical approach and those based on the clinical-inferential approach.

5. Discuss the impact of a phonological deficit on reading and spelling

6. Discuss six problems with written language in children with learning and/or reading disabilities.

▥ **INTRODUCTION**

It is estimated that children with language disorders make up 50 to 80% of the cases seen by speech-language pathologists who serve the preschool- and school-age population. In some school districts, eligibility for language therapy is expressed as a gap between the mental age (MA) of the child, as measured by standardized psychoeducational batteries (such as the Wechsler Intelligence Scale for Children–Revised), and the child's language age (LA), as measured by norm-referenced languages tests (such as the Test of Language Development). The school district will set criteria such as an MA/LA gap of 18 months for a child to qualify for language therapy. In other districts, placement in school-based therapy often hinges on the labeling of the child's problem as a language disorder or language delay, so this chapter will be structured to reflect the assessment and treatment of language disorders based on a diagnostic label in school-age children.

A speech-language pathologist is a critical member of the educational team responsible for assessing and treating language-based **learning disabilities.** It is important to note that not all learning disabilities are language-based. Children with nonlanguage-based learning disabilities should be referred to professionals in occupational therapy, physical therapy, psychology, or

Learning disability. Any one of a heterogeneous set of learning problems that affect the acquisition and use of listening, speaking, writing, reading, mathematical, and reasoning skills.

education for remediation. However, if the learning disability is based on a language disorder, the speech-language pathologist should be involved in the child's educational process. Most language-based learning disabilities will be manifested as reading or spelling difficulties, or both. Many of these **language-based learning disabilities** are extensions of speech and language disorders occurring during the preschool years.

Early semantic and syntactic skills are predictors of later reading success in children, but most researchers agree that the best predictor is phonological awareness. In fact, when the impact of three phonological processing skills— phonemic awareness, rapid serial naming, and phonological coding in working memory—is assessed, phonemic awareness emerged as the best predictor of later reading (Torgensen, Wagner, & Rashotte, 1994).

Other risk factors and red flags for the development of a language-based learning disability include being a late talker, familial patterns, and premature and/or difficult birth. Brain studies indicate that children with a language-based learning disability possibly have a breakdown along the neural pathways that facilitate communication between the frontal cortex and the midbrain (Owens, 2004). Such a breakdown would affect the individuals' executive abilities such as planning, attending, and regulating.

A second category of language-based disorders seen by clinicians serving school-age children results from traumatic brain injury and other disorders acquired in childhood. Finally, children who exhibit signs of attention deficit disorder (with or without hyperactivity) often have an accompanying language-based learning disability. This section of the book addresses these labels and the interaction they have with language.

Many of the children who are diagnosed as having a language-based learning disability have very subtle deficits that may elude even the most astute clinician. Nelson (1993) describes a category of children as being ABNQ children: They "almost but not quite" manage to keep pace with their classmates, particularly in the language-based portions of the academic curriculum. These children have relatively normal cognitive ability and remain somewhat competitive with their age-level peers. They do not have moderate to severe cognitive limitations or language delays that persist from the preschool years into older childhood. "Almost but not quite" children do not have physical or sensory impairments that interfere with acquisition of language and social interaction skills. They do have specific language and learning disabilities that interfere with their educational and social progress. Frequently, teachers will refer to these children as children who "are not performing up to their potential," yet their deficits are so subtle that many times they do not perform poorly enough on tests to be easily identified as having a language-based learning disability.

Language-based learning disability. A single disorder that manifests itself in different ways at various points in development as communicative contexts and learning tasks change.

In addition to the fact that many of these disorders are relatively subtle, and therefore difficult to identify, another problem in identifying school-age children with language-based learning disabilities is that there is no homogeneous definition of language disorders in the school-age population. At school age, delays may persist as disorders either because of the nature of the delay or because of ineffective remediation during the preschool years. However, because most developmental charts stop at approximately 10 years of age, it becomes more difficult to determine if a child has a delay or a disorder in his or her language. At this point, language is less universal and more dependent on individual interests and experiences. Also, disorders due to etiologic factors, such as Down syndrome and fetal alcohol syndrome, do not disappear and need continued intervention during the school-age years.

Owing to the inherent differences among individuals, language disorders will have varying effects on a child, with the impact being determined by the clinician's best judgment. This judgment is often based on the degree to which the language delay or disorder impacts on the child's socialization and academic progress. Larson and McKinley (1995) took all of these factors into consideration and concluded that the clinician's primary job is to judge the child's abilities and disabilities based on the impact the problem or problems have on the child's social environment, academic environment, and vocational environment. It is also important to pay attention to how language delays and disorders affect reading and writing in school-age children.

■ CURRICULAR DEMANDS BASED ON LANGUAGE

Incidental learning.
Learning that results
from normal, routine
interactions with the
environment.

In the preschool years, the curricular emphasis is on language development and social-emotional growth. Activities focus on motor skills, visual-spatial skills, and visual and auditory perceptual skills. Torgesen (1977) writes that preschoolers experience **incidental learning** that results from normal, routine interactions with the environment. In addition, during the preschool years, children learn the value of the printed word and develop a sense of story structure as a result of exposure to books. As toddlers and preschoolers participate in book-reading routines, they learn to answer simple questions, which forms the basis for replying to questions in the school setting. In fact, through having the same story read and reread, many preschoolers learn to repeat the story as they flip the pages, giving the appearance of reading (Kamhi & Catts, 1989).

In kindergarten through second grade, children develop the basic skills needed for reading and writing. According to Chall (1983), children in this age bracket learn about phoneme-grapheme correspondences. That is, they begin to learn associations between the sounds they speak and hear and the printed letters. They also begin to learn about spelling, both oral and written, and begin to learn basic mathematical operations.

When the child reaches the middle grades (grades 3 and 4), he or she experiences a curricular leap from decoding to reading for comprehension. As expressed by Kamhi and Catts (1989), children in these grades read to learn instead of learning to read. In fact, basic skills are only reviewed; they are no longer the curricular focus. In grades 3 and 4, content areas such as English, social studies, and science are introduced. Also, mathematics includes word problems, so that even this subject area can be affected if a child has a reading disability. In addition to the shift in the curricular emphasis, around the third and fourth grades children develop "attention-demanding control processes" and learn information that must be recalled at a later time. In fact, this "controlled attentional learning" becomes a critical measure of achievement in the later school years (Torgesen, 1977).

In the upper elementary grades (grades 5 and 6), the curricular emphasis is on the acquisition of knowledge in the content areas that were introduced in grades 3 and 4. During this time, decoding skills should be fully automatic so that the child can focus his or her attention on comprehension (Kamhi & Catts, 1989).

By the time the child reaches middle school (seventh through ninth grades), he or she should be able to read popular magazines, *Reader's Digest,* the newspaper, and popular fiction. At this point, cognitive development and its impact on reading is a bigger focus than reading development per se (Kamhi & Catts, 1989). The curriculum continues to focus on content areas, but the number of content areas expands to include more subjects. "English" includes literature, study skills, composition, and language arts. Social studies encompasses world geography, American and world history, and economics; science expands to biology, chemistry, and physics. In high school, foreign languages also become part of the curriculum, as does vocational education and other life-skills coursework. Students this age develop cognitive skills, including abstract reasoning, analysis, synthesis, and judgment. They learn to develop alternate hypotheses and to create strategies to test these hypotheses. They are capable of dealing with more than one point of view and glean more from their reading because they have increased ability to think abstractly.

■ IDENTIFICATION OF CHILDREN AT RISK

Many "almost-but-not-quite" students are identified as academic underachievers. However, before taking this label lightly, it is important to look at the long-term impact of academic underachievement. As identified by Larson and McKinley (1995), academic underachievement can have devastating effects.

Thirteen percent of high school students in the United States read below the sixth grade level, and one of every four high school students drops out of school. In addition, the impact of functional illiteracy is well documented as outlined in Table 6–1.

Even more devastating are the findings of the Los Angeles Suicide Prevention Center showing that 50% of the suicide victims between the ages of 10 and 14 years are diagnosed as being hyperactive, perceptually impaired, or dyslexic. Through suicide notes and conversations with their families and peers prior to the suicide, these children cited a lack of friends (see Figure 6–1)

TABLE 6–1. Demographics of functional illiteracy.

85% of teens in juvenile court are functionally illiterate

79% of welfare recipients are functionally illiterate

85% of school drop-outs are functionally illiterate

72% of the unemployed are functionally illiterate

Source: From *Making the Grade: A Report Card on American Youth,* by R. Schubert and M. Gates, 1990, p. 9. Washington, DC: National Collaboration for Youth.

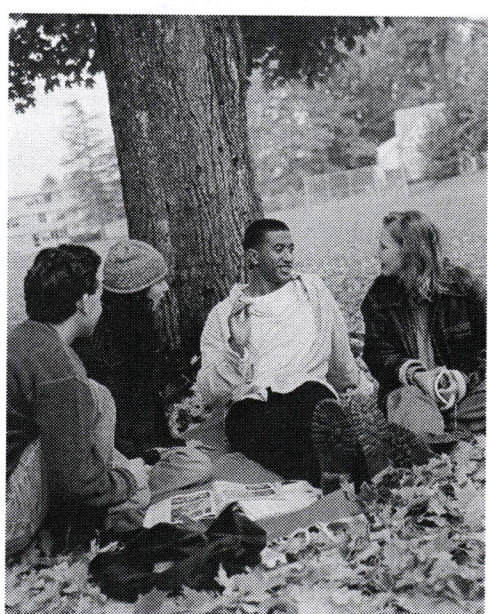

FIGURE 6–1. During the adolescent years, the value of friendship cannot be underestimated, particularly since many adolescent suicide victims claim to have no friends in whom they can confide.

and having no one to talk to as contributors to their depression and low self-esteem. In addition, they cited the presence of communication problems that interfered with making and keeping friends and expressing feelings as factors affecting their decision to commit suicide (Larson & McKinley, 1995). The statistics are strong enough to suggest that learning disabilities are accompanied by low self-esteem and that these children should be considered at risk for devastating academic and social problems (Peck, 1982). Even more compelling evidence that speech-language pathologists need to be involved in the assessment and treatment of language-based learning disabilities is offered by Nelson (1994), who noted that 24.4% of youth in the general population fail to complete high school. In addition, 36.1% of youth with learning disabilities fail to complete high school, as do 32.5% of youth with speech impairments. Furthermore, 54.8% of youth with severe emotional disturbances fail to complete this level of schooling. Given Peck's finding that low self-esteem places children at risk for suicide, this last statistic is particularly disturbing. Table 6–2 provides more information on children who are at risk for not completing high school.

The presence of attention deficit disorder (ADD) is another risk category that warrants attention from the speech-language pathologist. Although ADD in and of itself is not a language-based problem, it can have serious consequences on students' social interactions, so pragmatic issues need to be addressed in this population. Also, many children who exhibit ADD with hyperactivity (ADHD) have reading underachievement without the phonological and linguistic deficits seen in children with reading disabilities (Lombardino et al., 1997).

There is no question that a wide variety of concerns relates to identifying school-age children who are at risk for academic problems because of language-based difficulties. The question becomes how to identify these children. In most schools, screening programs serve as the first line of identification. Screenings are done in a variety of ways, including paper and pencil tasks that are administered to whole classrooms at one sitting. In other situations, teams of volunteers give simple screening tests, which take anywhere from 5 to 15 minutes to administer. These screenings are typically done in kindergarten when the child begins school, in first grade, in third grade (when the curricular emphasis shifts to reading for comprehension), and in the last year in elementary school. Regardless of the type of screening or when it is done, the speech-language pathologist typically follows up with those who fail the screening by giving more complete test batteries to identify the presence or absence of a language delay or disorder that may have an effect on the child's academic, social, and vocational career. These tests are discussed more thoroughly in Chapter 10.

As listed in Table 6–3, Hynd (1991) has identified a series of **soft signs** seen in early childhood that may be indicators of a learning disability. By itself,

Soft signs. Possible early indicators that, taken as a group, could be warning signs for a possible language-based learning disability.

TABLE 6–2. Risk factors that precipitate dropping out of school.

Many absences

Frequent tardiness

Poor grades

Low math and reading scores

Failure in one or more grades

Limited participation in extracurricular activities

Boredom with classes

Failure to see relevance of education to life goals

Disciplinary problems

Verbal and language deficiencies

Low family income/financial difficulties

Poorly educated mother

A fatherless home

A parent or sibling who dropped out

Low self-esteem

Poor social adjustment

Lack of friends

Lack of rapport with teachers

Chronic illness

Teenage pregnancy

Presence of learning disabilities

Source: Adapted from "Failure: Why Schools Must Help Children at Risk," by Sunburst Communications, 1988, *Solutions: News from Computer Educators, 3*(2), p. 1 © 1988 by Sunburst Communications.

TABLE 6–3. Soft signs that may be indicative of a learning disability.

Left-handedness

Visual-motor deficits

Letter and number reversals

Damage to supplementary motor areas of brain

Phonological deficits

History of ear infections

Higher rate of allergies and autoimmune disorders in the family

Complaints of headaches

Developmentally delayed in speech onset

Source: From G. Hynd, (1991, March). Brain Morphology As It Relates to Learning Disabilities. Lecture at the 1991 G. Paul Moore Symposium. Gainesville, FL.

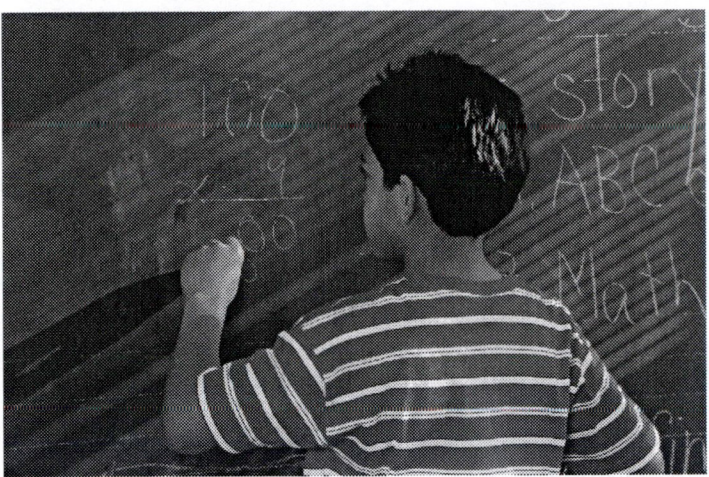

FIGURE 6–2. Left-handedness is a soft sign that, when combined with other soft signs, may predispose a student to have reading and spelling disabilities.

each of these soft signs would be of little concern. However, if a child exhibits more than one of these signs, the child should be tested and closely monitored to be sure that a language-based learning disability is not present.

The prevalence of left-handedness as seen in Figure 6–2, in the general population is 10 to 15%, but in the population of people with learning disabilities, the percentage rate is 30 to 45%. Children with damage to supplementary motor areas of brain often have characteristics similar to those who demonstrate elective mutism. They also will have problems with reading silently. Approximately 60 to 70% of all children who have reading problems have a history of developmental articulation problems. This may be tied to a higher prevalence of otitis media (OM) and otitis media with effusion (OME), which correlates with language-based learning disabilities. It is possible that whatever puts the child at risk for ear infections may also preordain children to language-based learning disabilities.

A review of the family history may show a higher rate of allergies and autoimmune disorders, such as rheumatoid arthritis, lupus erythematosus, myositis, and scleroderma. In addition, children who are eventually found to have a language-based learning disability tend to have a larger number of complaints related to headaches. Parents also typically report that the child was developmentally delayed with regard to speech onset in the preschool years (Hynd, 1991).

Historically, children who are at risk for language-based learning disabilities are described by their teachers as being socially adequate on entering school, but quickly showing poor performance in language-based activities in the classroom.

Other children with the same risk factors may do well in school initially but their performance may degenerate in late elementary or middle school as the curricular demands rely more on reading for comprehension. Many of the children are identified in third grade when, as written earlier, they are expected to read for comprehension. This presents a problem because their struggle to decipher individual words interferes with their comprehension of text. In other cases the children are identified in grades 4 to 5 and 8 to 9 when word problems become a set part of the mathematics curriculum. Regardless of when a child's disorder is identified, early and appropriate intervention is critical to help the child keep pace with his or her peers in the academic world. Extra concern should be given older children with learning disabilities because they tend to internalize the disorder, which results in severe depression. In fact, serious depression and suicide among older children with a learning disability is six times the national rate (Larson & McKinley, 1995).

■ DEFINITIONS OF LEARNING DISABILITIES

The National Joint Committee on Learning Disabilities (NJCLD, 1991) defines learning disabilities as a "heterogeneous group of disorders manifested by significant difficulties in the acquisition and use of listening, speaking, reading, writing, reasoning, or mathematical abilities" (p. 18). This committee further states that these disorders are intrinsic to the individual and may be due to central nervous system dysfunction. The group also points out that learning disabilities may coexist with other conditions but not be the direct result of these conditions or influences.

In contrast, the legally accepted definition of learning disabilities is the one provided by the United States Office of Education (USOE, 1991) in the Individuals with Disabilities Education Act (IDEA). This organization defines learning disabilities as a disorder in "one or more of the basic psychological processes involved in understanding or in using language, spoken or written, which disorder may manifest itself in imperfect ability to listen, think, speak, read, write, spell, or do mathematical calculation." The definition includes perceptual deficits, brain injury, minimal brain dysfunction, dyslexia, and developmental aphasia, but it does not include learning problems due primarily to visual, hearing, or motor disabilities, mental retardation, or environmental disadvantage.

Even though the USOE definition is the legal definition, the NJCLD definition is the one preferred by educators. Educators criticize the USOE definition as being a list of diagnostic labels without describing behavioral characteristics associated with learning disabilities. Furthermore, the USOE definition does not give precise criteria for determining if a child fits into the category. We also know that perceptual-motor ("basic psychological processes") problems are not at the root of all learning disabilities. The NJCLD definition also acknowledges the heterogeneous nature of learning disabilities and respects the fact that they are not limited to children but also may persist into adulthood. It points out the strong possibility of central nervous system dysfunction as playing a role in the existence of learning disabilities (Shames, Wiig, & Secord, 1994).

Similarly, it is important to differentiate between language disorders and learning disabilities. They are separate problems, and a child can have either or both. In some children the language disorder causes the learning disability, and these children are the focus of this chapter. Language-based learning disabilities constitute a single disorder that manifests itself in different ways at various points in development as communicative contexts and learning tasks change. At the preschool level, language disorders are considered as demonstrated in a child's communicative functioning and in his or her receptive and expressive language skills. In the school-age child, it is important to look at the child's metalinguistic abilities, narrative and classroom discourse, figurative language use, and written language skills.

Learning disabilities can be classified in a variety of ways. One approach is the historical approach that classified language-learning disabilities according to the age of the child when the problems were first observed. In 1986, Donahue described three categories based on the historical approach:

1. Children diagnosed during the preschool years with obvious language learning problems or evidence of attention deficit hyperactivity disorder (ADHA) (Blackman, 2000; Connor, 2002).

2. Children who enter school with adequate interpersonal communication skills but who show poor performance.

3. Children who initially fare well in school but eventually exhibit problems (Reed, 2005, p. 136).

Another approach to the classification of learning disabilities is the clinical-inferential approach in which profiles of children with language-based learning disabilities are developed based on the review of test scores. The first profile in this approach is those children who have "difficulty on language and language-related tasks" (Reed, 2005, p. 135). According to Reed, this group constitutes 40 to 60% of the children with learning disabilities. When considering language-based learning disabilities, the role that language expression and use problems and word-finding difficulties play in the child's learning problems must be considered. It is also important to pay attention to the existence of possible auditory processing problems and difficulties with speech discrimination.

A second clinical-inferential profile of learning disabilities consists of articulatory and graphomator deficits which occur in 10 to 40% of the learning disabled population (Reed, 2005). This group of learning disabilities is characterized by articulation, writing, and drawing difficulties. These children are often labeled as having developmental apraxia, or identified as having "clumsy child syndrome."

A third, and less common, categorization is identified as a visuospatial perceptual deficit syndrome (5 to 15% of the population) (Reed, 2005). These children have deficits in visual discrimination and visual memory and exhibit problems with spatial orientation. They may confuse similar looking letters or they may have problems orienting themselves in space, or both (Shames et al., 1994). Regardless of the type of learning disability the child exhibits, he or she typically performs within normal or near normal limits on neuropsychological tests, although a discrepancy may occur between performance on language-based tasks and tasks that require visual-spatial and other nonlinguistic skills.

In addition to the historical and the clinical-inferential approaches to classification of language-based learning disabilities, five categories based on statistical analysis have been proposed. As listed in Reed (2005), these categories are as follows:

1. Those with global language impairment (30% of the population)

2. Those with selective impairment of naming (16%)

3. Those with a mixed deficit of language impairment and difficulty on visual-perceptual-motor tasks (11%)

4. Those with impairment only on nonlanguage visual-perceptual-motor tests (26%)

5. Those with normal performance on all the neuropsychological tests (13%) (pp. 135–136).

■ CLINICAL FINDINGS

Phonological Deficits

Children with language-based learning disabilities frequently have trouble with phonological aspects of speech and language. Some of these children have speech that is difficult to understand due to a simplification of the manner in which sounds are produced. Children who have this type of deficit may fall into the category described above as being comprised of children with articulatory and graphomotor deficits. In other children the phonological problem is related to phonological awareness problems. That is to say, they have trouble processing the grapheme-phoneme association that helps them couple the auditory signal of the phoneme with the written letter that represents the sound. They also tend to have inferior performance on segmentation tasks. **Segmentation** tasks are the skills needed to break words into syllables and syllables into phonemes. This includes poor letter-by-letter decoding strategies (phonological deficits contribute to this problem) (Reed, 2005). In some children, poor accuracy at distinguishing sentence forms based on prosodic cues, such as pitch, stress, and pauses, is also symptomatic of language-based learning disabilities.

Segmentation. The breaking down of sentences into words, words into syllables, and syllables into phonemes.

Although these children typically perform within normal limits on neuropsychological testing, it is not uncommon for the verbal IQ to be lower than the performance IQ. This is because most of the verbal segments of IQ tests require reading, decoding, and spelling skills.

Writing Skills in Children with Language-Based Learning Disabilities

Children who have difficulties with reading, spelling, and conversational speech often will have problems with writing. Children who have articulatory-graphomotor problems and children with visuospatial deficits will have problems writing legibly. Children who have poor language and learning skills will also exhibit difficulties with the content and form of their written language. Based on the work of several researchers (Espin et al., 1999; Parker, Tindal, & Hasbrouck, 1991; Scott, 1991; Scott & Windsor, 2000; Treiman, 1997; Watkinson & Lee, 1992), Reed (2005) listed the following problem areas with written language in individuals with learning and/or reading disabilities:

1. Productivity problems (they typically use fewer words, have decreased MLU, and use fewer sentences).

2. Text structure (poor use of cohesion devices, poor organization of text).

3. Sentence structure (lack of grammatical complexity and poor use of conjunctions).

4. Spelling (use of many nonphonetic spelling errors).

5. Lexicon (tendency toward repetitive use of words).

6. Handwriting (poor letter formation, mixture of uppercase and lowercase), and uneven spacing.

Bourassa and Treiman (2001) summarized the research on spelling difficulties in individuals with specific learning disabilities in written language. When these individuals spell, there is a high frequency of spellings that are not phonologically structured. The errors that are made can be divided into "phonetic" misspellings and "nonphonetic" errors. The authors provide the following examples:

Phonetic   "plad" for plaid
Nonphonetic   "pad" for plaid

               "doo" for door

               "wom" for warm

               "foz" for past

               "jry" for dry

These spellings would be consistent with the phonological deficit hypothesis which states that "these individuals compensate for their phonological weaknesses by relying heavily on visual memorization of orthographic patterns" (Bourassa & Treiman, 2001, p. 177). There are mixed reviews as to the accuracy of this hypothesis, however. Bourassa and Treiman suggest that it may be more productive to look at the misspellings in terms of how people with spelling disabilities and controls at the same spelling level differ on specific types of linguistic stimuli. Taking this approach, the authors found that students with spelling deficits were more likely to omit the internal consonants of word-initial clusters. An example they cite is "bot" for "blot."

Another theory based on the linguistic foundations of spelling deficits is the morphological deficit hypothesis. Carlisle (1987) compared morphologically based spelling of ninth graders with language-based learning disabilities with that of nondisabled fourth graders. An example of an item was, "Warm. He chose the jacket for its ___" with the expectation that the children would write "warmth." On standard spelling tests, the ninth graders performed similarly to or worse than the fourth graders. However, on oral morphological spelling, the ninth graders performed similarly to sixth and eighth graders; that is to say, oral spelling was better than written spelling. However, the gap between oral and written spelling was greater for the ninth graders than it was for the normal children. The results "are consistent with the morphological deficit hypothesis, for they suggest that individuals with spelling difficulties have particular difficulty appreciating the way in which the English writing system reflects the morphological structure of the language" (Bourassa & Treiman, 2001, p. 178). It is suggested that the phonological systems of children with spelling deficits be assessed, and that phonological awareness training that addresses the specific phonological deficits will help these children with their reading and spelling abilities.

Semantic Deficits

Tiegerman-Farber (1997) writes about the semantic-feature hypothesis, saying it "proposes that children establish meaning by combining features (characteristics) that are present and observable in the environment. As children continue to experience reality, their ideas and concepts about objects and events change" (p. 77). In addition, children use overextensions when learning the labels and meanings of objects. This overextension has a broader meaning than does the adult's meaning. For example, a child may refer to all four-legged animals as dogs because the child does not use as many semantic features as the adult does when defining a word. Children normally use a variety of hypotheses and concepts to develop their lexicon. However, children with language-based learning disabilities may not be able to develop these hypotheses and concepts and, hence, have an underdeveloped lexicon.

With regard to specific language features, children with language-based learning disabilities show some distinctive semantic characteristics. Often these children have difficulty in organizing word meanings, particularly when multiple meanings exist for the same word. The children also have trouble in retrieving lexical items in naming tasks and spontaneous speech. This is possibly due to underdeveloped lexical systems that result in poor vocabulary and poor metalinguistic skills, such as difficulty with synonyms, antonyms, and metaphors. Children with language-based learning disabilities also tend to define words in a very concrete manner. For example, they may define the word banana as "something you eat" and geography as "something you study at school."

Research shows that some children have difficulty differentiating semantic and retrieval deficits (Leonard, 1998). In other words, it is difficult to determine if the child has a problem with encoding the words so that the lexicon is never stored into memory or if the child has retrieval problems, in which case the information was encoded but cannot be retrieved from the short- or long-term memory. In studying **confrontational naming** and spontaneous speech in these children, researchers have found several skills to be different or higher in frequency.

Confrontational naming. The naming of items as the child is confronted with the item by the clinician.

One difficulty is in retrieving the name of an item. Instead of naming an item that is shown to the child, he or she describes it. This is called **circumlocution** because the child "goes around" naming an item by describing it instead.

Circumlocution. The use of an indirect manner of expression to describe an object or event when the name cannot be recalled; e.g., saying "that thing you use to unlock the door" instead of "key."

Second, the use of word substitutions for the target word has been noted. Third, a lack of specificity as seen in the language of children with language-based learning disabilities, with the frequent use of low information words such as pronouns and indefinite adverbs such as "somewhere," "it," and "sometime" instead of more specific information. These children also may demonstrate verbal hesitancies and the use of extra verbalizations such as "um" and "uh" to cover for delays in producing target words.

It has been noted that children who have language-based learning disabilities have greater difficulties in naming what has been described than do their peers. For example, if the teacher asks, "What animal has four legs and black and white stripes?" the child with a learning disability will have more difficulty providing the answer than his or her peers. These children also tend to overuse functional definitions, describing items according to their use instead of particular and distinguishing features.

The concern as to whether the issue is one of encoding or decoding may be unsolvable, so it may be more important to focus on the more immediate concern: the inability to use semantic information in a useful manner.

Syntactic Deficits

Children should be combining words by 18 to 24 months of age, and failure to do so is one of the first delays observed in the syntactic development of children with specific language impairment (Paul, 1996; Rescorla, Roberts, & Dahlsgaard, 1997). Children with language-based learning disabilities typically have a lower mean length of utterance (MLU) than their peers, leading to more immature and less imaginative sentence structure. They have difficulty with bound morphemes (-s, -ed), auxiliary verbs (is, be), and closed-class morphemes such as "a" and "the" (Paul, 2001). Normally, children learn syntax in short, rapid bursts of development. However, children with language-based learning disabilities typically have a constant slow rate of learning syntax, and they show a poorer command of morphological items.

As a rule, children with language-based learning disabilities will exhibit reading deficits. Although they may have difficulties with mature syntax in their expressive language, they may not necessarily have trouble comprehending syntax in reading. However, they do have poorer sentence comprehension. This may be explained by an inadequate ability to hold a representation of the sentence in the short-term memory.

Pragmatic Deficits

Many children with language-based learning disabilities will exhibit pragmatic deficits that are worse than their deficits in form and content. Indeed, some children with normal linguistic abilities may have pragmatic deficits; that is, they are unable to use language in an appropriate manner for a variety of purposes (Roth & Spekman, 1984a).

Roth and Spekman (1984b) posit that discourse organization, a segment of pragmatics, can be tested by implementing discourse within activities familiar to the child. By testing discourse in familiar activities, a scaffolding for dialogue can be set up. As part of this scaffolding, the speech-language pathologist can create opportunities for the child "to initiate conversation, to take turns, and to repair in response to self-feedback or the feedback of others in different situations" (Owens, 2004, p. 132). While playing, preschool-age children often have nonsocial dialogues while older children engage in social monologues and in social dialogues. Thus, as the child matures, he or she becomes more aware of the use of speech and language in a social manner.

Pragmatic deficits in children with language-based learning disabilities are more likely to be linguistic problems than social delays. The children exhibit poor conversational repair strategies, and they tend to be passive in groups and to ask fewer questions. The questions they do ask are simple and typically require uncomplicated answers. They also tend to have topical discontinuity, meaning that they have difficulty maintaining a topic of conversation. They may exhibit an overuse of meaningless starters such as, "Now, you see."

Children with language-based learning disabilities also face problems with **survival language**, particularly when they reach middle school age. Survival language basically refers to knowing the "lingo" associated with peer language but also involves knowing how to be a part of a peer group through appropriate actions. As stated earlier, many children with language disorders or language-based learning disabilities have low self-esteem and do not feel as if they are part of a peer group. Thus, it is possible they will agree to participate in an inappropriate behavior if they believe it will make them an accepted member of a peer group. Thus, the survival language needed to "just say no" instead of participating in an inappropriate activity may be absent.

Survival language. Knowing the "lingo" associated with peer language, and knowing how to be a part of a peer group through appropriate actions and communication styles.

■ SPECIFIC LANGUAGE IMPAIRMENT

Questions regarding the etiology of specific language impairment (SLI) still persist. In some children, there may be a familial history of language problems, and a central nervous system deficit cannot be ruled out as a causative factor. SLI is a difficult category to track in terms of causative agents due to the diversity of the problems exhibited from one child to the next, and the fact that many of these children never have a causative factor identified. In fact, some researchers even question the advisability of having a label of SLI. In short, it is a heterogeneous disorder with a multiplicity of possible etiological factors.

Children who fail a screening and subsequent testing may have a specific language impairment. Leonard defines SLI as "significant limitations in language functioning that cannot be attributed to deficits in hearing, oral structure and function, or general intelligence" (Leonard, 1987, p. 1). This is an interesting diagnostic category because there is not one apparent cause, and the child does not have perceptual deficits one might see in language-based learning disabilities or cognitive deficits associated with mental handicaps. When given a nonverbal test, their language performance scores are "significantly lower than their intellectual performance scores"

(Owens, 2004, p. 37). Typically, the performance IQ is above 85, but the child has a low verbal score, with the child's expressive skills being significantly below his or her receptive skills.

Rescorla (1989) estimated that 10 to 15% of children do not have 50 single words, or combine words by 24 months of age. While many of these children will develop normally, approximately 20 to 25% of these children with early language problems have their difficulties persist into the preschool and school-age years (Paul, 1996; Rescorla, 1990; Thal, 1989). Tomblin and colleagues (1997) cite an SLI prevalence figure of 7.4% of all children in kindergarten. The language problems in these children frequently persist as language problems when the children become adolescents, especially as the language problems related to phonological and literacy abilities (Owens, 2004). Also, usage of verbs tends to be more problematic than use of nouns. One particular deficit area in children with SLI is a limit in the use of finite verb morphemes (Goffman & Leonard, 2000). A description of semantic difficulties of children with SLI is found in Table 6–4.

In addition to the written and oral language deficits found in many children with SLI, there is documentation of difficulties with math, particularly beyond the second grade. Fazio (1999) looked at mathematical abilities in low-income children with SLI over a five-year period. The subjects were 10 children who were 9 to10 years of age, and who had been diagnosed with SLI during the

TABLE 6–4. Several areas of semantic difficulties experienced by children with SLI.

Area of Semantic Difficulty	Problems
Size of the lexicon	Smaller vocabularies
Rate of growth of the lexicon	Slower vocabulary acquisition
	Less lexical diversity
Robustness of word meaning	Less depth of knowledge about word meanings
	Less known about the meaning of individual words
	Only partial meanings of a word known
Speech of new word learning	Difficulties learning new lexical items quickly
	More exposures to a new word in context needed to abstract the meaning of the word
Word finding	Difficulties retrieving words from the cognitive store to use them in quick flow of connected speech
	The word on the "tip of the tongue"

Source: From *An Introduction to Children with Language Disorders* (3rd ed.) by V. A. Reed, 2005, p. 107. Boston: Allyn and Bacon. Reprinted with permission.

preschool years. In a 1996 study by Fazio, she found that children with SLI had delays in counting and basic mathematical knowledge, but they did fairly well in simple calculations in first and second grades. However, in fourth and fifth grade, these children had difficulties with math. Possible reasons for this difficulty in later elementary and subsequent years include the following:

1. The necessity of completing several steps in order to perform the calculations

2. An increase in the amount of domain-specific mathematical vocabulary

3. The need to engage in automatic retrieval of math facts instead of simply counting

4. A difficulty with rote retrieval of previously memorized material

5. A lack of active participation in group discussion of the math problems and solutions

6. Problems with underlying mechanisms such as conceptual knowledge, memory retrieval, and procedural knowledge

One of the findings of the 1999 study was that the performance of the subjects on written calculation tasks improved when they were given extra time. The children who did worst on tasks requiring working memory and language had the most difficulty with timed math tasks.

Children with SLI do not appear to have efficient problem-solving skills, in part due to the demands of working memory that hinder the automatic retrieval of math facts that results from extensive practice and the need for fewer resources. However, the children with SLI showed slow but steady growth in their math abilities over the five-year period of the study. "Despite early delays in counting, the SLI group was not using counting as the primary means of solving calculation problems. However, learning a new set of rote material is still a formidable task for these children" (Fazio, 1999, p. 427). Children with SLI have inefficient processing of information which places a heavier demand on verbal working memory than it does in normally developing children. This, in turn, negatively impacts working memory and interferes with the child's ability to efficiently perform on mathematical problems.

Mercer and Miller (1992) have suggested that children in third or fourth grade need "automatic basic fact retrieval" for increased efficiency in solving math problems. Children with SLI frequently cannot solve math problems rapidly and accurately, and counting speed is slow in children with SLI. All of these factors contribute to weak performances in math by children with SLI.

Obviously, SLI can impact multiple areas of language and academic performance in school-age children. Owens (2004) has summed up the impact of SLI on the primary features of language as seen in Table 6–5.

TABLE 6–5. Language characteristics of children with specific language impairment.

Pragmatics	May act like younger children developing typically.
	Less flexibility in their language when tailoring the message to the listener or repairing communication breakdowns.
	Some pragmatic functions as chronological-age-matched peers developing typically but expressed differently and less effectively.
	Less effective than chronological-age-matched peers in securing a conversational turn. Those with receptive difficulties most affected.
	Inappropriate responses to topic.
	Narratives less complete and more confusing than those of reading-ability-matched peers developing typically.
Semantics	First words and subsequent vocabulary development occur at a slower rate, with occasional lexical errors seen in younger children developing typically.
	Naming difficulties may reflect less rich and less elaborate semantic storage than actual retrieval difficulties. Long-term memory storage problems are probable.
Syntax/Morphology	Co-occurrence of more mature and less mature forms.
	Similar developmental order to that seen in children developing typically.
	Fewer morphemes, especially verb endings, auxiliary verbs, and function words (articles, prepositions) than younger MLU-matched peers. Learning related to grammatical function as in children developing typically.
	Tend to make pronoun errors, as do younger MLU-matched peers, but tend to overuse one form rather than making random errors.
Phonology	Phonological processes similar to those of younger children developing typically, but in different patterns, i.e., occurring in units of varying word length rather than in one- or two-word utterances.
	As toddlers, vocalize less and have less varied and less mature syllable structures than aged-matched peers developing typically.
Comprehension	Poor discrimination of units of short duration (bound morphemes).
	Reading miscues often unrelated to text graphophonemically, syntactically, semantically, or pragmatically.

■ AUDITORY PROCESSING DISORDERS

In 1996, the ASHA Task Force on Central Auditory Processing Consensus Development attempted to develop a definition of auditory processing disorders. The members of the task force believed that central auditory processes were mechanisms and processes of the auditory system and produced several behavioral patterns. The processes they identified included

1. Sound localization and lateralization

2. Auditory discrimination

3. Auditory pattern recognition

4. Temporal aspects of audition, including

   a. Temporal integration

   b. Temporal masking

   c. Temporal resolution

   d. Temporal ordering

5. Auditory performance decrements with competing acoustic signals (including dichotic listening)

6. Auditory performance decrements with degraded acoustic signals (ASHA, 1996; ASHA, 2005; Keith, 1999)

They defined CAPD as "an observed deficiency in one or more of a group of mechanisms and processes related to a variety of auditory behaviors" (ASHA, 1996, p. 43). They went on to note that there are "four issues related to the diagnosis and management of children and adults with central auditory processing disorders:

1. What does basic science tell us about the nature of central auditory processing and its role in audition?

2. What constitutes an assessment of central auditory processing and its disorders?

3. What are the developmental and acquired communication problems associated with central auditory processing disorders?

4. What is the clinical utility of a diagnosis of central auditory processing disorder? (ASHA, 1996, p. 43)

Current terminology is auditory processing disorder (APD), as opposed to central auditory processing disorder (CAPD). In 2005, the ASHA Working Group on Auditory Processing Disorders met to define the role of the au-

audiologist in the assessment and treatment of APD. As part of their report, the working group proposed the following definition of (C)APD:

> Broadly stated, (Central) Auditory Processing [(C)AP] refers to the efficiency and effectiveness by which the central nervous system (CNS) utilizes auditory information. Narrowly defined, (C)AP refers to the perceptual processing of auditory information in the CNS and the neurobiologic activity that underlies that processing and gives rise to electrophysiologic auditory potentials. (ASHA, 2005, p. 2)

It is important to note that the working group determined that the deficiencies in auditory processing are not caused by psychological, language, learning, communication, ADD/ADHD, and cognitive deficits, even though individuals with APD frequently have problems that coexist in these areas. Also, it is important to realize that auditory processing and language processing are not the same, even though they share many characteristic symptoms (ASHA, 2005). APD must include a diagnosis of deficit(s) in the central auditory nervous system. According to the ASHA task force established in 1996, "the brain lesions associated with CAPD may be situated cortically in the left and right temporal and parietal lobes or subcortically in the thalamus, basal ganglia, and brain stem structures" (p. 45). However, they go on to say that some diseases and injuries lead to a broader distribution of damage. Some of these diseases and injuries include traumatic brain injury, cerebrovascular accident, tumors, multiple sclerosis, epilepsy, and Alzheimers.

Assessment of Auditory Processing Disorders

As with many other language disorders, assessment of auditory processing disorders should involve a team consisting of audiologists, speech-language pathologists, teachers, psychologists, and neurologists in the testing of an individual with difficulty processing auditory information. In fact, the 1996 ASHA Task Force on CAP Consensus Development implicitly states that a multidisciplinary approach to auditory processing disorders should be addressed using a multidisciplinary approach. This multidisciplinary team should take the following into account when diagnosing an auditory processing disorder:

- The physical structure of the acoustic stimulus

- The neural mechanism that encodes the stimulus

- The perceptual dimensions that arise from the encoding

- The interactions that occur between perceptual processes and the activation of the higher level resources

- The nature of the pathological process (ASHA, 1996, pp. 41–42)

Each team member has a unique set of tests that can be used to help define the patient's ability to process information using the auditory channel. For example, the speech-language pathologist should employ tests of language across modalities, paying particular attention to performance of skills that are tested using the auditory channel only, then of the same skills using the visual modality only. It should be noted here that due to the neurological organization of processing language, the child may demonstrate problems with visual processing as well, but the deficits are more pronounced in the auditory modality (ASHA, 2005). Receptive and expressive abilities should also be analyzed, as well as standardized and functional assessment of form, content, and use of language.

The educator should provide information as to how the child functions in the classroom setting, and a description of the environment. For example, does the teacher use an FM system and are there visual and acoustic distractions in the classroom. The teacher can also provide insight regarding the child's personality and performance in groups, his or her ability to follow directions, and how the child is performing academically. Some behaviors that teachers (and family members) can provide insight into include the following:

> difficulty understanding spoken language in competing messages, noisy backgrounds, or in reverberant environments; misunderstanding messages; inconsistent or inappropriate responding; frequent requests for repetitions, saying "what" or "huh" frequently; taking longer to respond in oral communication situations; difficulty paying attention; being easily distracted; difficulty following complex auditory directions or commands; difficulty localizing sound; difficulty learning songs or nursery rhymes; poor musical and signing skills; and associated reading, spelling, and learning problems. (ASHA, 2005, p. 5)

The audiologist should use assessment procedures designed to demonstrate the integrity of the central auditory nervous system and central auditory processes. These procedures would include evaluation of the integrity of the peripheral auditory system, clinical observation, and electrophysiological measures (Friel-Patti, 1999; Keith, 1999). The task force specifically recommended the following auditory tests:

1. Case history (medical, social, and educational)

2. Observation in a variety of sound environments

3. Thorough basic auditory battery, including pure tones, speech recognition, and immitance

4. Analysis of temporal processes

5. Ability to localize and lateralize to sound

6. Monaural low redundancy speech tests

7. Dichotic stimuli

8. Binaural interaction procedures

9. Speech and language assessment (ASHA, 1996; Keith, 1999)

The psychologist can provide invaluable information on the status of the patient's cognitive and learning skills, and the neurologist can provide information regarding the integrity of the neurological system with regard to auditory signal and language processing through the use of MRI and CT scans and neurochemical analysis.

Over the years, there have traditionally been at least two methods of identifying children who need further evaluation for a possible auditory processing disorder. These are

1. Using checklists of auditory performance to determine categories of performance

2. Referring a child based on behavioral observations

In 1999, Keith compiled a list 10 characteristics frequently seen in children with APD:

1. Normal pure-tone hearing thresholds

2. Inconsistent responses to auditory stimuli

3. Difficulty with auditory localization skills

4. Difficulty with auditory discrimination

5. Deficiencies in remembering phonemes and manipulating them

6. Difficulty understanding speech in the presence of background noise

7. Difficulty with auditory memory, either span or sequence, and poor ability to remember auditory information or follow multiple instructions

8. Poor listening skills

9. Difficulty understanding rapid speech or persons with an unfamiliar dialect

10. Frequent requests for information to be repeated

Other indications of a possible APD include problems with reading, spelling, and handwriting, as well as articulation and/or language disorders. However, it would be necessary to rule out speech language and cognitive deficits as being causative of an APD.

Treatment of Auditory Processing Disorders

Given the impact an auditory processing disorder can have on an individual's social, educational, and academic success, early identification and intervention are critical. Early intervention will enable the clinician to take advantage of the plasticity and cortical reorganization abilities of the brain. In most cases, treatment will include environmental analysis and modification through the use of devices such as personal FM systems and classroom/workplace/home amplification. Environmental manipulation is critical in the treatment of APD because the language deficit most affected by APD is the comprehension of spoken language (ASHA, 1996).

In addition, treatment should include training in the interhemispheric transfer of information activities such as "using interaural temporal offsets and intensity differences, as well as other unimodal (e.g., linking prosodic and linguistic acoustic features) and multimodal (e.g., writing to dictation, verbally describing a picture while drawing) interhemispheric transfer exercises" (ASHA, 2005, p. 11).

Keith (1999) writes that management of APD should consist of modification of the environment, perceptual training, compensatory training, and cognitive training. Modification of the environment would include, as previously mentioned, the use of assistive listening devices as well as classroom amplification. Other environmental changes can include improving the acoustics of the classroom, providing preferential seating, and assigning a "listening buddy" to assist the child with APD.

Auditory training including "procedures targeting intensity, frequency, and duration discrimination; phoneme discrimination and phoneme-to-grapheme skills; temporal gap discrimination; temporal ordering or sequencing; pattern recognition; localization/lateralization; and recognition of auditory information presented within a background of noise or competition" should be incorporated into any treatment plan for an individual with APD (ASHA, 2005, p. 11). Computer games that provide training in fundamental temporal processing can also be used.

Compensatory strategies can be used to develop auditory skills that will improve the academic skills and perceptual processes. These would include training in auditory figure-ground and auditory memory, phonemic synthesis, speech sound discrimination, auditory analysis, and training in prosody.

Cognitive therapy should focus on monitoring and self-regulating skills needed for message comprehension and problem solving. Included in cognitive therapy would be activities that address language training, organizational skills, and development of the lexicon. These would also incorporate the following skills: following directions, using written notes, listening and anticipating what will be said, asking relevant questions, and answering questions (Keith, 1999).

■ SUMMARY

An understanding of the role of language is critical in dealing with learning disabilities. By clarifying the role played by phonological awareness in the development of reading and spelling skills (discussed in Chapter 7), more children can be identified at an early age and appropriate interventions can be developed. Neuroimaging techniques have contributed to our understanding of brain morphology as it relates to language-based learning disabilities and has had an impact on the diagnostic and therapeutic process. Because language-based learning disabilities can carry over into adulthood, this understanding is assuming increasing importance in educational literature. With the focus in IDEA on transition, preparing individuals with language-based learning disabilities for the work place places further emphasis on the importance of studying the role of language in learning disabilities.

CASE STUDY

History

In November 2002, C, a 9-year-old boy, was referred to Shands Hospital in Gainesville, Florida by his third grade teacher for a psychological evaluation because of academic problems and hyperactivity. He was referred to our clinic (University of Florida Speech and Hearing Clinic) in October 2003 by his teacher and the speech-language pathologist at his school to address language and academic problems possibly related to his ADHD.

Previous Testing

Between November 21, 2002 and December 19, 2002, C was evaluated at Shands in three different departments: the Pediatric Neurology clinic, the Department of Clinical Psychology, and the Communicative Disorders department.

C was initially seen in the Pediatric Neurology clinic on November 21, 2002 because of his parents' and teacher's concerns about his short attention span and hyperactivity. They referred C to the Department of Clinical Psychology where he was tested using the Weschler Intelligence Scale for Children-Revised (WISC-R). On the WISC-R, he received a full scale IQ of 79, a verbal IQ of 87, and a performance IQ of 73. They also noted that he had academic weaknesses in reading, spelling, and math. Reading and spelling were at the first grade level, and math was at the second grade level.

On December 5, 2002, C was evaluated in the Communicative Disorders department. The results were that he had (1) a moderately severe language disorder for skills such as sentence formulation and repetition, (2) poor problem-solving skills, (3) difficulties with auditory processing and auditory sequencing, (4) pragmatic problems, and (5) difficulties with topic maintenance and appropriate topic switching.

On December 19, 2002, C returned to the Pediatric Neurology clinic for a cumulative diagnosis. They determined that C had ADHD, and prescribed 5 mg of Ritalin to be taken each morning.

At school, C is repeating the third grade, and he was pulled out for supplemental instruction in reading, writing, and math. He is not receiving speech-language therapy at school.

Initial Evaluation at the University of Florida Speech and Hearing Clinic (UFSHC)

In October 2003, C was seen at the UFSHC. In their initial interview, his parents reported that all developmental milestones were within normal limits, and that his problems did not begin until he was in kindergarten. In kindergarten, he would hug and kiss the other children, and he was teased by his classmates until he would cry. In first grade, he had surgery for a "lazy eye" and began to wear corrective glasses. His parents agreed to the referral for a speech-language evaluation in the UFSHC because they were concerned about his low self-esteem and his frequent temper tantrums. They were also worried about the fact that he would not establish eye contact with them, and that he always "forgets what he was told to do."

On The Token Test, C scored within an average performance range. He had difficulty with two step commands with two modifiers ("Touch the small blue circle and pick up the small green circle."). Results of the Wide Range Achievement Test-Revised (WRAT-R) indicated that C's reading was at the first grade level. He would sound out the letters, and sometimes read the same word twice. However, he would read the words differently on each try. He constantly asked for feedback about his correctness. Spelling results on the WRAT-R also were at the first grade level. He would spell quickly, using some self-corrections.

C was also given the Illinois Test of Psycholinguistic Abilities (ITPA-3). The ITPA-3 is a relatively short multimodality test (when compared to the Woodcock Johnson Psychoeducational Battery), so it was used to assess C's cognitive skills and to compare performance when the input is auditory versus visual, and output is graphic versus oral versus gestural. This testing revealed strengths in grammatic closure (which addresses morphology), and sound blending. His weaknesses were auditory closure, manual expression, and auditory association (analogies). On the ITPA-3, C received a developmental age of 6 years 8 months. It was extremely difficult keeping him on task.

Articulation was within normal limits based on observation. No formal testing was done in this area.

Behavioral observations included the following: (1) C frequently perseverated on one topic, making it difficult to shift from one subtest to another on testing, and from one topic to another in conversation; (2) C needed structure, so the session was divided into periods of work time and periods of play time that were used as breaks; (3) C frequently interrupted the testing with tangential comments, and (4) C was in constant motion.

Summary and Recommendations

C is a 9-year, 11-month-old boy who was referred to this clinic for language and cognition testing due to concerns about academic performance in school, low self-esteem, and frequent temper tantrums. C has previously been diagnosed with ADHD at Shands Hospital. He has been tested in the pediatric neurology, clinical psychology, and communicative disorders clinics at Shands.

At the UFSHC, C was tested using the Revised Token Test, the Wide Range Achievement Test-Revised, and the Illinois Test of Psycholinguistic Abilities-3. Performance on the Revised Token Test was in the average range. On the WRAT-R, spelling and reading were at the first grade level. On the ITPA-3, he achieved a developmental age of 6 years, 9 months (3 years 2 months below his chronological age). The conclusions are that C has a language processing disorder complicated by his ADHD. A summary of his strengths and weaknesses is as follows.

	Strengths	Weaknesses
Communicative	Average intelligence	Poor eye contact
	Interactive	Poor pragmatic skills
	Can concoct stories	Tangential conversations
	Relates events	Poor reading skills
	Likes therapy	Poor spelling skills

	Good articulation	ADHD
		Poor topic maintenance
		Poor auditory processing skills
Noncommunicative	Supportive family	Socially frustrated
	Supportive teacher	Academically frustrated
	Determined to improve	Parents functionally illiterate
	Can delay gratification	Poor reasoning skills
		Poor math skills
		Temper
		Poor affect control
		Poor focal control
		Poor visual memory
		Poor sequencing skills
		Poor handwriting

It is recommended that C enroll in therapy to address auditory processing skills, pragmatics, auditory and visual memory skills, grapheme/phoneme association, following directions, and topic maintenance.

Addendum to Original Report

Further Testing. In July 2004, at age 10 years 9 months, C was given the Woodcock-Johnson Psychoeducational Battery. On the Test of Cognition, he received the following scores:

Assessment Area	Grade Score	Age Score	Percentile Rank
Full Scale Cluster	1.8	7-4	2
Verbal Ability Cluster	5.6	10-8	50
Reasoning Ability	1.0	3-10	Below 1st
Perceptual Speech Cluster	3.0	8-4	9

On the Tests of Achievement, which measure academic performance, he performed as follows:

Cluster	Grade Score	Age Score	Percentile Rank	Functioning Level
Reading	2.3	7-6	4	Severely deficient
Mathematics	1.7	1-7	Below 1	Severely deficient
Written Language	1.8	1-8	2	Severely deficient
Knowledge	4.7	4-7	38	Average

The clinicians were encouraged by C's improvement in reading and found it not surprising that C's knowledge was in the low average range. As is typical with many children with ADHD and language-based learning disabilities, C had relatively normal intelligence, but he had trouble in specific academic areas that required concentration and adequate attending to the task.

To address the deficits in reasoning, we used "deduction puzzles" to help C chart information as a story was read to him. These deduction puzzles were eventually incorporated into his classroom activities to help him organize his school notes. Work continued on all the original goals.

Behavior management included a token economy and response-cost system. C earned pennies for remaining in seat and on task, and pennies were removed from the jar when off-task behaviors occurred. He could exchange the pennies for X-Men comic books and action figures. His parents were also taught this system of behavior management and they followed through with it at home.

▓ REVIEW QUESTIONS

1. At what grades do children make the leap from decoding to read to reading for comprehension?

   a. Kindergarten–2nd grade
   b. 3rd–4th grade
   c. 5th–6th grade

2. Children who present in clinic with difficulty in organizing word meanings, underdeveloped lexical systems, and word retrieval problems would be exhibiting a _____ deficit.

   a. Semantic
   b. Syntactic
   c. Pragmatic
   d. Morphological

3. Which of the following are considered soft signs that may be indicators of a language-based learning disability?

   a. Left-handedness   e. a, b, c, d
   b. Visual-motor deficits   f. b, c, d
   c. Letter and number reversals   g. a, b, d
   d. Phonological deficits   h. a, b, c

4. Children with SLI frequently have difficulties with math in the later elementary years because
   a. It takes more steps to perform the calculations.
   b. They have difficulty retrieving previously memorized material.
   c. They have problems with underlying mechanisms such as conceptual knowledge.
   d. All of the above.
   e. None of the above; children with SLI don't have trouble with math.

5. Which of the following are typically indicative of children with specific language impairment?
   a. Difficulty with bound morphemes
   b. Increased mean-length of utterance due to tangential conversations
   c. Failure to combine words by 18–24 months of age
   d. All of the above
   e. a and b
   f. b and c
   g. a and c

6. Children typically outgrow language-based learning disabilities by the time they are adolescents.
   a. True
   b. False

7. At school age, delays may persist as disorders either because of the nature of the delay or because of ineffective remediation during the preschool years.
   a. True
   b. False

8. Children who have difficulties with reading, spelling, and conversational speech will rarely have difficulties with writing because this taps a different part of the brain.
   a. True
   b. False

9. Children with language-based learning disabilities frequently have poor conversational repair strategies.
   a. True
   b. False

10. Children with auditory processing disorders typically have normal pure-tone hearing thresholds.
    a. True
    b. False

■ REFERENCES

American Speech-Language-Hearing Association (ASHA) Task Force on Central Auditory Processing Consensus Development. (1996, July). Central auditory processing: Current status of research and implications for clinical practice. *American Journal of Audiology, 5*(2), 41–54.

American Speech-Language-Hearing Association (ASHA) Working Group on Auditory Processing Disorders. (2005). (Central) auditory processing disorders. ASHA Technical Report, February 2005.

Blackman, J. A. (2000). Attention-deficit / hyperactivity disorder in preschoolers. *Pediatric Clinics of North America, 46,* 1011–1025.

Bourassa, D. C., & Treiman, R. (2001, July). Spelling development and disability: The importance of linguistic factors. *Language, Speech, and Hearing Services in the Schools, 32* (3), 172–181.

Carlisle, J. F. (1987). The use of morphological knowledge in spelling derived forms by learning-disabled and normal students. *Annals of Dyslexia, 27,* 90–108.

Catts, H. W., & Kamhi, A. G. (1999). *Language and reading disabilities.* Boston: Allyn and Bacon.

Chall, J. (1983). *Stages of reading development.* New York: McGraw-Hill.

Connor, D. F. (2002). Preschool attention deficit hyperactivity disorder: A review of prevalence, diagnosis, neurobiology, and stimulant treatment. *Journal of Developmental and Behavioral Pediatrics, 23,* 51–59.

Donahue, M. (1986). Linguistic and communicative development in learning-disabled children. In C. Ceci (Ed.), *Handbook of cognitive, social, and neuropsychological aspects of learning disabilities,* Vol. 1. Mahwah, NJ: Lawrence Erlbaum.

Espin, C. A., Scierka, B. J., Skare, S., & Halverson, N. (1999). Curriculum-based measures in writing for secondary students. *Reading and Writing Quarterly, 15,* 5–27.

Fazio, B. (1996). Mathematical abilities of children with specific language impairment: A 2-year follow-up. *Journal of Speech and Hearing Research, 39,* 1–10.

Fazio, B. (1999). Arithmetic calculation, short-term memory, and language performance in children with specific language impairment. *Journal of Speech, Language, and Hearing Research, 42*(2), 420–431.

Friel-Patti, S. (1999, October). Clinical decision-making in assessment and intervention of central auditory processing disorders. *Language, Speech, and Hearing Servcies in the Schools, 30*(4), 345–352.

Goffman, L., & Leonard, J. (2000, May). Growth of language skills in preschool children wit specific language impairment: Implications for assessment and intervention. *American Journal of Speech-Language Pathology, 9*(2), 151–161.

Hammill, D. D., & Newcomer, P. L. (1997). *Test of language development-I:3.* Austin, TX: Pro-Ed.

Hynd, G. (1991, March). Brain morphology as it relates to learning disabilities. Lecture at the 1991 G. Paul Moore Symposium, Gainesville, FL.

Kamhi, A. B., & Catts, H. W. (1989). *Reading disabilities: A developmental language perspective.* Austin, TX: Pro-Ed.

Keith, R. W. (1999). Clinical issues in central auditory processing disorders. *Language, Speech, and Hearing Services in Schools, 30*(4), 339–344.

Larson, V. L., & McKinley, N. (1995). *Language disorders in older students: Preadolescents and adolescents.* Eau Claire, WI: Thinking Publications.

Leonard, C. M. (1998). Language. In H. Cohen (Ed.), *Neuroscience for rehabilitation* (2nd ed., chap. 17). Philadelphia: Lippincott-Raven.

Leonard, L. B. (1987). Is specific language impairment a useful construct? In S. Rosenberg (Ed.), *Advances in applied psycholinguistics,* Vol. 1 (pp. 1–39). Cambridge: Cambridge University Press.

Lombardino, L. J., Ricco, C. A., Hynd, G., & Pinheiro, S. B. (1997). Linguistic deficits in children with reading disabilities. *American Journal of Speech-Language Pathology, 6*(3), 71–78.

Lyon, R. (1995). Toward a definition of dyslexia. *Annals of Dyslexia, 45,* 3–30.

Mercer, S. P., & Miller, S. P. (1992). Teaching students with learning problems in math to acquire, understand, and apply basic math facts. *Remedial and Special Education, 13,* 19–35, 61.

National Joint Committee on Learning Disabilities (NJCLD). (1991). Learning disabilities: Issues on definition (a position paper). *Asha, 33* (Suppl. 5), 18–20.

Nelson, N. W. (1993). *Childhood language disorders in context: Infancy through adolescence.* New York: Merrill/Macmillan Publishing Company.

Nelson, N. W. (1994). School-age language: Bumpy road or super-expressway to the next millennium? *American Journal of Speech-Language Pathology, 3*(3), 29–31.

Nelson, N. W. (1998). *Childhood language disorders in context: Infancy through adolescence.* New York: Merrill/Macmillan Publishing Company.

Owens, R. E. (2004). *Language disorders: A functional approach to assessment and intervention* (4th ed.). Boston: Allyn and Bacon.

Parker, R., Tindal, G., & Hasbrouck, J. (1991). Countable indices of writing quality: Their suitability for screening-eligibility decisions. *Exceptionality, 2,* 1–17.

Paul, R. (1996). Clinical implications of the natural history of slow expressive language development. *American Journal of Speech-Language Pathology, 5*(2), 5–22.

Paul, R. (2001). *Language disorders from infancy through adolescence: Assessment and intervention* (2nd ed.). St, Louis, MO: Mosby.

Peck, M. (1982). Youth suicide. *Death Education, 6,* 29–47.

Reed, V. A. (2005). *An introduction to children with language disorders* (3rd ed.). Boston: Allyn and Bacon.

Rescorla, L. (1989). The language development survey: A screening tool for delayed language in toddlers. *Journal of Speech and Hearing Disorders, 54,* 587–599.

Rescorla, L. (1990, June). Outcomes of expressive language delay. Paper presented at the Symposium for Research in Child Language Disorders, Madison, WI.

Rescorla, L., Roberts, J., & Dahlsgaard, K. (1997). Late talkers at 2: Outcome at age 3. *Journal of Speech and Hearing Research, 40,* 556–566.

Roth, F. & Spekman, N. (1984a, February). Assessing the pragmatic abilities of children; Part 1: Organizational framework and assessment parameters. *Journal of Speech and Hearing Disorders, 49,* 12–17.

Roth, F., & Spekman, N. (1984b, February). Assessing the pragmatic abilities of children; Part 2: Guidelines, considerations, and specific evaluation procedures. *Journal of Speech and Hearing Disorders, 49,* 12–17.

Schubert, R., & Gates, M. (1990). *Making the grade: A report card on American youth.* Washington, DC: National Collaboration for Youth.

Scott, C. M. (1991). Problem writers: Nature, assessment, and intervention. In A. G. Kamhi & H. W. Catts (Eds.), *Reading disabilities: A developmental language perspective* (pp. 303–344). Boston: Allyn and Bacon.

Scott, C. M., & Windsor, J. (2000). General language performance measures in spoken and written narrative and expository discourse of school-age children with language learning disabilities. *Journal of Speech, Language, and Hearing Research, 43,* 324–339.

Shames, G. H., Wiig, E. H., & Secord, W. A. (1994). *Human communication disorders: An introduction* (4th ed.). New York: Merrill/Macmillan Publishing Company.

Sunburst Communications. (1988). *Solutions: News from Computer Educators, 3*(2), 1.

Thal, D. J. (1989). *Language and gestures in late talkers.* Paper presented at the Biennial Meeting of the Society for Research in Child Development, Kansas City, MO.

Tiegerman-Farber, E. (1997). The ecology of the family: The language imperative. In D. K. Bernstein and E. Tiegerman-Farber (Eds.), *Language and communication disorders in children* (pp. 60–96). Boston: Allyn and Bacon.

Tomblin, J. B., Records, N. L., Buckwalter, P., Zhang, X., Smith, E., & O'Brien, M. (1997). Prevalence of specific language impairment in kindergarten children. *Journal of Speech, Language, and Hearing Research, 40,* 1245–1260.

Torgesen, J. (1977). The role of nonspecific factors in the task performance of learning disabled children: A theoretical assessment. *Journal of Learning Disabilities, 10,* 24–34.

Torgesen, J., Wagner, R., & Rashotte, C. (1994). Longitudinal studies of phonological processing and reading. *Journal of Learning Disabilities, 27,* 276–286.

Treiman, R. (1997). Spelling in normal children and dyslexics. In B. Blachman (Ed.), *Foundations of reading acquisition and dyslexia* (pp. 191–218). Mahwah, NJ: Lawrence Erlbaum.

United States Office of Education (USOE). (1991). Thirteenth annual report to Congress on the implementation of the Individuals with Disabilities Act. Washington, DC: Government Printing Office.

United States Department of Health and Human Services. (n.d.) *International classification of diseases.* Washington, DC: Author Publication No. (PHS) 80-1260. Washington, D.C.: Author.

Watkinson, J. T., & Lee, S. W. (1992). Curriculum-based measures of written expression for learning-disabled and nondisabled students. *Psychology in the Schools, 29,* 184–191.

Wiig, E. H. & Semel, E. (1984). *Language assessment and intervention for the learning disabled* (2nd ed.). New York: Merrill.

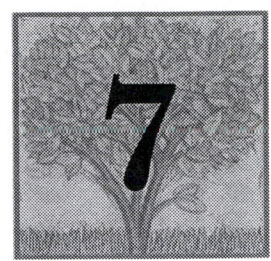

Spelling and Reading Disorders

■ LEARNING OBJECTIVES

After completion of this chapter, the reader will be able to

1. Discuss acquisition and skills that determine the development of normal reading.

2. Discuss early indicators of reading disability, and problem areas for readers identified as having a reading/spelling disability.

3. Discuss the roles of genetics and the central nervous system as causative factors in dyslexia.

4. Delineate the criteria for being diagnosed with a reading impairment, and discuss assessment strategies for reading disabilities.

5. Discuss how cultural diversity affects the diagnosis of a reading and/or spelling disability.

6. Differentiate between the different approaches to remediation of reading and/or spelling deficits.

■ NORMAL READING

Reading disability is the most prevalent learning disability, accounting for 75% to 80% of all learning disabilities (Livesay, 1995). Reading has phonetic, semantic, syntactic, and memory components, all of which must be integrated if a person is to be a successful reader. Therefore, to determine a child's status with regard to reading, it is necessary to assess his or her visual and auditory modalities to determine if there is a problem, and, if so, where the problem lies. Auditorily, an emphasis should be placed on phonics, phonetics, and linguistic information. The child must be able to decode letters to form an accurate phonological image of each word, then retrieve the definition of each word from memory. He or she must then combine syntactic and semantic information from the definitions into proper representation of a sentence. Finally, the child must combine the representations of individual sentences to comprehend the passage.

Perceptual-cognitive skills. The integration of thinking and organizing sensory input.

Preoperational skills. Skills needed to emerge into conceptual thinking leading to prelogical thought.

These skills are all taught in the first three years of elementary school, with the expectation that the child will integrate the knowledge and be a successful reader by third grade. In kindergarten through second grade, the emphasis is on **perceptual-cognitive skills**, which permit the integration of thinking and organization of sensory imput, and **preoperational skills**. Preoperational skills typically develop between ages 2 and 7 and represent the emergence into conceptual development. In the third and fourth grades, the emphasis shifts to require a child to exercise his or her linguistic and symbolic language skills.

TABLE 7–1. Stages of reading.

Stage	Ages	Primary Development
0	Birth to 5–6 years	Accumulation of knowledge about letters, words, & books
1	5–7 years	Initial reading or decoding
2	7–9 years	Decoding becomes more automatic; beginning of reading for comprehension
3	9–14 years	Reading to learn; decoding skills become fully automatic
4	14–18 years	Multiple viewpoints due to increased cognitive skills, which enable abstract thinking
5	18+ years	Construction and reconstruction in critical reading; development of hypothetical-deductive reasoning

Source: Adapted from *Stages of Reading Development* by J. Chall, 1983, New York: McGraw-Hill. Copyright 1983 by McGraw-Hill.

The content of all subject areas requires the child to abstract, analyze, and synthesize the information with the expectation that the child can read for content and no longer needs to focus on decoding each word because word recognition and understanding have become internalized operations. Furthermore, the child is faced with a higher level of vocabulary, more complex sentence structure, and more abstract concepts.

Chall (1983) sums up this academic progression in reading by dividing the development of reading into six stages (Table 7–1).

Stage 0 is the longest stage and the one with the most changes. During this period, children accumulate knowledge about letters, words, and books. They learn to produce syntactically correct utterances and develop early metalinguistic skills. These early metalinguistic skills involve "the awareness that language consists of discrete phonemes, words, phrases, and sentences" (Kamhi & Catts, 1989, p. 26). At this point, the children do not understand letter order and **phoneme-grapheme correspondences**, meaning they can "make the link" between the printed letter and the sound it makes. However, they do show interest in initial sounds and word shapes.

Phoneme-grapheme correspondence. The association of a printed letter with the sound it makes.

In stage 1, children who are 5 to 7 years old learn about phoneme-grapheme correspondences and learn to decode words. The children decode to read, and they read for comprehension once they are beyond the single-word level in their reading. During stage 2, decoding becomes more automatic so they can begin to focus on meaning. They also use their knowledge of **scripts** and story structure to assist in reading for meaning as they develop reading fluency. Decoding skills becomes fully automatic by stage 3, which covers ages 9 to 14 years.

Scripts. Scenarios designed to facilitate language development and the application of language skills to reading.

Finally, in stages 4 and 5, children become mature readers. They also develop cognitive skills that enable them to become critical readers (Chall, 1983).

In 1973, K. S. Goodman suggested that miscue analysis is a method normal readers use to analyze errors they make when reading aloud. Goodman suggests that nondisabled, mature readers implement three types of cues to predict the meaning of the text: semantic, syntactic, and graphophonemic. Nelson (1998) writes the following:

> Because mature readers have considerable knowledge about language, they continually form hypotheses as they read about what they expect the texts to say. First, they use semantic cues to predict words that fit textual meaning; second, they use syntactic cues to predict words that fit syntactic contexts; and third, they use graphophonemic cues to check whether the words they have predicted fit visual perceptual information sampled from the print. (p. 409)

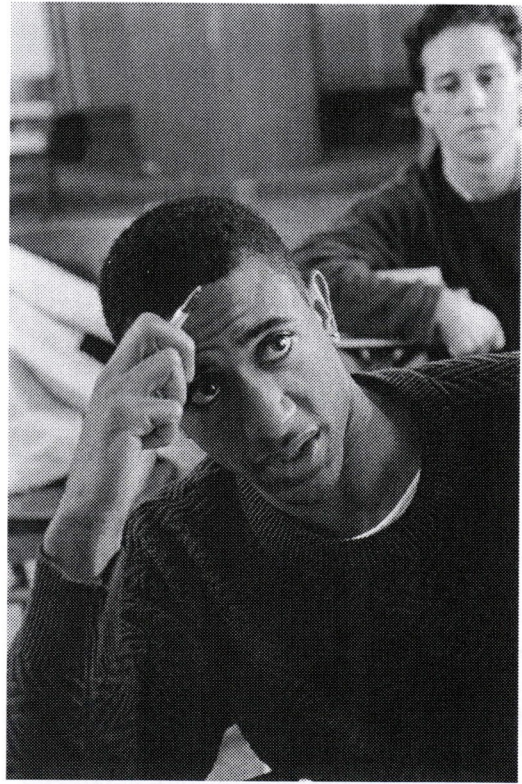

FIGURE 7–1. School-age children who have a reading and/or spelling deficit that impacts their academic progress often show signs of frustration when attempting school work and homework.

Individuals who have reading disabilities will have trouble invoking syntactic, semantic, and graphophonemic cues into their reading, thus impeding comprehension of read material. As illustrated in Figure 7–1, students who have reading and/or spelling deficits frequently become frustrated or discouraged when attempting academic material in school.

EARLY INDICATORS OF READING AND SPELLING DISABILITIES

Shaywitz (2003) makes the point that clues that may indicate a potential reading problem for a child can often be determined by listening to the child speak. Children who are late in saying their first words (i.e., after 15 months of age) and who do not combine words until after 24 months of age may be exhibiting warning signs of a potential reading problem. This does not occur in all children with reading disabilities, but they warrant attention, particularly if there is a history of reading problems in the family. Another early indicator is the persistence of difficulty pronouncing words beyond the normal period of "baby talk." Normally, children are able to pronounce most words by age 6 years. Typically developing children may mispronounce new words as their vocabulary expands, but these mispronunciations are easily overcome as the child increases his awareness and understanding of the word. In addition, around ages 3 to 4 years, most children delight in rhyming verses, repetitions of sounds, but children with reading problems "have trouble penetrating the sound structure of words and as a result are less sensitive to rhyme. Sensitivity to rhyme implies an awareness that words can be broken down into smaller segments of sound and that different words may share a sound in common; it is a very early indicator of getting ready to read. Children's familiarity with nursery rhymes turns out to be a strong predictor of their later success in reading" (Shaywitz, 2003, p. 95).

PROBLEM AREAS FOR READERS IN TROUBLE

According to Wiig and Semel (1984), readers in trouble experience difficulty with the skills outlined in Table 7–2.

Children who experience reading difficulties will frequently have trouble encoding the information, retrieving it from memory, and using phonological memory codes to decode the words (Catts & Kamhi, 2005). It is also important to analyze the child's visual and auditory skills because successful reading requires a high level of integration of both sets of skills. The integration of these skills is critical for the child to associate written language with underlying meanings and structures.

TABLE 7–2. Trouble areas for poor readers.

Visually decoding the printed, graphic words

Integrating auditory-visual inputs

Associating printed words, phrases, concepts, and other relations with their underlying meaning

Processing the surface structure of the printed sentences and relating it to the underlying meaning

Difficulty integrating graphophonemic, syntactic, and semantic information

Generating a tentative, anticipatory hypothesis about subsequent printed messages

Verifying, rejecting, or revising the anticipatory hypothesis with reference to the actual printed, graphic representation

Trouble with developmental sensitivity to grammar in written language

Source: From E. H. Wiig and E. M. Semel, *Language Assessment and Intervention for the Learning Disabled.* Published by Allyn and Bacon, Boston. Copyright © 1980 by Pearson Education. Reprinted by permission of the publisher.

Children who exhibit deficits in reading often have difficulties with oral language and impoverished environments. Justice and colleagues (2003) have summed up relevant literature and state that preschool children who have oral language impairments "consistently show depressed performance relative to their peers on an array of emergent literacy tasks addressing both written language and phonological awareness" (p. 321). In 1990, Scarborough found that many second grade children who were having reading problems also had significant problems in developing oral language skills. In a 1999 study with 183 children who were classified as poor readers, Catts and colleagues found that 57% had receptive language difficulties as kindergartners, including problems with narrative comprehension, vocabulary, and understanding of grammar.

A major problem area for many poor readers is grammar. Children with difficulty in reading will have problems correcting incorrect grammar. Regular and irregular morphemes are particularly problematic for these children. It is also known that poor readers typically have poor short-term memory for various sentence structures, which increases the problems they have because they have difficulty processing complex sentences.

Gough and Tunmer (1986) proposed a reading theory called the Simple View of Reading. There is tremendous variance in children with reading disorders, and the simple view posited is that listening comprehension and word recognition can be used to explain this variance. They developed a matrix that created four subgroups of reading disabilities based on listening

TABLE 7–3. Subtypes based on word recognition and listening comprehension.

Listening Comprehension	Word Recognition: Poor	Word Recognition: Good
Good	Dyslexia	Non-specified
Poor	Mixed	Specific Comprehension Deficit

Source: From Catts, Hugh, and Kamhi, Eds., *Language and Reading Disabilities*, 2nd ed. Published by Allyn and Bacon, Boston. Copyright © 2005 by Pearson Education. Reprinted by permission of the publisher.

comprehension and word recognition. This matrix is seen in Table 7–3. The individuals who have good listening comprehension but poor word recognition are defined as being dyslexic. Those who have poor listening comprehension and poor word recognition are listed as being language-learning disabled. Poor listening comprehension and good word recognition skills define the group labeled as **hyperlexia**.

Hyperlexia. Recognizing and reading words exceeding one's cognitive and language levels, yet having no comprehension of what is said or read.

Hyperlexia is frequently seen in children with autism. Finally, there is an "other" category in which word recognition and listening comprehension are good, but subtle language-based disabilities exist. The individuals in the dyslexic, hyperlexic, and language-learning disabled groups all have problems with reading comprehension, but for different reasons. The children with hyperlexia have difficulty because they have language and cognitive deficits. The children with reading and spelling difficulties have difficulty because they have poor decoding skills, often being slow and/or inaccurate in their decoding (Catts & Kamhi, 2005).

Catts and Kamhi (2005) further differentiate between subtypes of reading impairment by determining whether the individuals were rate-disabled or accuracy-disabled readers. Rate-disabled readers were defined as children who, despite having decoding skills at grade-appropriate levels, still had a markedly poor reading. Accuracy-disabled readers were defined as those children who had significant deficits in decoding accuracy. In order for a child to be classified as accuracy-disabled, he or she had to score at least 18 months "below grade level expectations on at least four of five different measures of word recognition" (Catts & Kamhi, 2005, p. 85). To be labeled as rate-disabled, the children "had to perform close to, at, or above grade level on four or more measures of work recognition and at least one and half years below grade-level on four of five measures of reading speed" (Catts & Kamhi, 2005, p. 85). A graphic representation of subtypes of reading disabilities is found in Table 7–4.

TABLE 7–4. Subtypes of reading disabilities.

Subtype	Listening Comprehension	Word Recognition
Dyslexia	Good	Phonological
		Surface
		Rate Disabled
Mixed	Poor	Phonological
		Surface
		Rate Disabled
Specific Comprehension Deficit	Poor	Good

Source: From Catts, H. and Kamhi, A., *Language and Reading Disabilities*, 2nd ed. Published by Allyn and Bacon, Boston. Copyright © 2005 by Pearson Education. Reprinted by permission of the publisher.

In a study done to validate these subgroups, Lovett (1987) administered oral and written language tests to 96 children. There were 32 children in each of three categories: accuracy-disabled, rate-disabled, and normal. The subjects were matched for sex, IQ, and chronological age. The results of the testing were as follows.

1. For children who were accuracy-disabled, errors made while reading nonwords reflected basic deficits in sound-letter correspondence rules;

2. Accuracy-disabled students had deficits in syntactic and morphological knowledge in their oral language skills;

3. In analyzing individual speech sounds, accuracy-disabled students were significantly slower than were the rate-disabled students;

4. In naming serial-letter arrays, accuracy-disabled students were significantly slower than were the rate-disabled students;

5. There were no differences in identifying regular and exception words (phonetic decoding and sight words) between the rate-disabled and the normal readers;

6. The rate-disabled students had significant deficits in word recognition speed, particularly in connected text;

7. The rate-disabled students were similar to the normal children with regard to oral language skills, but on tasks designed to measure rapid automatic naming, the rate-disabled students were significantly slower than the normals.

■ DYSLEXIA

Originally referred to over 65 years ago as "congenital word blindness," **dyslexia** is a developmental reading disorder. Hynd (1991) defines dyslexia as a definable and diagnosable form of primary reading retardation with some form of central nervous system dysfunction. There is evidence that dyslexia runs in families (Leonard, 1998; Owens, 2004). Children with dyslexia have unexpected reading failures that often are accompanied by tendencies toward atypical spelling and handwriting. In addition, evidence exists to support the concept that the difficulties with phonologic awareness originate in "the phonologic component of the larger specialization for language" (Shaywitz et al., 1998).

Dyslexia. Difficulty learning to read, often due to a neurological deficit.

As outlined in Table 7–5, the American Psychiatric Association's *Diagnostic and Statistical Manual-IV* (1994) lists very specific criteria for the diagnosis of a reading disorder.

The International Classification of Diseases—10 diagnostic criteria for the diagnosis of a specific reading disorder—are outlined in Table 7–6 (Lyon, 1995). With regard to the IQ discrepancy in the ICD-10 codes, questions have been raised as to whether or not IQ-reading discrepancies are a valid measure to determine the presence of dyslexia (Siegel, 1992; Stanovich, 1991). Historically, a discrepancy between IQ scores on neuropsychological tests and reading achievement scores on reading tasks has been used to

TABLE 7–5. Characteristics of dyslexia as outlined in the *Diagnostic and Statistical Manual-IV (DSM-IV-R)*.

A.	Reading achievement, as measured by individually administered standardized tests of reading accuracy or comprehension, is substantially below that expected given the person's chronological age, measured intelligence, and age-appropriate education.
B.	The disturbance in Criterion A significantly interferes with academic achievement or activities of daily living that require reading skills.
C.	If a sensory deficit is present, the reading difficulties are in excess of those usually associated with it.

Source: Reprinted from "Toward a Definition of Dyslexia," *Annals of Dyslexia, 45* (1995) by R. Lyon with permission of the International Dyslexia Association.

TABLE 7–6. International Classification of Diseases (ICD-10; 1993) diagnostic criteria for the diagnosis of specific reading disorder.

A.   Either of the following must be present:

(1)   a score on reading accuracy and/or comprehension that is at least 2 standard errors of prediction below the level expected on the basis of the child's chronological age and general intelligence, with both reading skills and IQ assessed on an individually administered test standardized for the child's culture and educational system;

(2)   a history of serious reading difficulties, or test scores that met criterion A(1) at an earlier age, plus a score on a spelling test that is at least 2 standard errors of prediction below the level expected on the basis of the child's chronological age and IQ.

B.   The disturbance described in Criterion A significantly interferes with academic achievement or with activities of daily living that require reading skills.

C.   The disorder is not the direct result of a defect in visual or hearing acuity or of a neurological disorder.

D.   School experiences are within the average expectable range (i.e., there have been no extreme inadequacies in educational experiences).

E.   Most commonly used exclusion clause: IQ is below 70 on an individual administered standardized test.

*Children who have an IQ below 70 are excluded from the classification of learning disabled.
Source: Reprinted from "Toward a Definition of Dyslexia," *Annals of Dyslexia, 45* (1995) by R. Lyon with permission of the International Dyslexia Association.

determine or confirm the presence of dyslexia. However, this discrepancy is now seen as an inappropriate and invalid marker. Recent research studies do not support the use of a discrepancy-based definition of developmental dyslexia. In fact, when looking at the reading impaired population, minimal differences are observed between reading-disabled children who meet discrepancy criteria and reading-disabled children who do not show a wide IQ-reading achievement gap (often referred to as "garden variety" poor readers). Measures of phonological awareness provide the most robust difference in performance between normal and impaired readers, making phonological awareness, not IQ-reading discrepancies, a better tool for diagnosing reading problems such as dyslexia.

Causative Factors in Reading Disabilities

Catts and Amhi (2005) explored the causes of reading disabilities and divided the various factors into **extrinsic** and **intrinsic causes**. Extrinsic causes included lack of exposure to the printed word, lack of instruction as to how print works, and lack of opportunity to practice reading skills. It should be

Extrinsic causes. Factors in the environment of the child that interfere with development.

Intrinsic causes. Factors within the child such as neurological damage.

noted that these extrinsic factors are not included in the definition of reading disabilities, but they deserve further attention in the literature.

More support is available for the role of intrinsic factors in reading disabilities. There is an apparent inherited basis, with reading disabilities often seen in siblings and throughout generations of a family. Catts and Kamhi (2005) sum up the extensive research in this area by noting that 30 to 40% of parents of a child with reading disabilities will also have a history of reading deficits, and that the sibling of a child with reading disabilities has about a 40% chance of having a reading problem as well. Twin studies have been done to solidify the argument that reading disabilities have a genetic basis. Light and DeFries (1995) studied identical and fraternal twins and documented the existence of reading disabilities in each set. Among the fraternal twins, when one twin had a reading disability, 40% of the other twins also had a reading disability. Among identical twins, when one twin had a reading problem, 68% of the twin partners also had a reading disability. It is believed that other factors contribute to the development of reading because these figures are not 100%. It is apparent that one can carry the gene for reading disabilities but not develop the disorder, although the chances are increased. Further research on which chromosomes carry the gene for reading disabilities is ongoing. Shaywitz (2003) expresses the belief that reading is such a complex process that no single dominant gene results in dyslexia. Early indicators show that sites on chromosomes 6 and 15 are the most likely areas associated with reading ability (Catts & Kamhi, 2005).

In addition to possible genetic and hereditary factors, there is evidence of neurological bases for reading disabilities. Early studies indicated that there may be an issue with hemispheric dominance for language, with individuals who have reading disabilities having mixed dominance or right hemisphere dominance for language. This has led some to believe that left-handedness may be a marker for reading disabilities. However, there is no consistency in the literature in associating reading disabilities and handedness (Catts & Kamhi, 2005).

Much of the literature on reading supports the belief that brain abnormalities observed in people with dyslexia are an atypicality of development, just as if one extremity were larger than the other. That is to say, brain abnormalities are structural, not physiological, anomalies. It is most likely that the central nervous system deficits are in the left temporal lobe, the right frontal lobe, and/or in the **subcortical pathways** that connect the left and right hemispheres (Riccio & Hynd, 1996; Owens, 2004). Leonard and colleagues (1993) used MRI studies and found that family members of individuals with dyslexia demonstrated atypical anatomical findings.

These findings included a shift of parietal tissue to the right plenum temporale, a long Sylvian **fissure** (a furrow within the brain) in the left hemisphere,

Subcortical pathways. Interconnections in the brain that lie below the cerebral cortex.

Fissure. A deep furrow in the brain; also known as a sulcus.

Gyrus. A rounded elevation in the cerebral hemispheres.

an extra supramarginal **gyrus**, an elevated, rounded area in the brain, and multiple Heschl's gyri in the left and right hemispheres. Dyslexia is not part of a disease process that would involve progressive weakness or deterioration of brain structures and functions. Also, some disorders that appear to be developmental may in actuality result from acquired lesions in early stages of development, with possible accompanying central nervous system dysfunction. Furthermore, significant deficits in social skills are sometimes reported in children with reading disorders. This may relate to the difficulty with increasing complexity of sentences and the general language difficulties experienced by some children who have language-based learning disabilities.

Shaywitz (2003) writes that, in developmental dyslexia, there may not be a specific lesion that results in the reading disability. Rather, the problem is most likely in the neural pathways that develop a "glitch" during the development of the brain in the fetus. As a result, the

> neurons carrying the phonologic messages necessary for language do not appropriately connect to form the resonating networks that make skilled reading possible. . . . Most likely as a result of a genetically programmed error, the neural system necessary for phonologic analysis is somehow miswired, and a child is left with a phonologic impairment that interferes with spoken and written language. Depending on the nature or severity of this fault in the wiring, we would expect to observe variations and varying degrees of reading difficulty. (Shaywitz, 2003, p. 68)

Functional magnetic resonance imaging (fMRI). An MRI of the brain done while the patient performs specific tasks so the radiologist can visualize the mechanisms of the brain activated with specific tasks.

Using **functional magnetic resonance imaging (fMRI)**, Shaywitz and her colleagues (2003) are progressing in efforts to map out the neural pathways for reading. They have found that there are at least two neural pathways for reading. One of these pathways is activated in the early efforts associated with beginning reading, and in particular the efforts to slowly sound out words. The second pathway is faster and is more involved in skilled reading. There is a breakdown in these pathways (especially those in the back of the brain) in individuals with dyslexia.

As the field of brain pathophysiology advances, we will have better answers to the questions on the identification of structural abnormalities in the brains of individuals with dyslexia. Galaburda (1989) reported abnormalities in brain structures and symmetries post mortem. Recent advances in the use of neuroimaging techniques such as fMRI have contributed significantly to our knowledge of the morphology of the brain (Hynd et al., 1990; Leonard, 1998).

Shaywitz and colleagues (1998) used functional MRI techniques to study brain activation patterns in people with dyslexia. They designed a set of tasks that required their subjects to decide whether two stimuli presented simultaneously were the same or different. Their subjects included 29 dyslexic readers and 32 nonimpaired readers, all completing the tasks as outlined in

TABLE 7–7. Tasks performed by subjects in the study by Shaywitz and colleagues (1998).

Task	Example	Adds the Demand of
Line orientation	Do [\\V] and [\\v] match?	Visual-spatial processing
Letter case	Do [bbBb] and [bbBb] match?	Orthographic processing
Single letter rhyme	Do the letters [T] and [V] rhyme?	Phonologic processing
Nonword rhyme	Do [leat] and [jete] rhyme?	Difficult phonological processing
Semantic category	Are [corn] and [rice] in the same category?	Retrieval from lexicon

Table 7–7. They found that the reading performance of the subjects with dyslexia were significantly impaired compared with that of the nonimpaired readers. The biggest discrepancies were on the single-letter rhyme and non-word rhyme tasks, both of which require phonological processing. Using fMRI imaging, Shaywitz and colleagues (1998) found that the portions of the brain responsible for segmenting words into their phonological components functioned imperfectly in the subjects with dyslexia. Thus, the cognitive and behavioral deficits commonly associated with dyslexia were linked to problematic activation patterns in posterior and anterior language regions of the brain.

Although MR imaging had been used extensively to study brain morphology in individuals with dyslexia, it had not been used to study brain morphology in children with specific language impairment (SLI). Using the MRI scans, Gauger, Lombardino, and Leonard (1997) studied brain morphology in 11 children with SLI. They found that (a) pars triangularis was significantly smaller in the left hemisphere of children with SLI, and (b) children with SLI were more likely to have rightward asymmetry of language structures (Gauger et al., 1997, p. 1272).

Catts and Kamhi (2005) are careful to point out that while many differences have been found in the function and structure of the brain in individuals with reading disabilities when compared to normals, there is tremendous variability in these differences. Also, the differences are more diffuse in nature than those associated with acquired reading disabilities such as those found in patients with aphasia. Thus, it is probable that "individual differences in neurological development, not neurological deficits, contribute to many cases of developmental reading disabilities" (Catts & Kamhi, 2005, p. 101).

Other factors have been explored throughout the years, including the role of visual perception and processing deficits, attention deficit disorder with hyperactivity, and language problems. Language problems identified in early childhood are apparently causal factors in the development of later reading disabilities. In fact, the "research indicates that 50 percent or more of children with language impairment in preschool or kindergarten go on to have reading disabilities in primary or secondary grades" (Catts & Kamhi, 2005, p. 108).

■ ASSESSMENT AND DIAGNOSIS OF READING DISABILITIES

The differential diagnosis of language-based learning disabilities, dyslexia, ADHD, and auditory processing disorders can be a difficult task because there is co-morbidity among these disorders. In addition to a variety of language and cognitive tests, assessment of behavior and pragmatics should be included in a test battery for the differential diagnosis of reading disabilities and language-based learning disabilities (LLD). Some children will be inappropriately labeled as dyslexic instead of LLD, especially if the language testing (lexicon, syntax, morphology, and text-level processing) reveals that the deficits in language are relatively mild. In addition, some people include a **discrepancy criterion** for the labeling of an individual as dyslexic. In these cases, there needs to be a discrepancy between the child's achievement and his expected achievement based on IQ.

Catts and Kamhi (2005) argue against the use of discrepancy criteria because a child with poor language skills will score a lower verbal IQ which in turn lowers the overall IQ. Sometimes this lowered IQ score does not adequately reflect the difference between IQ and achievement needed in order to be diagnosed as dyslexic. It has been suggested that nonverbal IQ tests be given to children who are dyslexic; however, Stanovich (1991) has found that there is little relationship between reading achievement and performance on nonverbal IQ tests. Children who do not meet the discrepancy criterion are often labeled as underachievers. Catts and Kamhi (1999) suggest that these children should be labeled as LLD since "this term focuses attention on the central role that language-learning difficulties play in these children's reading, writing, and other learning problems" (p. 66). They suggest that an extensive battery of language tests that encompass semantics, syntax, language processing, **phonological processing**, and reading be given.

Children who have reading disabilities and score within normal limits or high on the language-based tests would be labeled as dyslexic, whereas those children who score below age limits would be diagnosed as language-learning disabled (LLD). In other words, children who have dyslexia will perform within normal limits or higher than normal on language tests; their only problem is reading. Children with LLD will have a poorer performance

Discrepancy criterion. The measurable difference between a child's achievement and his expected achievement based on IQ.

Phonological processing. Understanding of the sound system of a language.

in language tests as well as in reading, often creating a sense of frustration as seen in Figure 7–1. Phonemic awareness is at the heart of dyslexia, so it should be tested as part of a reading battery.

Torgesen (1999) defines **phonemic awareness** as "a more or less explicit understanding that words are composed of segments of sound smaller than a syllable, as well as knowledge, or awareness, of the distinctive features of individual phonemes themselves" (p. 129). Phonemic awareness is embedded in the more general construct of phonological awareness. Phonemic awareness is assessed for two primary reasons: (1) to identify children at risk for reading failure prior to receiving reading instruction, and (2) to assess the level of phonological impairment in individuals who have been diagnosed with a reading disorder.

Phonemic awareness. Recognition of the fact that words are made up of sounds, and understanding the differences between phonemes.

Catts and his colleagues (1997) categorize assessment tasks for phonemic awareness in three categories. The first category is **phonemic segmentation** tasks that include counting, pronunciation, deletion and adding of sounds to words, or reversing phonemes in words.

Phonemic segmentation. The act of breaking down a word into sounds.

Phoneme synthesis is the second category. In this task, sounds are presented is isolation and the child is asked to blend them into a word. Sound comparison tasks are the third category. On sound comparison tasks, the child is asked to compare the sounds of different words. In an example of this task, the clinician presents a target word, and the child is asked to indicate which in a series of words begins with the same sound as the target sound.

Phoneme synthesis. The act of combining sounds presented in isolation into a single word.

All these areas should be tested as part of the diagnostic process for reading impairment. A list of tests that can be used to assess phonemic awareness is found in Table 7–8.

TABLE 7–8. A list of tests that can be used to assess phonemic awareness.

Name of Test	Author
Rosner Test of Auditory Analysis	Rosner (1975)
Lindamood Auditory Conceptualization Test	Lindamood and Lindamood (1979)
Test of Invented Spelling	Mann, Tobin, Wilson (1987)
Test of Phonological Awareness	Torgesen and Bryant (1993)
Yopp-Singer Test of Phoneme Segmentation	Yopp (1995)
The Phonological Awareness Test	Robertson and Salter (1995)
The Comprehensive Test of Phonological Processes in Reading	Wagner and Torgesen (1997)

Source: Adapted from "Assessment and Instruction for Phonemic Awareness and Word Recognition Skills" by J. K. Torgesen. In H. Catts and A. G. Kamhi, *Language and Reading Disabilities* (2nd ed.), pp. 133–135. Copyright 2005 by Allyn and Bacon (Boston).

TABLE 7–9. A list of tests that can be used to assess word recognition.

Task	Name of Subtest	Name of Test
Sight Word Reading	Word Identification	Woodcock Reading Mastery Test-Revised (Woodcock, 1987)
	Reading	Wide Range Achievement Test-3 (Wilkinson, 1995)
Phonetic Decoding	Word Attack	Woodcock Reading Mastery Test-Revised (Woodcock, 1987)
Word Recognition Fluency	All 13 Subtests	Gray Oral Reading Test, 3rd ed. (Wiederholt & Bryant, 1992); Word Reading Eficiency (Torgesen & Wagner, 1997);
		Nonword Reading Efficiency (Torgesen & Wagner, 1997)

Source: Adapted from "Assessment and Instruction for Phonemic Awareness and Word Recognition Skills" by J. K. Torgesen. In H. Catts and A. G. Kamhi, *Language and Reading Disabilities*, pp. 133–135. Copyright 1999 by Allyn and Bacon (Boston).

Word recognition skills should be tested in addition to phonemic awareness. Children with reading disabilities have difficulty with orthographic processing, which enables the child to retrieve sight words from memory, and with phonetic decoding that involves applying alphabetic strategies when reading new words (Torgesen, 1999). Tests that can be used to assess word recognition skills are listed in Table 7–9.

The Assessment of Literacy and Language (ALL) is a test developed by Lombardino, Lieberman, and Brown (2005). It can be used to assess oral and written language skills for prekindergarten through first grade students. The ALL consists of a Caregiver Questionnaire and an individually administered test with 11 norm-referenced and 6 criterion-referenced subtests. Examiners can screen, diagnose, and prescribe treatment for emergent literacy and language deficits for young children who are at risk for developing reading disabilities. The subtests target six areas that match Early Reading First and Reading First initiatives for development of effective reading skills, including oral language, phonological awareness, phonics knowledge, print awareness, fluency, and comprehension.

At the University of Florida Speech and Hearing Clinic, a battery of tests has been assembled to test the reading, writing, and spelling skills of children with suspected reading and spelling disorders. It is particularly important to assess the student's knowledge of sound-letter correspondences. This battery is outlined in Table 7–10.

TABLE 7-10. Protocol for assessment of reading and spelling disorders used at the University of Florida Speech and Hearing Clinic.

Test	Subtest
Comprehensive Test of Phonological Processing (Wagner, Torgesen, & Rashotte, 1999)	Phonological Awareness Composite
	Rapid Naming Composite
	Phonological Memory Composite
Woodcock-Johnson III Test of Achievement (RD book)(Woodcock, McGrew, & Mather, 2001)	Written Language (computer scored)
	Word Identification—Test 1
	Reading Fluency—Test 2
	Math Calculation—Test 5
	Math Fluency—Test 6
	Applied Problems—Test 10
	Word Attack—Test 13
	Picture Vocabulary—Test 14
	Spelling—Test 7
Woodcock-Johnson Achievement Tests (SP Book)	Oral Language (computer scored)
	Story Recall—Test 3
	Oral Comprehension—Test 15
Woodcock-Johnson III Tests of Cognition (Computer scored) (Woodcock, McGrew, & Mather, 2001)	Verbal Ability Composite
	Thinking Ability Composite
	Cognitive Efficiency
	General Intellectual Ability
	(GIA)(composite)
Gray Oral Reading Test-4 (Wiederholt & Bryant, 2001)	Fluency
	Comprehension
	Oral Reading Quotient (Composite)
Test of Word Recognition Efficiency (Torgesen, Wagner, & Rashotte, 1999)	Sight Word
	Phonemic Decoding
	Total Word Reading
Brief Language Samples	Spoken, Written Language Story Re-Tell

In summary, comprehensive testing of language and cognition, as well as phonological awareness skills and a hearing evaluation, needs to be done in order to differentially diagnose between an auditory processing disorder, a language-based learning disability, and dyslexia.

■ CULTURAL DIVERSITY ISSUES IN THE ASSESSMENT OF READING DISORDERS

Historically, there tends to be an overdiagnosis and an underdiagnosis of literacy problems in children who are from low socioeconomic, racially, and/or ethnically diverse backgrounds. This is problematic because there is not a wide variety of assessment tools available that are normed on these populations. It is especially problematic when taking into consideration the No Child Left Behind Act of 2001. Scarborough (2000) contends that socioeconomic status is a stronger predictor of a child's literacy abilities than are assessments of emergent literacy skills, home literacy experiences, nonverbal intellect, and oral language skills. Laing and Kamhi (2003) point out that many standardized tests have problems with linguistic bias, content bias, and with poor representation in norming samples. They write that linguistic bias may "be associated with the use of standardized tests and refers to a disparity between (1) the language or dialect used by the examiner, (2) the language or dialect used by the child, and (3) the language or dialect that is expected in the child's responses" (p. 45). If one adapts the test to account for these factors, the test is no longer valid in its administration and can lead to under- and/or overreferral of children who have a language difference, not a language disorder.

With regard to content validity, many tests derive their items based on the belief that most children are exposed to the same concepts and lexicon based on similar experiences in life. They also point out that literacy experiences such as being read to and pointing to pictures in story books may not be a traditional part of these children's experiences, thus they are ill-prepared for tasks such as the Peabody Picture Vocabulary Test-III (Dunn & Dunn, 1997) and others that require receptively and expressively identifying pictures. **Content bias** would occur when the response to an item on a test could be affected by a dialectal or cultural difference.

Content bias. The effect of a dialectal or cultural difference on the responses of an individual to a test item.

Test developers need to make a conscious effort to include culturally and linguistically diverse individuals in their norming samples. Laing and Kamhi (2003) point out that there has been improvement in this in recent years, but there are still many tests whose norming samples do not reflect the approximate percentages of subjects that are represented in the general population. Tests which have addressed the issue of representative sampling include the

Peabody Picture Vocabulary Test-III, the Test of Language Development-Primary-3 (Newcomer & Hammill, 1997), the Test of Language Development-Intermediate-2 & 3 (Newcomer & Hammill, 1988; Newcomer & Hammill, 1997), and the Test of Adolescent and Adult Language-3 (Hammill et al., 1994).

In addition to using tests with normative samples that include those of the child being tested, the clinician can use criterion-referenced tests. These types of tools were discussed in Chapter 3, but as a reminder, criterion-referenced tests allow a clinician to test a child's language skills in a more in-depth context than does standardized testing, and the child's performance is compared to criteria developed by the clinician that permits comparison with other children who have similar cultural, ethnic, or racial backgrounds.

Other assessment devices that can be used in addition to criterion-referenced tests include obtaining and analyzing a language sample from the child and interviewing the parents of the child to develop a more complete picture of the child's form, content, and use of language, as well as a description of the child's life experiences. Laing and Kamhi (2003) also discuss two additional procedures that can be used to determine the linguistic abilities of children from culturally diverse populations. These are processing-dependent techniques and dynamic assessment techniques. Laing and Kamhi (2003) describe processing-dependent tasks as being "minimally dependent on prior knowledge or experience. Examples of processing-dependent tasks include various memory tasks (e.g., digit span, working memory, nonword repetition), certain perceptual tasks (e.g., discrimination of rapidly presented tones, sequencing tones presented in rapid sequence), and competing stimuli tasks (filtered words, auditory figure ground, competing words)" (p. 46).

Dynamic assessment techniques are sometimes referred to as diagnostic therapy, and are based on the work of Vygotsky (1978). Vygotsky defined a zone of proximal development as being the difference between how well a child performed on an independent task, and how well the child performed when provided assistance on the same task. Thus, the clinician is able to determine the child's current level of performance as well as determine therapy methods that can improve the child's ability on the specified task. Other dynamic assessments include test-teach-retest, **graduated prompting**, and task/stimulus variability. In test-teach-retest, the child is given a test, then is provided with instruction on the information he or she missed, followed by retesting on the same test. Lidz and Pena (1996) did a case study based on dynamic assessment and found that standardized tests did not provide much information on children's learning potential.

In graduated prompting, assessment and treatment occur concurrently. The child is presented with a task, then is tested for **stimulability** on those items

Graduated prompting. In diagnostic therapy, the co-occurrence of assessment and treatment, with the child being tested for stimulability on a language construct.

Stimulability. The degree to which a child can imitate a language construct presented by the clinician. The less intervention is needed, the more the child is stimulable.

missed. "How well a child responds to graduated prompts can help determine which language forms and structures to target and the amount of improvement a child might be expected to make in intervention" (Laing & Kamhi, 2003).

In 1997, Laing, Kamhi, and Catts studied the predictive value of static versus dynamic tasks when using phonological awareness tasks to predict early reading achievement. Their study consisted of 72 normally developing children in kindergarten and first grade. During the fall and spring, each child was given a static and dynamic measure of segmentation skills, as well as an assessment of reading performance (the Woodcock Reading Mastery Test-Revised by Woodcock, 1997). Their findings indicated that the dynamic measures of phonological awareness were better at predicting reading success than were static tests.

Task/stimulus variability can be used to modify the method by which test items are presented. For example, the clinician could present the test items in the traditional static method, or he or she could present them in a more natural method based on experiential context. Several studies are cited by Laing and Kamhi (2003) as showing that African-American children tend to learn better in classrooms that are interactive and incorporate music, movement, and cooperative learning, and that these children do better on tests that are administered in their natural environment and focus on action-object orientations.

■ ADDRESSING READING DISORDERS IN THE SCHOOL SETTING

Using the Collaborative Model for Early Reading Instruction

Early and substantial exposure to books correlates with many verbal skills, including the acquisition of knowledge and growth in vocabulary (Stanovich, 1994). Direct and dedicated instruction on phonemic awareness can prevent the reading, spelling, and writing failures that are often associated with reading disabilities (Goldsworthy, 1996; Livesay, 1995). Using a consultative model, the speech-language clinician can provide a wealth of information on skills needed to be ready to read. Goldsworthy outlined several early interventions that can be used for children getting ready to read. These interventions are delineated in Table 7–11.

We know that children who are exposed to stories (e.g., those who are read to by their parents) have better language, reading, and spelling skills than those who are not read to by their parents or others. In fact, children who

TABLE 7–11. Activities to promote reading readiness.

Promoting Emergent Literacy	1. Play word games with letter sounds and syllables.
	2. Expose the child to the printed word, reading aloud to the child a variety of books and encouraging his or her participation.
	3. Have the child construct stories using household events and items, as well as by "reading" books without words.
	4. Encourage the child to draw and write.
Enhancing Listening Skills, Concentration, Memory, and Selective Attention	1. To encourage listening, have the child indicate by raising his hand, ringing a bell, etc. when he hears a specific word as a story is read to him or her.
	2. Have the child participate in activities such as finding hidden pictures or words, matching patterns, letters, words, and pictures.
	3. "Alert" the child when you are beginning to say something by saying the child's names and asking if he or she is ready to listen.
	4. Have the child retell a paragraph and answer specific questions about what he or she has heard and gradually increase the length and complexity of the auditory input.
	5. Have the child focus his attention on an interesting object and challenge him or her to see how long (s)he can concentrate on the object.
	6. Vary the rate of presentation of material, gradually try to increase the time interval between presentation of material and response from the child, introduce visual and auditory distractors through which a child must concentrate on the primary material, and vary directions.
	7. Play games with the child.
	8. Help the child organize his school work, homework, desk, room, etc.
	9. Encourage children to "stop, look, and listen" before providing a response to a question or request.
	10. Encourage memorization and recitation of songs, rhymes, riddles, story sections, and tongue twisters.

(Continued)

TABLE 7–11. (*Continued*)

Phonological Awareness	
	1. Read aloud to the child on a regular basis.
	2. Encourage story-telling and "reading" wordless books.
	3. Sing songs.
	4. Have the child answer questions about what has been read.
	5. Pose a question to the child prior to reading the story and then have the child listen for information needed to answer the question.
	6. Use puns, idioms, and riddles to enhance manipulating sounds and words.
	7. Teach the child to discriminate pitch, volume, and rhythms of auditory information.
	8. Point to words and letters as you read to the child.
	9. As you read to the child, omit words and have him or her guess what the word should be.
	10. Provide the child with word cards that can be arranged to formulate a sentence.

Source: Compiled from information in *Developmental Reading Disabilities: A Language-Based Treatment Approach* (pp. 127–170) by C. L. Goldsworthy. Copyright 1996 by Singular Publishing Group, Inc.

enter school with good narrative skills are more likely to succeed on tasks addressing comprehension and production of the decontextualized language of writing and reading (Owens, 1999).

Also, the role of phonological awareness cannot be overemphasized when looking at causative factors in reading and spelling disorders. Children should be taught to group words on the basis of common sounds. For example, a list of 10 to 15 words could be provided with approximately half of the words containing the sound /a/. The children would then be asked to write the words from the list that contain the /a/ sound. They should also learn to segment words into phonemes. Other phoneme games include rewriting words by reversing the phonemes and deleting phonemes. As an example, the child could be asked to rewrite a one-syllable word by reversing the first and last phoneme in the word, or to rewrite the words leaving out all the /b/ sounds (Blachman, 1994). Goldsworthy (1996) noted that

> Developing phonological awareness requires that one play with the sounds of the language by identifying and producing rhyme, segmenting sentences into words and words into syllables, and segmenting and blending sounds within syllables. (p. 147)

TABLE 7–12. A phonological awareness training program outline.

1. Program levels
   a. Level I. Increasing word awareness: dividing sentences into words
   b. Level II. Increasing syllable awareness: dividing words into syllables
   c. Level III. Increasing sound awareness: dividing syllables into sounds
2. Level sections
   a. Level I. Listening activities for increasing word awareness
   b. Level I. Deliberate manipulation of words in sentences
   c. Level II. Listening activities for increasing syllable awareness
   d. Level II. Deliberate manipulation of syllables in words
   e. Level III. Listening activities for increasing sound awareness
   f. Level III. Deliberate manipulation of sounds in syllables

Source: Developmental Reading Disabilities: A Language-Based Treatment Approach (p. 154) by
C. L. Goldsworthy. Copyright 1996 by Singular Publishing Group, Inc.

Goldsworthy also delineated a phonological awareness training program which is outlined in Table 7–12.

There is no doubt that phonemic awareness and exposure to books play a role in the literacy of school-age children. Thus, it makes sense that these activities would be a substantial part of early childhood education geared toward preparing children for school.

Treatment Methods for Students with Reading Disabilities

When a group of college students with reading disabilities was evaluated, the majority had problems with the speech production of complex phonological sequences. The authors concluded that speech processing, language processing, and speech and language production are affected by weak phonological connections (Catts, 1989). Thus, focusing on treatment methods that address phonological awareness is paramount. Catts and Kamhi (2005) make the point that children with dyslexia need therapy that targets primarily phonological processing and word recognition. Children with language-based learning disabilities also need to work on phonological processing and word recognition, in addition to language comprehension.

Numerous methods of reading intervention are documented in the education and speech-language pathology literature. There are several phonics computer programs that have had mixed reviews in the literature. Lombardino and colleagues (1997) stress the need for long-term instruction in phonemic decoding for reading, spelling, and rapid word recognition. They advocate that the first step in therapy be to teach phoneme-grapheme associations using a multimodality approach. The second step should focus on irregular spelling and reading words with irregular orthographies. This is to be followed by morphological manipulations in which the student learns to use sound segments to change meaning at the word level. Extensive practice is necessary to develop rapid and automatic word recognition that is needed to have increased reading comprehension.

The Orton-Gillingham Method

Alphabetic principle. The dictum governing how specific sounds in a language are represented by specific spelling patterns.

The Orton-Gillingham method of teaching reading, writing, and spelling is a philosophy of teaching that incorporates an integrated curriculum of language skills. The **alphabetic principle** is at the core of the Orton-Gillingham method.

The alphabetic principle governs the orthographic structure of many languages, including English. It requires knowledge of how specific sounds are represented by specific spelling patterns. Alphabetic-phonic associations are trained from the first lesson and reinforced through phonetically controlled reading and spelling activities to form the foundation of reading and writing in alphabetic language.

The Orton-Gillingham method also focuses on the role of cognition in reading, writing, and spelling. Children are taught to think about the rules that they have learned and to apply these rules in different contexts (e.g., syllabication). Using old information to draw inferences about new information is a skill that is necessary for continued independent learning (Lombardino, 1998).

Project Read

Developed by Greene and Enfield in 1991, Project Read is a modification of the Orton-Gillingham method that also stresses input through the auditory, visual, and tactile modes. Goldsworthy (1996) describes the method as a "systematic, structured, developmental approach based on the links of the language" (p. 184). It uses practice and generalization to move from the concrete to the abstract and from part to whole. The phonology component is intended for children in grades 1 to 3. It focuses on sound-symbol relationships, segmenting words into sounds, and learning syllabication patterns. The comprehension component is designed for students in grades 4 through 12. Its focus is on acquiring and organizing information using specifically designed report forms. The written expression component focuses on syntax in written language. It also includes clustering related information and editing procedures (Goldsworthy, 1996).

Lindamood Phoneme Sequencing Program (LiPS)

The Lindamood Phoneme Sequencing Program for Reading, Spelling, and Speech (LiPS) (Lindamood & Lindamood, 1998) was developed for students in prekindergarten to grade 12. It was formerly known as the Auditory Discrimination in Depth program. The first three levels are specifically recommended for kindergarten students to be used preventively as basic building blocks toward successful reading and spelling. These levels are also recommended for students and adults with learning disabilities. Stimuli include mouth-form cards depicting the oral production plus the label and corresponding phonemes, the vowel circles, colored blocks, and letter tiles. Syllable construction and reading charts also are provided.

The LiPS program was developed to facilitate the acquisition of reading and spelling skills through a **multimodality approach** that uses auditory, visual, tactile, and kinesthetic information to train the conceptual elements of phonemes and the corresponding graphemes. Initially, the basic auditory conceptual elements of consonant sounds are trained, followed by teaching the vowel sounds.

Multimodality approach. An approach to therapy that incorporates information from all sensory systems to teach a conceptual element.

Objectives of ear, eye, and mouth training are dependent on the following tenets:

1. Sensory input is required to pair the oral motor activity with the basic auditory element.

2. Conceptualization of the distinctive features of each phoneme is required.

3. Perception of same and different number and order of speech sounds in isolation is followed by perception of minimal changes between syllable units.

4. Storage and retrieval of the agreed upon representations for phonemes and graphemes are required for reading and spelling. (LeGrand, 1997)

The Barton Reading and Spelling System

Developed by Sue Barton in 1999, the Barton Reading and Spelling System is also based on the Orton-Gillingham program. It can be used in individual sessions with children and adults, and a series of videotapes are available to train practitioners, teachers, and parents who are interested in learning the Barton system. The Barton system also includes fully scripted lesson plans and reading materials, including color-coded letter tiles. It is divided into 10 levels, each of which contains between 10 and 15 lessons. A list of these levels is found in Table 7–13. It is anticipated that a student receiving instruction two times a week will need an average of three to five months to complete each level. According to Barton, individuals who complete all 10 levels of the

TABLE 7–13. Levels of the Barton System.

Level 1:	Phonemic Awareness
Level 2:	Consonants and Short Vowels
Level 3:	Closed Syllables and Units
Level 4:	Syllable Division and Vowel Teams
Level 5:	Prefixes and Suffixes
Level 6:	Six Reasons for Silent—E
Level 7:	Vowel—R Syllables
Level 8:	Advanced Vowel Teams
Level 9:	Influences of Foreign Languages
Level 10:	Greek Words and Latin Roots

program will be functioning at approximately the mid-ninth grade level of reading, spelling, and basic writing.

The Wilson Reading System

The Wilson Reading System was developed by Barbara Wilson in 1988. It was originally developed to provide reading instruction to children in the upper-elementary school grades as well as adults, but it is now also available for younger children. It is a 12-step program to remediate reading and writing problems in children who have language-based learning disabilities. It, too, is based on the Orton-Gillingham approach. The phonemic awareness program emphasizes strategies that can be used for spelling and decoding. The Wilson system uses visualization techniques to help with reading comprehension and also incorporates oral expression language development. It takes approximately one to three years to complete the program and can be used in small groups as well as one-on-one treatment sessions.

The Slingerland Approach

The Slingerland Approach (1977) is an example of yet another program based on the Orton-Gillingham program. An underlying philosophy of the Slingerland Approach is that individuals with dyslexia have difficulty linking the visual, auditory, and kinesthetic motor systems. According to the Learning Disabilities Association of America, "the Slingerland Approach starts with the smallest unit of sight, sound and feeling—a single letter. Expanding upon that single unit students are taught through an approach which strengthens inner-sensory association and enables the strong channel of learning to reinforce the weak" (2005, p. 2). The Slingerland Approach is a comprehensive language therapy system.

The Laubach Method

The Laubach method was developed by Laubach for the purpose of providing group instruction to high school dropouts, illiterate adults, and those for whom English is a second language. It can also be used with students in the intermediate grades in tutorial or group settings. The basic principle behind the method is the teaching of sound-symbol relationships. Consonant sounds are taught first, followed by the short vowels, then the long vowels. Irregular spellings are then addressed, followed by reading, writing, and grammar exercises with increasing complexity. The Laubach method uses picture association cards to teach letters, sounds, and key vocabulary words. Lowercase letters are taught before uppercase letters, but both are taught in alphabetic sequence (Buchanan, Weller, & Buchanan, 1997).

Montessori Reading Instruction

The Montessori method of reading instruction uses self-paced, multisensory input to teach the letters. Visual-motor activities are designed to facilitate letter recognition and are then modified to teach writing and reading. The children participate in activities such as tracing and identifying sandpaper letters with their eyes open, then with their eyes closed. While they are tracing the sandpaper letters, they say the letter's sound. The Montessori method uses phonograms that are alphabet cards to construct words. A unique feature of this method is that it does not allow oral reading. Teachers check reading comprehension by writing questions on a chalkboard, then eliciting answers to the questions (Buchanan et al., 1997).

The Whole Language Approach

Whole language is a discovery-based, informal method of integrating cognitive skills, language skills, and curricular goals (Goldsworthy, 1996). Hegde (1996b) described whole language as follows:

> Language teaching should not be broken down into speaking, reading and writing; instead, all aspects of literacy including speaking, listening, reading, and writing should be taught simultaneously as an integrated whole. (p. 189)

Children are encouraged to write on a daily basis, and often teachers use dialogue journals to monitor the child's progress in writing and integrating knowledge. Spelling is rarely corrected; invented spellings that are part of the normal process are allowed to stand uncorrected in many instances. Although certainly something is to be said for integrating the curriculum and encouraging writing, there is some concern about the absence of instruction in phonological awareness in the whole language curriculum.

Intervention with Stories

Use of prewritten narratives and the creation of novel scripts are valuable therapy tools to use with children who have language-based learning disabilities. Stories can be used to coordinate academic issues in the classroom with events happening in therapy. It is important that the stories use complete texts, events, and experiences so that children can learn the structure of stories (Naremore, Densmore, & Harman, 1995). This structure includes introducing the story, developing the components, and reaching a resolution.

By grade 2, a child should be able to get the main idea of a sentence. Thus, when reading with the child, it is helpful to point out that the first sentence in a paragraph typically reveals the general content of the entire passage. If the child can get the main idea of a sentence, he or she can move on to understanding the content of a paragraph. Reading written text from grade 3 and beyond requires the use of metalinguistic and metacognitive skills to comprehend the content of the story. Children can be taught to single out key words, then to use the repetition of those words to tie the sentences in the paragraph together (Naremore et al., 1995). Lexicon can be addressed by having the child think of synonyms for the key words. They can also make lists of the information words within the paragraph to help remember the key elements and sequence of events within the paragraph. Another strategy to help children remember the sequence of events is to type out the sentences of the paragraph, then cut the sentences apart into sentence strips. Then, after the child reads the paragraph, he or she can use the sentence strips to reconstruct the paragraph. This facilitates the learning of sequencing, which is critical to comprehension of a story (Naremore et al., 1995).

Stories can also be used to work on written expression. Naremore and colleagues (1995) advocate first teaching the child to state the main idea of his or her paragraph in one sentence. The child is then taught to tie each sentence back to the main idea through the use of repetition of words, pronouns, substitutions, and lists of the events. From that point, the child should be taught to make inferences and predictions using information in the paragraph and learning from past experiences. As part of this process, the child should be taught to organize his or her ideas using old and new information. This will require that the child tap into short-term and long-term memory banks.

Increasing Memory

Many activities and techniques can be used to improve the memory skills needed to be successful readers and writers. One way is to tell a story to the child and have him or her repeat it back in the proper sequence. For children who have difficulty with this initially, the story can be written down on note cards that the child can read and use to reconstruct the story. Memory and concentration games are also useful tools that can be used at home and in the classroom. Playing "20 Questions" and memorizing rhymes and songs are additional helpful activities. Games that require the duplication of visual and auditory patterns are good activities for improving memory. For example, the clinician can tap out a series of knocks on the table and then have the student repeat the pattern using appropriate pauses and cadences. Alternately, the clinician could repeat a series of verbalizations (words and sounds) that the student is then required to repeat. Telling "how to" sequences likewise can be useful (Goldsworthy, 1996). An example would be to make brownies with a child and have him or her reconstruct the sequence of events that led up to eating the brownies. These are activities that can easily be implemented in the therapy room, the classroom, and at home.

Increasing Metacognitive Skills to Enhance Reading Comprehension

The development of **metacognitive skills** has been found to be a valid marker for later reading development. Some strategies to help students learn metacognitive skills include using advance organizers such as having learning objectives provided prior to reading a passage, and the use of pretests and prequestions.

Metacognitive skills. Those skills that enable a child to solve problems, form hypotheses, analyze his or her thoughts, and make a decision.

Having advance organizers helps the student develop strategies that enable him or her to evaluate the information read, categorize the content, and generalize information (Nelson, 1998).

It is also important for the students to know that there is a purpose to reading. Tierney and Cunningham (1984) delineated four steps that could be utilized to increase reading comprehension:

Step 1: Establish purpose(s) for comprehending.

Step 2: Have students read or listen for the established purpose(s).

Step 3: Have students perform some task that directly reflects and measures accomplishment of each established purpose for comprehending.

Step 4: Provide direct informative feedback concerning students' comprehension based on their performance of that (those) task(s) (p. 625).

It may be necessary to teach students to develop a self-questioning approach to reading comprehension in order to implement the four steps. Wong and

Jones (1982) proposed five steps for developing self-questioning:

a. What are you studying this passage for? (So you can answer some questions you will be given later).

b. Find the main idea/ideas in the paragraph and underline it/them.

c. Think of a question about the main idea you have underlined. Remember what a good question should be like. (Look at the prompt).

d. Learn the answer to your question.

e. Always look back at the questions and answers to see how each successive question and answer provides you with more information (p. 231).

As the students learned to formulate good questions about the textual units, their reading comprehension increased.

■ ROLE OF THE SPEECH-LANGUAGE PATHOLOGIST IN DIAGNOSING AND TREATING DEVELOPMENTAL READING AND SPELLING DISORDERS

Children with reading and spelling disabilities need intervention that includes speaking, listening, reading, and writing because reciprocity appears to occur in oral-written language. Dyslexia is a specific deficit in the processing of phonological information, an area about which most speech-language pathologists are well versed with regard to assessment and remediation. The primary role of the speech-language pathologist should be early identification. A test battery (see Chapter 8) that is designed to evaluate language production and processing (including phonology, semantics, and syntax) should be administered to children who are at risk for problems in reading (Lombardino et al., 1997). In addition, all children in kindergarten and first grade should be given tests of phonological awareness that predict reading disabilities. Because of the interplay between auditory and visual processing, it also makes sense for a speech-language pathologist to be involved in remediation because many children with reading disabilities also show deficits in oral language. Likewise, many of the strategies speech-language pathologists use to treat auditory processing disorders can be used to treat developmental reading and spelling disabilities. With the understanding of the phoneme-grapheme information possessed by the speech-language pathologist, it is only logical that he or she be involved in the early identification and treatment of developmental reading and spelling problems. There is no doubt that the speech-language pathologist should work collaboratively with classroom teachers and specialists in reading or learning disabilities in modifying the curriculum to facilitate optimal academic success for children with reading and spelling disabilities.

■ SUMMARY

Reading and spelling disabilities are rapidly ascending to one of the most referred cases in speech-language pathology. Over the last decade, these disabilities have received much attention in the literature with the majority of these studies confirming that the speech-language pathologist assume an active role in the diagnosis and treatment of individuals with reading/spelling disabilities. There have been efforts to confirm the etiology of reading/spelling disorders, with more and more evidence showing that genetics may play a role as well as specific deficits in the central nervous system. The use of functional magnetic resonance imaging has enhanced the ability of researchers to determine which areas of the brain are active in normal readers and then to compare these images to those of individuals with reading/spelling deficits. The study of reading and spelling disabilities is an exciting area in our profession, and it is paramount that speech-language pathologists make known their ability to participate in the assessment and treatment of these disorders.

CASE STUDY

Author's Note: This report greatly exceeds in length the other case studies, but the exam is very comprehensive and multifaceted.

Background Information

W P, a 10-year-old male, was seen at the University of Florida Speech and Hearing Clinic (UFSHC) on May 31, 2005, for an assessment of his reading, spelling, and oral language skills (Diagnostic Procedure Code: 92506 Evaluation of Speech and Language). He was referred by a speech pathologist at the University of Florida Speech and Hearing Clinic at Shands Hospital in Gainesville, Florida. W also had a second referral from S, nurse practioner at the Family Psychiatry clinic in Gainesville, Florida. S diagnosed W with ADD. His mother, Mrs. P, says he has difficulty focusing. He is not on medication.

W is currently home-schooled by his mother who reported that he is at the fourth grade level. Mrs. P has been concerned with W's academic performance since he was in kindergarten, where he began showing signs of difficulty with writing and verbal communication skills. However, she reports that language comprehension seems to be one of W's strengths, and that he does not have much trouble with memorization. W has received treatment only from an occupational therapist for his difficulty with handwriting. His mother explains that W uses a four-finger grasp while writing, a problem that was never successfully corrected in therapy.

W's developmental history is unremarkable. He reached all his developmental milestones at the appropriate stages except for toilet training, which gave him some difficulty through kindergarten. During W's delivery there was meconium staining, and he had low blood sugar. W has asthma, which resulted in hospital visits on two occasions. He has a heart murmur. He has had no operations and his general health was noted to be average. There is a negative history for language learning disability in Ws immediate family; however, his second cousin has some language difficulties.

The purpose of this assessment was to evaluate W's oral and written language abilities in conjunction with his overall cognitive abilities to determine if he has a reading disability that requires academic accommodations and/or specific intervention strategies.

Reading and Spelling Achievement Measures

The following diagnostic tools were used:

- Woodcock-Johnson Tests of Cognitive Abilities-3rd Edition (WJ-COG-III, Woodcock, McGrew, & Mather, 2001)

- Comprehensive Test of Phonological Processing (CTOPP, Wagner, Torgesen, & Rashotte, 1999)

- Gray Oral Reading Mastery Test-4 (GORT-4, Weiderholt & Bryant, 2001)

- Test of Word Reading Efficiency (TOWRE: Wagner, Torgesen & Rashotte, 1999)

- Woodcock-Johnson Tests of Achievement-3rd Edition (WJ-III ACH, Woodcock, McGrew & Mather, 2001)

WJ-III Cognitive Battery

Seven subtests from the Woodcock-Johnson Tests of Cognitive Abilities-3rd Edition (WJ-COG-III) were used to assess W's cognitive processing skills. These subtests were as follows: Verbal Comprehension, Visual-Auditory Learning, Spatial Relations, Sound Blending, Concept Formation, Visual Matching, and Numbers Reversed. The mean score for each subtest is 100 with a standard deviation of +/−15. Combinations of WJ-COG-III subtests are used to derive Verbal Ability, Thinking

Ability, Cognitive Efficiency, and General Intelligence Ability composite scores.

W's Visual Auditory Learning and Concept Formation subtests scores were in the superior range for his age. His Verbal Comprehension and Sound Blending subtests scores were in the above average range, while his Spatial Relations subtest score was in the average range for his age. He scored at the lower end of the average range on the Numbers Reversed subtest. His score on the Visual Matching subtest was depressed.

W's Thinking Ability (intentional cognitive processing) was in the superior range. General Intellectual Ability and Verbal Ability composite scores were at the higher end of the average range for his age. However, his Cognitive Efficiency composite score was depressed. A discrepancy of this nature, where scores range from superior to depressed, is characteristic of a learning disability. The following table shows W's standard scores and percentiles for the WJ-COG-III.

Subtests	Standard Score	Percentile
Verbal Comprehension	110	76
Visual-Auditory Learning	125	95
Spatial Relations	109	73
Sound Blending	115	84
Concept Formation	134	99
Visual Matching	71*	3
Numbers Reversed	91	28
Thinking Ability Composite	132	98
Verbal Ability Composite	110	76
Cognitive Efficiency	76*	6
General Intelligence Ability	112	80

*Score is more than one standard deviation below the mean.

Phonological Awareness

The Comprehensive Test of Phonological Processing for ages 7 through 24 (CTOPP) was used to assess W's phonological awareness, phonological memory, and rapid naming skills. Six subtests of the CTOPP were given to W during this evaluation: Elision, Blending Words, Memory for

Digits, Rapid Digit Naming, Nonword Repetition, and Rapid Letter Naming.

The Elision subtest is a 20-item procedure that measures the extent to which an individual can say a word and then say what is left of that word after dropping out designated sounds. This test directly assesses phonemic awareness, a skill that is necessary for an individual to read and spell with accuracy. The Blending Words subtest is a 20-item procedure that measures an individual's ability to combine sounds to form words. The Memory for Digits subtest is a 21-item procedure that measures the extent to which an individual can repeat a series of numbers ranging in length from two to eight digits. The Nonword Repetition subtest measures an individual's ability to repeat nonsense words that range in length from 3 to 15 sounds. The Rapid Digit Naming subtest is a 72-item procedure that measures the speed with which an individual can name the numbers on two pages. The Rapid Letter Naming subtest measures the speed with which the examinee names letters of the alphabet. An individual's ability to rapidly name several items is often associated with reading accuracy and rate. The CTOPP has an average score of 10 and a standard deviation of +/−3 for each subtest. Composite scores are calculated for Phonological Awareness, Phonological Memory, and Rapid Naming. Each composite score is based on an average score of 100 and a standard deviation of +/−15.

W's scores on the phonological processing subtests ranged from average to the lower end of average. All of his composite scores, Phonological Awareness (combination of Elision and Blending Words subtests), Phonological Memory (combination of Memory for Digits and Nonword Repetition subtests), and Rapid Naming (combination of Rapid Digit Naming and Rapid Letter Naming subtests) were average for his age. However, his scores indicate a slight weakness in phonological memory. His CTOPP scores are shown in the following table.

Subtest	Standard Score	Percentile
Elision	11	63
Blending Words	10	50
Memory for Digits	10	50
Nonword Repetition	8	25
Rapid Digit Naming	11	63
Rapid Letter Naming	9	37
Phonological Awareness Composite	103	58
Phonological Memory Composite	94	35
Rapid Naming	100	50

Reading, Spelling, and Mathematic Skills

The Woodcock-Johnson-III Tests of Achievement (WJ-ACH-III) were administered to measure W's reading abilities for single-word reading, nonsense word decoding, and his math fluency and calculation. The Story Recall subtest measured W's ability to recall increasingly complex stories. The Word Attack subtest measured his ability to apply phonics skills in reading phonetically structured nonwords. The Reading Fluency subtest measured his ability to read and answer yes/no questions both quickly and accurately. The Spelling subtest evaluated W's knowledge of orthography and the Letter-Word Identification subtest measured his sight vocabulary. The Math Fluency subtest measured his automaticity in basic arithmetic while the Calculation subtest measured W's computational skills. The standard scores and percentile ranks reported for these tests are grade-based. The average score is 100 with a standard deviation of +/−15.

W's scores on the Letter-Word Identification and Word Attack subtests were in the high average range for his grade. His score on the Reading Fluency and Spelling subtests fell within the average range for his grade. However, spelling was significantly lower than all other achievement test scores. On the Story Recall subtest, W's score is in the superior range. An unexpected discrepancy is noted between W's performance on reading tests (first three tests) and his performance on story recall, a task of spoken language.

Subtest	Standard Score	Percentile Rank
Letter-Word Identification	113	81
Word Attack	112	79
Reading Fluency	106	66
Spelling	95	37
Story Recall	130	98

W's score on the Math Fluency subtest is in the average range while his score on the Calculation subtest is in the superior range for his grade. This unexpected discrepancy in math scores is likely due to the timed constraints of the math fluency test. W's scores are summarized in the following table.

Subtest	Standard Score	Percentile Rank
Math Fluency	97	41
Calculation	122	93

The Test of Word Reading Efficiency (TOWRE) was used to measure W's ability to pronounce printed words accurately and fluently in timed conditions. The Sight Word Efficiency subtest was used to measure W's ability to recognize familiar words as whole units (sight words). The Phonemic Decoding Efficiency subtest was used to measure W's ability to decode words. Both subtests assess the number of words read in 45 seconds. The average score is 100 with a standard deviation of +/–15.

W's scores on Sight Word Efficiency and Phonemic Decoding Efficiency ranged from average to above average. There was an unexpected discrepancy between sight words and phonemic decoding. The Total Word Reading score, converted from the sum standard scores, shows that W's overall word reading efficiency is average for his age and grade. The results are shown in the following table.

Subtest	Standard Score	Percentile Rank
Sight Word Efficiency	96	39
Phonemic Decoding Efficiency	112	79
Total Word Reading	**105**	**64**

On the Sight Word Efficiency subtest, W read 67 words correctly and 1 word incorrectly in 45 seconds. On the Phonemic Decoding Efficiency subtest, W read 43 words correctly and 5 words incorrectly in 45 seconds. For several words, W initially read the word incorrectly but was able to self-correct quickly. At the end of the 45-second time frame, when the words were increasing in difficulty, W was reading very few words correctly.

The Gray Oral Reading Test-4 (GORT-4) is a test used to assess reading Rate and Accuracy, Fluency (rate + accuracy), and Passage Comprehension. The GORT-4 consists of a series of stories beginning with the first grade level and progressing to advanced levels. W was asked to read a story aloud as quickly and accurately as possible. He was then asked to answer five multiple-choice questions related to the story. W's Fluency score was computed for the story by combining his scores obtained by rate (time taken to read the passage) and accuracy (the number of errors made). The mean score for these subtests is 10 with a standard deviation of +/–3.

W's score for reading Accuracy was within the average range for his age. His Rate, Fluency (rate + accuracy) and Passage Comprehension scores were in the higher end of the average range. W's scores are shown in the table below. The Oral Reading Quotient score (fluency + comprehension) of 115, which is a measure of W's overall reading ability, is high average, indicating that his reading fluency and reading comprehension are areas of strength.

Subtest	Standard Score	Percentile
Rate	12	75
Accuracy	11	63
Fluency (rate + accuracy)	12	75
Passage Comprehension	13	84
Oral Reading Quotient	115	84

Articulation

W did not exhibit any articulation errors in his speech.

Hearing Screening

W's hearing was not screened because his mother stated that he had been tested and his hearing was found within normal limits bilaterally. Mrs. P also notes that W prefers one ear over the other.

Observations

W was extremely cooperative during the evaluation. He displayed excellent attention to the tasks and he worked diligently throughout several hours of testing.

Evaluation Summary

W, a 10-year-old male, was seen at the University of Florida Speech and Hearing Clinic (UFSHC) on May 31, 2005, for an assessment of his reading, spelling, and oral language skills (Diagnostic Procedure Code: 92506 Evaluation of Speech and Language).

W's test percentiles range from the 3rd to 99th. He is extremely bright and clearly demonstrates this in his Thinking Ability (98th percentile) and Verbal Ability (76th percentile) composite scores on the WJ-III Test of Cognitive Abilities. In contrast, W's Cognitive Efficiency is depressed

(6th percentile). This lower composite score is due mainly to his slow processing speed on the task for Visual Matching.

W's reading scores, while in the normal range, were lower than expected when compared to his verbal and thinking ability scores on the WJ-III. Discrepancies between W's (1) average reading and high-average language scores and (2) high thinking and verbal ability scores and low cognitive efficiency score are typical of bright children who have a developmental history of difficulty with reading, spelling, and writing.

W's performance on the battery of tests suggests that his problems are consistent with a diagnosis of Developmental Dyslexia and Dysgraphia (Developmental Dyslexia Code: 315.02 and Dysgraphia Code: 315.4) (ICD-9-CM: World Health Organization International Classification of Diseases). W has compensated for these difficulties very well due, in large part, to his advanced reasoning skills and his excellent home instruction. Like many very bright individuals with dyslexia, W's reading scores do not fall outside the average range. The diagnosis is based on discrepancies between areas of strength and weakness that are characteristic of the individuals identified in the research literature as having "compensated dyslexia."

As reported in the *Annals of Dyslexia*, Volume 53, dyslexia is defined as

> a specific learning disability that is neurobiological in origin. It is characterized by difficulties with accurate and/or fluent word recognition and by poor spelling and decoding abilities. These difficulties typically result from a deficit in the phonological component of language that is often unexpected in relation to other cognitive abilities and the provision of effective classroom instruction. Secondary consequences may include problems in reading comprehension and reduced reading experience that can impede growth of vocabulary and background knowledge. (Lyon, Shaywitz, & Shaywitz, 2003)

As reported by the National Center for Learning Disabilities (www.ncld.org), dysgraphia is defined as "a learning disability that affects writing abilities. It can manifest itself as difficulties with spelling, poor handwriting, and trouble putting thought on paper."

A summary of W's scores for all tests administered on May 31, 2005 are presented in the next table followed by specific recommendations. Percentile rank scores indicate the percent of individuals his age that fall below the score reported for W. For example, a percentile rank of 25 on a test means that 25% of his peers have lower scores on this test, while 75% of his peers have higher scores.

Test	Subtest	Standard Score	Percentile Rank	Descriptive Rating
CTOPP	Elision	11	63	average
	Blending Words	10	50	average
Composite Score	**Phonological Awareness**	103	58	average
	Memory for Digits	10	50	average
	Nonword Repetition	8	25	lower end of average
Composite Score	**Phonological Memory**	94	35	average
	Rapid Digit Naming	11	37	average
	Rapid Letter Naming	9	63	average
Composite Score	**Rapid Naming**	100	50	average
WJ-III ACH	Spelling	95	37	average
	Word Attack	112	79	higher end of average
	Word Identification	113	81	high average
	Reading Fluency	106	66	average
	Math Fluency	97	41	average
	Math Calculation	122	93	superior
TOWRE	Sight Words	96	39	average
	Phonemic Decoding	112	79	higher end of average
	Total Word Reading	105	64	average
GORT-IV	Rate	12	75	higher end of average
	Accuracy	11	63	average
	Fluency	12	75	higher end of average
	Comprehension	13	84	high average
	Oral Reading Quotient	115	84	high average

WJ-COG-III	Verbal Comprehension	110	76	**average**
	Visual-Auditory Learning	125	95	**superior**
	Spatial Relations	109	73	**average**
	Sound Blending	115	84	**high average**
	Concept Formation	134	99	**superior**
	Visual Matching	71	3	**depressed**
	Numbers Reversed	91	28	**lower end of average**
Composite Score	**Verbal Ability**	110	76	**average**
Composite Score	**Thinking Ability**	132	98	**superior**
Composite Score	**Cognitive Efficiency**	76	6	**depressed**
Composite Score	**General Intelligence Ability**	112	80	**higher end of average**

Since W has a mild form of developmental dyslexia along with dysgraphia, academic accommodations and intervention will be extremely helpful in assisting him to achieve his full academic potential. W will continue to advance his reading, writing, and spelling skills, despite his developmental dyslexia and dysgraphia, if his educators understand the nature of his weaknesses and if appropriate accommodations are made to provide W with the optimal academic environment.

There is a high incidence of secondary emotional difficulties, such as frustration and depression, in students with learning disabilities who do not receive adequate accommodations. W would benefit from alternative instructional strategies and appropriate methods of reading and writing therapy, as well as appropriate support and further instruction in the areas in which he does well and enjoys. His noticeable difficulties certainly fit the pattern of mild dyslexia and dysgraphia. Therefore, intervention may be very beneficial.

In our clinic at the University of Florida, we have tested several gifted students with reading disabilities. We typically recommend that they

(a) be given extra time to take exams and to complete in-class assignments; (b) have access to a note-taker when in classes that require rapid recording of lecture material; and (c) be exempt from taking a foreign requirement (a most difficult task for persons with dyslexia) and take, instead, a comparable number of hours in courses with cultural content.

Below are some general guidelines that might be helpful in understanding how developmental dyslexia can impact the academic performance of students who are bright yet struggling to perform comparably with their peers.

- All of these students demonstrate depressed academic performance unexpectedly given their overall intellectual abilities. Even with academic accommodations, reading fluency, spelling, and writing fluency difficulties persist.

- These children typically do not show difficulty in listening (oral comprehension of language). Their problems are limited to processing language and other abstract symbols in the written form. Timed tests exacerbate their depressed academic performance. A much more accurate picture of their conceptual abilities will be expressed when they are tested orally as opposed to having them read material and then write their responses in a limited period of time.

- Many classroom assignments that require reading and writing will not be able to be completed in the amount of time given. We need to give these students extra time or allow them to complete their assignments at home.

- Often these children show inconsistent progress in subjects like math. Some math concepts, those that require less linguistic processing and greater visual-spatial processing, will be easier. It is expected that W will show stronger abilities in some math tasks than others. When gifted children are not learning a skill as quickly as expected, we need to find alternative ways to teach the concepts. They possess the conceptual ability to learn but need to have the information presented in an alternative manner.

- While they may squeeze through foreign languages with C grades, they always struggle with learning the symbols of a new language.

- Children who are gifted and insightful may internalize these difficulties and run the risk of moving away from careers in which they have a keen interest and an ability to function unless academic subject matter is presented appropriately and/or they are afforded the accommodations that are necessary for their academic success.

Based on our findings, we recommended that

1. W be allowed extra time on tests and other class work.

2. W could benefit from a multisensory phonics- and fluency-based instructional program.

Examples of programs are the Orton-Gillingham Program; Barton Reading and Spelling System.

A. The Orton-Gillingham approach is a comprehensive phonics-based language program that utilizes a multisensory approach including auditory, visual, and kinesthetic stimuli. This type of program would be beneficial in enhancing W's academic progress. This program will allow him to acquire advanced level phonics (sounds) and orthographic (spelling) skills that will improve his prognosis for academic success. W should attend therapy sessions implementing this program at least two to three times per week. Components of the Orton-Gillingham program are listed below:

- Reading and spelling vowels (long and short)

- Reading and spelling of basic syllable types

- Reading and spelling with common spelling rules

- Reading and spelling rules for syllabification

- Reading and spelling regular and irregular vowel teams

- Reading and spelling word roots and suffixes

- Applying this knowledge to oral reading and written composition

B. The Barton Reading and Spelling System is a tutoring program that parents, volunteer tutors, resource specialists, and professional tutors can use with children, teenagers, and adults who have a learning disability. It is an adapted and simplified version of the Orton-Gillingham approach to teaching reading and spelling. It includes fully scripted lesson plans, plus all reading material, spelling lists, homework pages and training videos.

Possible sources for these therapies include

1. A private speech-language pathologist trained in the Orton, Wilson, or Barton Reading Program in the Georgia area, W's new area of residence.

2. If entered in the regular school system, W should have a 504 plan developed for his academic needs.

3. W should spend time using the computer. The spell-check could be especially beneficial.

4. W's mother should read the information on developmental dyslexia and dysgraphia provided to her by the clinician.

5. W's mother should visit the Scottish Rite of Georgia Web site: http://www.gascottishrite.org.

* Report courtesy of Linda Lombardino.

■ REVIEW QUESTIONS

1. Which of the following statements characterizes learning syntax by a child with a reading disability?

   a. They have rapid bursts of learning followed by plateaus.
   b. They have a constant slow rate of learning syntax.
   c. Neither one of the above statements is true.

2. Which of the following statements is true?

   a. The parietal bank of the planum temporale translates sound into meaningful language.
   b. The temporal bank of the planum temporale processes visual and spatial information.
   c. The temporal bank of the planum temporale translates sound into meaningful language.

3. Which of the following methods of reading instruction is a multi-modality program of reading instruction that incorporates mouth form cards, the vowel circle, syllable construction, and reading charts?

   a. Lindamood Phoneme Sequencing Program
   b. Montessori Reading Method
   c. Barton
   d. Orton-Gillingham

4. Which of the following is not based on the Orton-Gillingham program of reading instruction?

   a. Lindamood Phoneme Sequencing Program
   b. Barton Reading and Spelling System
   c. Wilson Reading System
   d. Laubach Method of Reading Instruction

5. At what age do children typically learn about phoneme-grapheme correspondences and learn to decode?

   a. 3–5 years of age
   b. 5–7 years of age
   c. 8–10 years of age

6. Children's familiarity with nursery rhymes is a strong predictor of being a successful reader.

   a. True
   b. False

7. Accuracy-disabled readers are those children who, despite having decoding skills at grade appropriate levels, still have markedly poor reading.

   a. True
   b. False

8. There apparently is a genetic basis in reading disabilities.

   a. True
   b. False

9. Based on fMRI studies, cognitive and behavioral deficits commonly associated with dyslexia have not been linked to problematic activation patterns in posterior and anterior language regions of the brain.

   a. True
   b. False

10. In graduated prompting, assessment and treatment of reading disabilities occur concurrently.

    a. True
    b. False

■ REFERENCES

American Psychiatric Association. (1994). *Diagnostic and statistical manual of mental disorders-IV* (4th ed.). Washington, DC: Author.

Barton, S. (2000). *Barton Reading and Spelling System.* San Jose, CA: Bright Solutions for Dyslexia, LLC/.

Blachman, B. A. (1994). Early literacy acquisition: The role of phonological awareness. In G. P. Wallach & K. G. Butler (Eds.), *Language-learning disabilities in school-age children and adolescents: Some principles and applications* (pp. 253–274). New York: Macmillan Publishers.

Buchanan, M., Weller, C., & Buchanan, M. (1997). *Special education desk reference.* San Diego: Singular Publishing Group.

Catts, H. W. (1989). Speech production deficits and reading disabilities. *Journal of Speech and Hearing Disorders, 54,* 422–428.

Catts, H. W., Fey, M. D., Zhang, X., & Tomblin, J. B. (1999). Language bases of reading and reading disabilities: Evidence from a longitudinal investigation. *Scientific Studies of Reading, 3,* 331–362.

Catts, H. W., & Kamhi, A. G. (1999). *Language and reading disabilities.* Boston: Allyn and Bacon.

Catts, H. W., and Kamhi, A. G. (2005). *Language and reading disabilities* (2nd ed.). Boston: Allyn and Bacon.

Catts, H. W., Wilcox, K. A., Wood-Jackson, C., Larrivee, L. S., & Scott, V. G. (1997). Toward an understanding of phonological awareness. In C. K. Leong & R. M. Joshi (Eds.). *Cross-language studies of learning to read and spell: Phonologic and orthographic processing.* Dordecht: Kluwer Academic Press.

Chall, J. (1983). *Stages of reading development.* New York: McGraw-Hill.

Dunn, L., & Dunn, L. (1997). *Peabody Picture Vocabulary Test*-III. Circle Pines, MN: American Guidance Service.

Galaburda, A. M. (1989). Ordinary and extraordinary brain development: Anatomical variations in developmental dyslexia. *Annals of Dyslexia, 39,* 67–79.

Gauger, L. M., Lombardino, L. J., & Leonard, C. M. (1997, December). Brain morphology in children with specific language impairment. *Journal of Speech, Language, and Hearing Research, 40,* 1272–1284.

Goldsworthy, C. L. (1996). *Developmental reading disabilities: A language-based treatment approach.* San Diego: Singular Publishing Group.

Goodman, K. S. (1973). Analysis of oral reading miscues: Applied psycholinguistics. In F. Smith (Ed.), *Psycholinguistics and reading* (pp. 158–176). New York: Holt, Rinehart and Winston.

Gough, P., & Tunmer, W. (1986). Decoding, reading, and reading disability. *Remedial and Special Education, 7,* 6–10.

Greene, V. E., & Enfield, M. L. (1991). *Project Read.* Bloomington, MN: Language Circle Enterprise.

Hammill, D., Brown, V., Larsen, S., & Wiederholt. J. (1994). *Test of adolescent and adult language-3.* Austin, TX: Pro-Ed.

Hammill, D., & Newcomer, P. (1997). *Test of language development-intermediate-3.* Austin, TX: Pro-Ed.

Hegde, M. N. (1996a). *PocketGuide to assessment in speech-language pathology.* San Diego: Singular Publishing Group.

Hegde, M. N. (1996b). *A coursebook on language disorders in children.* San Diego: Singular Publishing Group.

Hynd, G. (1991, March). Brain morphology as it is related to learning disabilities. Lecture at the 1991 G. Paul Moore Symposium, Gainesville, FL.

Hynd, G., Semrud-Clikeman, M., Lorys, A., Novey, E., & Eliopulos, D. (1990). Brain morphology in developmental dyslexia and attention deficit disorder/hyperactivity. *Archives of Neurology, 47,* 919–926.

Justice, L. M., Chow, S., Capellini, C., Flanigan, K., Colton, S. (2003, August). Emergent literacy intervention for vulnerable preschoolers: Relative effects of two approaches. *American Journal of Speech-Language Pathology, 12*(3), 320–332.

Kamhi, A. G., & Catts, H. W. (1989). *Reading disabilities: A developmental language perspective.* Boston: College-Hill Press.

Laing, S. P., & Kamhi, A. (2003, January). Alternative assessment of language and literacy in culturally and linguistically diverse populations. *Language, Speech, and Hearing Services in the Schools, 34*(1), 44–66.

Laing, S., Kamhi, A. G., & Catts, H. W. (1997, November). Dynamic assessment of phonological awareness in school-age children. Paper presented at the annual convention of the American Speech-Language-Hearing Association. Boston.

LeGrand, H. (1997). Unpublished manuscript. Gainesville, FL.

Leonard, C. M. (1998). Language, In H. Cohen (Ed.), *Neuroscience for rehabilitation* (2nd ed., Chap. 17). Philadelphia: Lippincott-Raven.

Leonard, C. M., Voeller, K. K. S., Lombardino, L. J., Morris, M. K., Hynd, G. W., Alexander, A. W., Andersen, H. G., Garofalakis, M., Honeyman, J. C., Mao, J., Agee, F., & Staab, E. V. (1993). Anomalous cerebral structure in dyslexia revealed with magnetic resonance imaging. *Archives of Neurology, 50,* 461–469.

Lidz, C. S., & Pena, E. D. (1996). Dynamic assessment: The model, its relevance as a nonbiased approach, and its application in Latino-American preschool children. *Language, Speech, and Hearing Services in the Schools, 27,* 367–377.

Light, J. G., & DeFries, J. G. (1995). Comorbidity of reading and mathematical disabilities: Genetic and environmental etiologies. *Journal of Learning Disabilities, 28,* 96–106.

Lindamood, C. H. & Lindamood, P. C. (1979). *Lindamood auditory conceptualization test.* Allen, TX: DLM Teaching Resources.

Lindamood, P., & Lindamood, P. (1998). *Lindamood phoneme sequencing program for reading, spelling, and speech.* Circle Pines, MN: American Guidance Service Publishing.

Livesay, Y. (1995). Dyslexia and reading instruction: Presented to California educators, legislators, and advocates. *Answers, 1,* 1–8.

Lombardino, L. J. (1998). Unpublished manuscript. Gainsville, FL.

Lombardino, L. J., Lieberman, R. J., & Brown, J. C. (2005). *Assessment of literacy and language.* San Antonio, TX: Harcourt Assessment.

Lombardino, L. J., Ricco, C. A., Hynd, G., & Pinheiro, S. B. (1997), Linguistic deficits in children with reading disabilities. *American Journal of Speech-Language Pathology, 6*(3), 71–78.

Lovett, M. W. (1987). A development approach to reading disability: Accuracy and speed criteria of normal and deficient reading skill. *Child Development, 58,* 234–260.

Lyon, R. (1995). Toward a definition of dyslexia. *Annals of Dyslexia, 45,* 3–30.

Lyon, G. R., Shaywitz, S. E., & Shaywitz, B. A. (2003). A definition of dyslexia. *Annals of Dyslexia, 53,* 1–14.

Mann, V. A., Tobin, P., & Wilson, R. (1987). Measuring phonological awareness through the invented spellings of kindergarten children. *Merrill-Palmer Quarterly, 33,* 365–389.

Naremore, R. C., Densmore, A. E., & Harman, D. R. (1995). *Language intervention with school-age children: Conversation, narrative, and text.* San Diego: Singular Publishing Group.

Nelson, N. W. (1998). *Childhood language disorders in context: Infancy through adolescence.* New York: Merrill/Macmillan Publishing Company.

Newcomer, & Hammill (1988). *Test of language development-intermediate 2.* Austin, TX: Pro-Ed.

Newcomer, & Hammill (1997). *Test of language development-primary-3.* Austin, TX: Pro-Ed.

Owens, R. E. (1999). *Language disorders: A functional approach to assessment and intervention* (3rd ed.). Boston: Allyn and Bacon.

Owens, R. E. (2004). *Language disorders: A functional approach to assessment and intervention* (4th ed.). Boston: Allyn and Bacon.

Riccio, C. A., & Hynd, G. W. (1996). Neuroanatomical and neurophysiological aspects of dyslexia. *Topics in Language Disorders, 16*(2), 1–13.

Rosner, J. (1975). Rosner test of auditory analysis. In *Helping Children Overcome Learning Disabilities.* New York: Walker and Company.

Robertson, C., & Salter, W. (1995). *The phonological awareness test.* East Moline, IL: LinguiSystems.

Scarborough, H. S. (1990). Very early language deficits in dyslexic children. *Child Development, 61*, 1728–1743.

Scarborough, H. S. (2000, September). *Predictive and causal links between language and literact development: Current knowledge and future directions.* Paper presented at the Workshop on Emergent and Early Literacy: Current Status and Research Directions, Rockville, MD.

Shaywitz, S. E. (2003). *Overcoming dyslexia: A new and complete science-based program of reading problems at any level.* New York: Alfred A. Knopf.

Shaywitz, S. E., Shaywitz, B. A., Pugh, I. R., Fulbright, R. K., Constable, R. T., Mencel. W. E., Shankweiler, D. P., Liberman, A. M., Skudlarski, P., Fletcher, J. M., Katz, L., Marchione, K. E., Lacadie, C., Gatenby C., & Gore, J. C. (1998). Functional disruption in the organization of the brain for reading in dyslexia. *Neurobiology, 95*, 2636–2641.

Siegel, L. S. (1992). An evaluation of the discrepancy definition of dyslexia. *Journal of Learning Disabilities, 25*, 618–629.

Slingerland, B. (1977). *A multi-sensory approach to language arts for specific language disability children.* Cambridge, MA: Educators Publishing Service.

Stanovich, K. E. (1991). Discrepancy definitions of reading disability: Has intelligence led us astray? *Reading Research Quarterly, 26*, 1–29.

Stanovich, K. E. (1994). Romance and reality. *The Reading Teacher, 47*, 280–290.

Tierney, R. J., & Cunningham, J. W. (1984). Research on teaching reading comprehension. In P. D. Pearson (Ed.), *Handbook of reading research* (pp. 609–655). New York: Longman.

Torgesen, J. K. (1999). Assessment and instruction for phonemic awareness and word recognition skills. In H. W. Catts and A. G. Kamhi, *Language and Reading Disabilities.* Boston: Allyn and Bacon.

Torgesen, J. K., & Bryant, B. (1997). *The comprehensive test of phonological processes in reading.* Austin, TX: Pro-Ed.

Torgesen, J. K., & Wagner, R. K. (1997). *Test of word and nonword reading efficiency.* Austin, TX: Pro-Ed.

Vygotsky, L. (1978). *Mind in society: The development of higher psychological processes.* Cambridge, MA: Harvard University Press.

Wagner, R., Torgesen, J., & Rashotte, C. (1999). *Comprehensive test of phonological processing.* San Antonio, TX: The Psychological Corporation.

Wiederholt, J. L., & Bryant, B. R. (2001). *Gray oral reading tests,* 4th ed. Austin, TX: Pro-Ed.

Wiig, E. H., & Semel, E. (1984). *Language assessment and intervention for the learning disabled* (2nd ed.). New York: Merrill.

Wilkinson, J. S. (1995). *The wide range achievement test-3.* Wilmington, DE: Jastak Associates.

Wilson, B. (1988). *Wilson language training.* Millbury, MA: Author.

Wong, B. Y., & Jones, W. (1982). Increasing metacomprehension in learning disabled and normally achieving students through self-questioning training. *Learning Disability Quarterly, 5,* 228–240.

Woodcock, R. W. (1997). *Woodcock reading mastery test-rev.* Circle Pines, MN: American Guidance Service.

Woodcock, R. W., McGrew, K. S., & Mather, N. (2001). *Woodcock-Johnson tests of cognitive abilities-3rd ed.* Itasca, IL: Riverside Publishing.

Yopp, H. K. (1999). A test for assessing phonemic awareness in young children. *The Reading Teacher, 49,* 20–29.

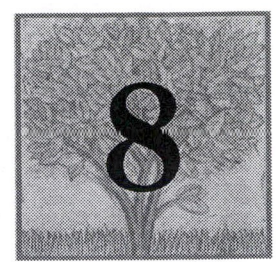

Attention Deficit Disorder and Attention Deficit Disorder with Hyperactivity

■ LEARNING OBJECTIVES

After completion of this chapter, the reader will be able to

1. Explain the relationship between attention deficit disorder (ADD)/ attention deficit with hyperactivity disorder (ADHD) and language-based learning disabilities.

2. Explain some of the brain activities typically associated with the areas believed to be damaged in children with ADD/ADHD.

3. Explain the statement, "ADHD is not about paying attention; rather, it is about controlling attention."

4. Explain the role of cognition and processing in the assessment and treatment of ADD/ADHD.

5. Explain why achievement testing is considered part of the assessment process in children with ADD/ADHD.

6. Discuss why problems with focal and associative control would impact problem solving.

7. Describe the typical language skills of children with ADD/ADHD.

8. Explain the behaviors and symptoms associated with each of the seven types of control systems.

■ INTRODUCTION

Hyperkinetic. Persistent and exaggerated motor movements.

Up until 1980, attention deficit hyperactivity disorder (ADHD) was known by a variety of terms such as Still's syndrome, Strauss syndrome, **hyperkinetic** syndrome, and hyperkinetic impulse syndrome.

It is estimated that 3% to 5% of school children in North America are diagnosed as having attention deficit disorder with hyperactivity (ADHD). The prevalence in adults is unknown. ADD and ADHD are nine times more common in boys than in girls (Sattler, 1988), although in adults, the sex ratio of identified ADHD is almost equal (Nelson, 1993; Arnold, 2002).

The relationship of ADD/ADHD to language disorders in children is receiving much attention in the literature. There are not any clear-cut relationships between the two disorders, yet some children are being seen who have a co-morbidity of language-based learning disabilities, auditory processing disorders, and ADD/ADHD. In fact, it is estimated that 20% to 30% of children with confirmed ADD/ADHD "have at least one type of learning disability in math, reading, or spelling" (Barkley, 2000, p. 98). However, it should be noted that ADHD does not cause the reading problem; rather, they are two separate problems, each with their own causative agents (Catts & Kamhi, 1999). The ADHD may impact reading, particularly silent reading comprehension, but, again, the ADHD is not the cause of the reading problem (Shaywitz et al., 1995).

Rutter, Tizard, and Whitmore (1970) studied the presence of learning, neurological, and psychiatric disorders in a group of children on the Isle of Wight and found that children who had "overt behavior disorders" had significant learning problems, particularly in the area of reading. Twenty-five percent of the children in their study who had reading disabilities also had a psychiatric behavioral disorder such as ADHD, ADD, or oppositional disorders. The effects of ADD/ADHD on language and learning can clearly make an impact on a child's academic and social success in school.

In the classroom, teachers rely on students' being able to attend to what is being taught. Therefore, teaching students to pay attention and process information as it is presented is critical to learning. For most children, this is learned through incidental teaching as teachers make comments like, "I like the way you are listening." However, for many children with learning disabilities, learning to control attention becomes almost a subject in and of itself. This is particularly true for children who have ADD or ADHD.

If a child is unable to attend in class, his or her schoolwork will fall behind and the child may face adverse ramifications in terms of academic and social progress. As stated in Chapter 6, poor academic and social adjustment often lead to low self-esteem in school-age children, particularly in the late elementary and middle school years. Therefore, it is even more critical that these children be afforded instruction that focuses on developing their ability to learn internal control and organization so that they can attend to the task at hand in academic and social settings.

While attending to the task at hand and overactivity are the most frequently assigned symptoms of various forms of ADHD, Arnold (2002) writes that impulsivity is the unifying symptom of all types of ADHD. He further notes the following:

> Patients with the disorder act before they think, react before they think, speak before they think, and even think before they think, jumping to conclusions prematurely. (p. 8)

Arnold goes on to say that there is some preliminary evidence that ordinary activities are not as inherently rewarding as they are for the patient's peers.

■ DEFINITION OF ADD AND ADHD

ADHD is best defined in terms of what it is and what it is not. ADHD is not just a behavior management problem. It is not a learning disability, nor is it an auditory processing disorder. Most importantly, it is not a label to be randomly applied to any child who has trouble sitting still or paying attention.

Children with ADD without hyperactivity are typically described as not having as many problems with aggression, hyperactivity, and impulsivity as do children with ADHD. Also, children with ADD do not usually have as many relationship problems with other children when compared to children with ADHD. In a study reported by Barkley and his colleagues, it was found that children with ADD "performed much worse on tests involving perceptual-motor speed or eye-hand coordination and speed. They also made more mistakes on a memory test. In particular, they had more trouble consistently recalling information they had learned as time passed" (Barkley, 2000, pp. 137–138).

ADD/ADHD is an inability to maintain focused, selected attention. It is thought to be related to disruptions in transmission and metabolism along subcortical pathways connecting the midbrain to the prefrontal cortex. These are the areas of the brain that play roles in executive functioning tasks such as directing attention, self-regulation, organizing information, making and executing an action plan, and inhibiting inappropriate actions. These skills are problematic in children with ADD/ADHD and frequently lead to a misdiagnosis of the child as being lazy, unmotivated, and disruptive.

Children with ADHD have more conduct and behavior problems than do children with ADD. They also are more impulsive and are reported to be less anxious than children with ADD. Children with ADD tend to be more shy and withdrawn than children with ADHD. Problems with social status and peer acceptance are critical areas of concern about children with ADHD. Socialization is hindered by "intrusiveness and sometimes aggression resulting from hyperactivity and impulsiveness, coupled with inattentiveness to social cues" (Arnold, 2002, p. 18).

Learning differences also exist between the two groups. According to Arnold (2002), 20% to 25% of children who have ADHD also have learning disorders. Children with ADD show higher co-morbidity of learning disabilities and more underachievement, particularly in mathematics. They are also slower on rapid naming tasks than are children with ADHD (Cantwell & Baker, 1992; Edelbrock, Costello, & Kessler, 1984; Hynd et al., 1991; Lahey et al., 1984; Lahey et al., 1987).

■ ADD/ADHD AND OTHER LABELS

Children with ADHD historically were labeled as having hyperactive child syndrome, as being hyperkinetic, or as having minimal brain dysfunction. Often, children with ADD have many features in common with children who are learning disabled; in fact, in many children with ADD, learning disabilities coexist (Hynd et al., 1991). Regardless of whether a child is learning disabled or has ADD or ADHD, multiple professions are involved in diagnosing and treating the child. The participation of more than one professional in diagnosis is often due to the fact that the child with ADD or ADHD typically presents a multiplicity of problems. The child's impulsivity may be misinterpreted as a behavior management problem. Problems with affective control and delayed gratification can be mislabeled as immaturity and/or noncompliance. Therefore, many negative labels can be applied to a child who is not properly diagnosed as having ADD or ADHD and can lead to disruption in the child's home and academic life.

In addition, as with learning disabilities, ADD and ADHD have complex effects on families. The parents are frequently called to the school because the child is not living up to the expectations of the academic system. It should be pointed out that some children with ADD can be so retiring that they "blend into the wallpaper" and are mislabeled as overly shy (Edelbrock, Costello, and Kessler, 1984; Hynd et al., 1991). However, these children will also suffer socially and academically because of the same types of problems demonstrated in children in whom the ADD or ADHD is more overt. The "wallpaper children" are often found to have only a few friends and to be at risk academically even though they are not "troublemakers," which is how many children with ADHD are labeled. Parents are confused as to why the child does not try harder or why the child continues to misbehave in the presence of negative consequences of the misbehaviors. Some parents feel embarrassed because their child causes a problem in the classroom, and others are ashamed because their child is not living up to the expectations of the teacher or performing at a level appropriate to his or her age, education, and family background. Thus, the time prior to the diagnosis of ADD or ADHD can be more frustrating for families than knowing the child's diagnosis. As upsetting as the diagnosis of ADD or ADHD can be, the definitive diagnosis at least offers an explanation for the child's academic and/or social difficulties.

Uncertainties regarding the cause and prognosis of ADD and ADHD can also have a debilitating effect on families. The parents tend to blame themselves or each other, which can produce tension in a home that is, most likely, already experiencing a high level of stress because of the child's difficulties. Also, fear about the future can create emotional turmoil in the families. It is absolutely critical that families receive adequate counseling regarding ADD and ADHD so that they have an understanding of the symptoms of the disorders and learn methods of managing the ADD or ADHD.

Parent support groups can be helpful. In one parent support group meeting, several parents complained that the worst part of the day was the time between when the child woke up and when he or she walked out the door to go to school. Frequently, there were delays in getting dressed, the child forgot to brush his teeth, and got half-way to school only to realize that something (lunch, homework, coat) had been left at home. The parents shared strategies that they had found helpful, and they all benefited from this type of sharing. One parent recorded morning instructions for her child on a WalkMan. The child was able to listen to the tape with its constant reminders regarding what he should be doing guiding him through the morning activities. Both parents found it much easier to provide the constant reminders via the audiotape than it was to keep going to the child's room to remind him of what he was supposed to be doing. Another mother made a checklist that hung in the child's room. Once everything was checked off, the child went to the kitchen for breakfast and then checked another list by the front door to be sure he had done all he was supposed to do, and that he had everything he was supposed to take to school.

It is important to keep the lines of communication open between the families and the school personnel and with any other professionals who may be providing therapy for the child. When a strategy is found that is effective with a child, everyone involved should share in its implementation to ensure consistency in how the child's problems are handled in different settings. This consistency is essential in developing the internal control that many children with ADD and ADHD lack.

■ WHAT CAUSES ADD/ADHD?

Although it is difficult to pinpoint one cause of ADHD, there are several factors under consideration as being causative. For example, there is some evidence to suggest that a mother who smokes or drinks during her pregnancy will have a child with increased risk of inattention and hyperactivity. Some children who suffer from a traumatic brain injury or other neurological events may also show signs of ADHD (Barkley, 2000). This is particularly true in instances where the brain injury occurs in the frontal lobe which regulates many of the behaviors and executive functions that are typically problematic for individuals with ADHD.

Although most children who have signs of ADHD do not have a history of significant brain injuries, one cannot help but be struck by the fact that for many children with ADHD there is a history of pregnancy and/or birth complications. However, not all children who have a history of pregnancy and/or birth complications will develop ADHD. In fact, less than 10% of children with ADHD have any history of brain injury; disruptions in the development of the brain, particularly the frontal cortex, seem to be a more likely explanation (Barkley, 2000). According to Arnold (2002), there is a high incidence of genetic predisposition in most cases of ADHD. Problems associated with two dopamine genes (the dopamine transporter gene (DAT1) and the D4 dopamine receptor gene have been noted in many cases of ADHD. Clinical evidence of the involvement of these genes is supported by the fact that individuals who have ADHD and are treated with drugs to enhance the neurotransmission of dopamine typically show some resolution or lessening of the symptoms (Arnold, 2002).

■ THREE CATEGORIES OF SYMPTOMS OF ADD/ADHD

There are three categories of symptoms of ADD/ADHD: control and regulation of attention, impulsivity, and activity. Following is a discussion of each of these categories (American Psychological Association, 1994).

Control and Regulation of Attention

In ADD and ADHD, controlling attention, not paying attention, is the problem. Paying attention implies the presence or absence of attention, or both; controlling attention refers to the ability to stay on task by focusing selectively on the appropriate stimuli. Everything is equally important to the child with ADD or ADHD, and he or she cannot isolate and focus on the important issues.

The academic impact of being unable to focus attention is that the child cannot determine what the important facts and activities are and channel his or her attention accordingly. As discussed previously, this also leads to free-flight associations and the answering of questions in an unexpected manner. It can also be problematic for these children because when they know the answer, they are likely to burst out with the reply without following the traditional rules of raising their hands and waiting to be called on. In the time children with ADD or ADHD spend waiting to be called on, they will probably forget the answer. Therefore, in an attempt to answer correctly, they blurt out the answer without waiting.

With regard to the social impact, the child who is labeled as having ADD or ADHD is often perceived as rude and uncaring by his or her peers. Because of the problems with associative control, he or she is likely to have pragmatic problems that interfere with being a good communication partner. These pragmatic problems include speaking out of turn, failing to maintain a topic, and topic switching inappropriately.

Impulsivity

Impulsivity is defined as the neurological inability to sustain inhibition. Impulsivity, then, has no premeditation or malicious intent. The child does not think before acting. Behaviors "just happen" and the child usually is unable to explain why they occurred or demonstrate understanding of the consequences of the action. Academically, impulsivity results in the child's being disorganized in his or her overt academic activities and in his or her thought processes. Socially, impulsivity makes the child always want to be first—to always be the winner. Because of affective control problems, this child is likely to act out inappropriately when he or she loses, which, as with so many aspects of this disorder, affects the child's interaction with his or her peers. In fact, many children with ADD or ADHD are described by their parents as having no friends. Impulsivity also impacts negatively on the child's ability to delay gratification.

Activity

Some children with ADD are underactive and the ADD may go undetected until fourth or fifth grade. At that time, their academic and social frustrations are likely to be expressed through behavior problems and failure to succeed in school. These children would benefit from having teachers who are aware of possible warning signs of ADD and can monitor them as soon as any soft signs indicative of ADD are noticed. These soft signs would include not finishing school work, crying excessively, laughing excessively, not living up to the academic potential, and not having many friends.

In contrast, the child who is overactive may be labeled a "motor mouth" and described as fidgety and being unable to sit still. The child with ADHD is identified much earlier than the child with ADD because of the hyperactive component. However, it is important for the child to be tested carefully before the label of ADHD is applied. As stated previously, ADHD is not a label to be applied automatically to all children who have difficulty sitting still in school.

■ SEVEN FRAGILE CONTROL SYSTEMS

For a child to attend to a task, he or she must develop internal control and organization, much as was discussed in Chapter 2 in the section on babies born to mothers who are drug abusers. Twelve control systems have been documented, but this discussion will be limited to seven systems.

Focal control. The ability to select what is important and attend to that over all other distractions and information.

A major problem for children with ADD and ADHD is **focal control**. Focal control is the ability to select what is important and attend to that over all other distractions and information (Heyer, n.d.). For example, in a traditional classroom, noises include paper shuffling, pencils tapping, and students moving around. Children with ADD cannot focus their attention on what is important (i.e., the teacher's talking) and tune out the insignificant noises. Also, when they do pay attention to the correct stimulus, it is likely that, as the teacher is talking, they will not attend to what the teacher is saying even though it may be important. That is to say, everything is of equal importance to the child with ADD/ADHD.

As a result of poor focal control, the child has to work hard at concentrating on what is being said in the classroom. This effort is called **mental effort control**. Because it takes so much mental effort to focus on what is important, may children with ADD or ADHD experience mental fatigue. Then, the tiredness coupled with the lack of focal control compounds the child's difficulties in learning in the classroom (Heyer, n.d.).

A third control system that poses problems for the child with ADD or ADHD is **associative control**. Associative control is what enables people to maintain a conversation by stating issues that are relevant to the conversation (Heyer, n.d.). A child with ADD or ADHD will have free-flight ideas during conversational exchanges, with these free-flight ideas being tangential to the content and intent of the conversation.

Table 8–1 contains a transcript of a child with ADD. The conversation started with the clinician's asking the child about her red fingernail polish. As can be seen from the transcript, most of what the child said was somewhat related to the color red, but each contribution to the conversation was a tangential thought. We can see the tangential relationships with the red possibly reminding her of the tomato sauce on the pizza, and the sauce reminding her of the tomatoes in her grandmother's garden. Similarly, watering the garden reminded her of the river, and the river is associated with the boat and swimming lessons. However, the original conversation, which was to be about the fingernail polish, never developed.

Children who have problems with associative control are also likely to answer questions correctly, but not as expected. For example, if the child is asked,

Mental effort control. Work at concentrating, resulting in mental fatigue when excess energy is expended on focal control.

Associative control. Control that enables a person to maintain a conversation by stating issues that are relevant to the conversation.

TABLE 8–1. Conversation with a child with deficits in associative control.*

T:	I really like your red fingernail polish. Who painted them for you?
C:	Mom
T:	Your mom fixed your fingernails. Were you playing dress up?
C:	We had pizza for supper.
T:	You had pizza for supper. Was it good?
C:	My grandmother has a garden with tomatoes in it.
T:	Did your grandmother eat pizza with you?
C:	No, she has a garden with tomatoes and she waters the garden. She lives at the river.
T:	Your grandmother lives on the river. That must be fun.
C:	My grandpa has a boat and we took swim lessons.

*T, therapist; C, child.

Appetite control. The ability to delay gratification, which is typically problematic for children with ADHD.

"What is your name?" the child is likely to say, "The same as my mother's," which may be correct, but it not what is expected in the way of an answer.

The fourth type of control is called **appetite control**, but it does not have anything to do with eating! Rather, appetite control is the ability to **delay gratification**, which is difficult for individuals with ADD or ADHD.

Delayed gratification. The ability to continue providing the correct and expected behaviors even when a delay exists between the response and the provision of reinforcement.

Delayed gratification refers to the ability to continue providing the correct and expected behaviors even when a delay exists between the response and the provision of reinforcement. Children with ADD expect immediate reinforcement, and this can be problematic in the classroom. Many times, children with appetite control problems are considered noncompliant because they have so much difficulty following rules when gratification is not offered immediately (Heyer, n.d.). Problems with peers also may develop because the child with ADD or ADHD may not be able to meet behavioral criteria that have been set for the class to receive positive reinforcement. For example, a teacher may say that the class will have a party on Friday if all the students complete their work in a timely manner on Wednesday and Thursday. The child with ADD or ADHD may not be able to complete the work, and furthermore, he or she may not be able to delay the gratification for two days if the work is complete. Thus, the party is at risk for his or her classmates, with the child with ADD or ADHD becoming a culprit if he or she does not complete the work in the specified time period.

Behavior control. Impulsive behavior due to a poorly organized central nervous system.

Behavior control is another control system that creates difficulty for a child with ADHD. A child with ADHD may be totally impulsive (Cantwell & Baker, 1992; Heyer, n.d.; Lahey et al., 1987). This, again, is due to a lack of organization of the central nervous system, particularly the parts of the nervous system that control impulsivity.

Complicating the issue is the fact that many children with ADD or ADHD cannot predict the consequences of their actions (Heyer, n.d.). Thus, telling a child he or she should not perform a certain behavior because of the resultant negative reactions may be futile, which makes behavior management techniques very difficult. ADD and ADHD are not diagnosed solely on the basis of behavior management problems. Due to the other symptoms of ADD and ADHD, such as impulsivity, poor quality control, and poor internal control systems, the use of traditional behavior management techniques often is ineffective with these individuals.

Affective control. Inappropriate affect and expression of emotions.

A sixth type of control issue for children with ADD and ADHD is **affective control**. Many of these children have inappropriate affect; they laugh too much and cry too much (Heyer, n.d.; Weintraub & Mesulam, 1983).

When a joke is told, or something funny happens in class, the child is likely to laugh out of proportion to the silliness or to laugh inappropriately at incidental behaviors. Likewise, when something sad or disappointing occurs, the child is likely to cry uncontrollably. A fifth grade boy who was in therapy at the University of Florida Speech and Hearing Clinic had particular difficulty with uncontrollable crying when he became frustrated with the task. Compounding the problem for him was his embarrassment at crying in front of the student clinician. Therefore, a system was worked out whereby he would put his head down on the table when he was going to cry, the student clinician would excuse herself, and the supervisor would help the child work through his frustration. Eventually, the crying subsided and he was able to deal with his frustrations in a positive manner with the student clinician.

The final control system to be discussed in the context of ADD/ADHD is **quality control**, which refers to a person's ability to provide an explanation for his or her own actions.

Quality control. A person's ability to provide an explanation for his or her own actions.

Many children with ADD or ADHD cannot explain their actions, particularly those that occur impulsively. Frequently reminding a child of the potential consequences of his or her behavior is ineffective because the child cannot predict the consequences of that behavior. Also, children with ADD or ADHD often cannot control their behavior, so it becomes difficult for them to explain whey they behaved in a particular way (Heyer, n.d.). For example, the child with ADD or ADHD typically likes to be first at everything, including lining up. If another child gets in front of him or her, he or she is likely to push the other child. When asked why he or she pushed the other child, the child with ADD or ADHD most likely will respond with, "I don't know—I just did it." These kinds of responses are very frustrating for parents and teachers to hear, but the truth is that the child truly does not know why he or she pushed the other child because it was an impulsive action.

It is easy to see how problems with these seven control systems can interfere significantly with the academic and social progression of a child with ADD or ADHD. They also lead to labeling and mislabeling.

■ DIAGNOSING ADD AND ADHD

The diagnosis of ADHD in a child requires the input of a diagnostic team made up of psychiatrists, psychologists, educators, and speech-language pathologists. Newhoff (1986, 1990) supported the participation of speech-language pathologists on the team due to the co-morbidity previously mentioned. Psychiatrists should be involved in the diagnosis of ADHD since many of these children will receive medications to help control the symptoms, and as many as 45% of children who are diagnosed with ADHD will also have another psychiatric problem such as depression, anxiety, and/or low self-esteem. Psychologists are involved in the diagnosis through the administration of tests such as the Weschler Intelligence Scale for Children-Revised

(1974). They have found that while children with ADHD earn scaled scores of 10 to 13 on most subtests, they typically score 6 or 7 on those subtests that relied on selective attention (digit span, arithmetic, coding, and mazes) (Newhoff, 1986). Educators and parents can provide information on the child's behavior and attitudes that may result from ADHD and are observed in the child's natural settings.

The *Diagnostic and Statistical Manual of Mental Disorders-IV* (American Psychiatric Association, 1994) suggests that ADD has two dimensions: (1) hyperactivity with impulsivity and (2) inattention. The DSM-IV describes three subtypes of ADD and ADHD:

1. ADHD with inattention, in which a child must have six of the nine inattention symptoms listed in Table 8–2. This classification does not include the specified number of hyperactivity or impulsivity symptoms;

2. ADHD with hyperactivity and impulsivity, in which the child must have four of the six hyperactivity or impulsivity symptoms, but not the specified number of inattention symptoms;

3. ADHD combined type, in which the child meets the criteria for hyperactivity or impulsivity and inattention (Morgan et al., 1996).

Objectives of the Evaluation

The child who comes to the speech-language pathologist is probably being seen to determine if a language-based learning disability is present. Therefore, the evaluation of the child by the speech-language pathologist is exclusionary. That is, the speech-language pathologist is trying to determine if the child's academic and social problems are due to the presence of a language-based learning disability. If no language-based learning disability is present, the clinician can make observations based on the child's performance in the evaluation session that can help to confirm or reject a possible diagnosis of ADD or ADHD.

As with all other evaluations, the first question to be asked of the referral source is, "What do you want me to answer as a result of this evaluation?" If the answer is, "I want to know if my child has ADD," it is necessary to explain to the parent or referral source that you, as the speech-language pathologist, will not be able to make the definitive diagnosis of ADD. What you can do is determine if the child has a language-based learning disability and analyze the child's learning style and behaviors to see if signs and symptoms of ADD or ADHD are present. If necessary, appropriate referrals can then be made to other professionals who should be involved in the diagnosis of ADD or ADHD.

TABLE 8–2. DSM-IV criteria for attention deficit/hyperactivity disorder.

A Either (1) or (2)

(1) Six (or more) of the following symptoms of inattention have persisted for at least 6 months to a degree that is maladaptive and inconsistent with developmental level:

Inattention

(a) Often fails to give close attention to details or makes careless mistakes in school work, homework, or other activities

(b) Often has difficulty sustaining attention in tasks or play activities

(c) Often does not seem to listen when spoken to directly

(d) Often does not follow through on instructions and fails to finish schoolwork, chores, or duties in the workplace (not due to oppositional behavior or failure to understand instructions)

(e) Often has difficulty organizing tasks and activites

(f) Often avoids, dislikes, or is reluctant to engage in tasks that require sustained mental effort, such as schoolwork or homework

(g) Often loses things necessary for tasks or activities (e.g., toys, school assignments, pencils, books, or tools)

(h) Often is easily distracted by extraneous stimuli

(i) Often is forgetful in daily activities

(2) Six (or more) of the following symptoms of hyperactivity-impulsivity have persisted for at least 6 months to a degree that is maladaptive and inconsistent with developmental level:

Hyperactivity

(a) Often fidgets with hands or feet or squirms in seat

(b) Often leaves seat in classroom or in other situations in which remaining seated is expected

(c) Often runs about or climbs excessively in situations in which it is inappropriate (in adolescents or adults, may be limited to subjective feelings of restlessness)

(d) Often has difficulty playing or engaging in leisure activities quietly

(e) Is often "on the go" or often acts as if "driven by a motor"

(f) Often talks excessively

Impulsivity

(a) Often blurts out answers before questions have been completed

(b) Often has difficulty waiting turn

(c) Often interrupts or intrudes on others (e.g., butts into conversations or games)

(continued)

TABLE 8–2. *(continued)*

B　Some hyperactive-impulsive or inattentive symptoms that caused impairment were present before age 7 years.

C　Some impairment from the symptoms is present in two or more settings (e.g., at school [or work] and at home).

D　There must be clear evidence of clinically significant impairment in social, academic, or occupational functioning.

E　The symptoms do not occur exclusively during the course of a pervasive developmental disorder, schizophrenia, or other psychotic disorder and are not better accounted for by another mental disorder (e.g., mood disorder, anxiety disorder, dissociative disorder, or a personality disorder).

Source: From *Diagnostic and Statistical Manual of Mental Disorders,* 4th ed., pp. 83–85 by American Psychiatric Association, 1994. Washington, DC: American Psychiatric Association. Copyright 1994 by the American Psychiatric Association. Reprinted with permission.

A second objective is to provide a baseline from which to monitor progress and judge the effectiveness of treatment. This also involves identifying the child's strengths that can be utilized to enhance his or her performance in academic and social settings.

A third objective is to determine the child's eligibility for school services. As stated in Chapter 5, to qualify for special education services in the schools, the child's condition frequently must be labeled. Therefore, determining if the child's disorder should be labeled needs to be studied from a fiscal, an emotional, and an academic perspective. Fiscally, if the child qualifies for a special education service, the funding will be different than it would be for a regular education student who is not receiving any special education services. Emotionally, it can be devastating to a parent, and to the child, to have the condition labeled as ADD or ADHD. After a staffing conference in which her child was identified as having ADD and placed into some special education services, a mother said, "You know, I have been trying to convince his teachers! But, to sit here and hear three professionals from different disciplines say that my child has ADHD was very hard. I wanted to stop the labeling, even though I know he needs this extra help to succeed in school."

Similar to describing the strengths the child has, the evaluation process should also describe deficits needing management. To minimize the stigmatizing of the student, careful consideration needs to be given to determine what management strategies can be incorporated into the classroom to help the child be more successful academically and socially. Also, if the child is to be removed from class (termed "pull-out"), this needs to be scheduled carefully so that the child does not miss the same academic subjects every time he or she goes to a therapy session outside of the classroom.

Eight Diagnostic Categories

When evaluating a child to determine if he or she has ADD or ADHD, it is important to address eight diagnostic categories to have a complete picture of the child's status with regard to possible ADD or ADHD, academic achievement, and social aptitude.

Cognition

The first category is cognition. As discussed in Chapter 10, cognition is assessed using multimodality testing. This means that the subtests are varied in terms of stimulus input (auditory or visual) and response modality (oral, written, or gestural). What is critical is to determine the modalities through which the child best responds to the provision of information, then to capitalize on that information to design the child's academic program. For example, the same young man who had problems with affective control had tremendous difficulty on spelling tests. He was punished at home for poor spelling grades, and his classmates made fun of him for his low grades on spelling tests (the students graded each other's papers). In therapy, it was determined that he spelled much better orally than he did when he had to write his answers. Therefore, the clinician approached the teacher and asked whether the child could take his spelling tests orally in the future. The teacher agreed to a trial run, and over the next four weeks his spelling grade improved from an F to a B. More important than the grade was the change in the child's self-esteem. Further explanation of this child's spelling difficulties can be found in the case history at the end of this chapter.

Processing

Processing is the second category that needs to be assessed. Processing determines how the child handles information that is presented to him visually and aurally.

Processing. How the child handles information that is presented to him visually and aurally.

Children can have normal vision and hearing but have a breakdown in the neurological connections that permit them to process and understand the information that is presented. Just as with cognition, it is important to determine if the child processes better when information is presented visually or aurally. Then, if necessary, teaching strategies can be modified to accommodate the child's best learning modalities which may, in turn, assist him or her in using focal control.

Achievement

The assessment of achievement is particularly important when the child has already completed two or more years of school. Achievement testing enables the clinician to determine what the child has learned, or achieved, during his or her academic career. Achievement testing is often done annually in

TABLE 8–3. Areas of focus in language testing for children suspected of having ADD or ADHD.

1. Problem-solving skills
2. Auditory skills
3. Visual skills
4. Sequencing
5. Pragmatic skills
6. Extracting detail
7. Story schema
8. Associative responses
9. Topic maintenance
10. Topic switching

schools but is also frequently done by school psychologists when a child's academic performance is a cause for concern.

Language

Language testing should include a variety of skills, such as those outlined in Table 8–3. Problem-solving skills require higher level cognitive skills that are frequently associated with the development of metalinguistic, metacognitive, and metapragmatic skills. In other words, the child needs to know how to analyze language and develop sequenced plans of actions to solve problems. Because of problems with focal and associative control, problem solving is usually a source of difficulty for children with ADD or ADHD.

Socially, children with ADD or ADHD usually have poor pragmatic skills. They typically do not respond to environmental cues that serve as regulators for pragmatic interactions with other individuals. They frequently ignore social rules, which further impedes their social adaptations and can result in lowered self-esteem owing to the lack of friends. Therefore, it is important to assess the child's pragmatic skills, looking at subareas such as topic maintenance and topic switching.

Metanarrative skills. Ability to analyze stories, extract appropriate details from a story, and comprehend a story.

Involving the child in a story-telling scheme is a critical part of the diagnosing of language problems that may be contributing to academic problems associated with ADD or ADHD. **Metanarrative skills** are of particular concern.

Special attention should be paid to how well the child extracts detail from a story, primarily because of the problems ADD or ADHD children have with focal control. It is also important to help a child stay focused on the story and to minimize the tangential remarks that may occur owing to problems with associative control. Finally, the clinician should look at the child's ability to hypothesize about what is going to happen as the story progresses.

Attention

Many people believe that having ADD or ADHD means that the child cannot pay attention. However, it is the controlling of attention, not paying attention, that is problematic for children with ADD or ADHD. Therefore, the child's abilities with regard to focal and associative control need to be assessed carefully to determine if the child can control his or her attention sufficiently to benefit from traditional academic instruction (Heyer, n.d.).

Behavioral

As mentioned earlier, ADD and ADHD are not behavior management problems per se. They do, however, present challenges to traditional methods of behavior management. Classroom observations, teacher feedback, and parental reports are critical in assessing the behavior of children with ADD or ADHD. All must work together to develop a plan of action that will enable the child to succeed academically and socially without frustrating the child in his or her efforts to participate in classroom lessons and social interactions.

Medical

Children who have a hyperactive component associated with their ADD frequently benefit from the use of **psychostimulants**. In fact, one way it is known that ADHD is related to central nervous system dysfunction is the fact that the children with this disorder typically respond positively to the use of psychostimulants to help control their ability to maintain appropriate attending skills. Therefore, it is mandatory for teachers, parents, and any specialists working with the child to make careful, controlled observations of the child's behavior to determine if the medicine is having a positive effect on the child. The child also needs to be monitored to be sure the levels of medication are not so high that the child is too sedated to respond appropriately in the academic setting.

Psychostimulants. Medications that have antidepressant effects and stimulate the production of dopamine that acts on the frontal lobe to improve executive functions.

Social and Environmental Interaction

As with the medical aspects of the evaluation, it is important to have multidisciplinary and parental reports on the child's social interactions. Many children with ADD or ADHD are considered class clowns or viewed as loners. Either way, it is likely that the child has negative social interactions with most of his or her peers. This can lead to lowered self-esteem and elevated levels of depression in the child with ADD or ADHD. The social and environmental interactions of the child need ongoing monitoring, with appropriate intervention to prevent additional problems related to poor self-esteem and/ or depression.

■ TREATMENT OF ADD/ADHD

Arnold (2002) delineates three goals that should be addressed when developing the initial treatment plan for an individual with ADHD.

1. Give the patient and family the necessary information (explain the nature of the disorder, expected effects of the prescribed medication, including "side effects, the expected duration of treatment, possible alternatives, and the targets of treatment") (pp. 107–108).

2. Facilitate acceptance of the plan and future compliance (debunk misinformation the family may have, and cite scientific evidence).

Placebo effect. An inactive treatment that has a suggestive effect on the individual's symptomology.

3. Optimize **placebo effect** (for some patients, just knowing the prescription is available can lead to improvement of symptoms).

In addition, the speech-language pathologist should bear in mind the role of language in a cognitive-behavioral treatment paradigm that is frequently employed when providing intervention for children with ADHD. According to Vail (1987), children need a combination of four factors in order to focus their attention: arousal, a filter, language, and appropriate work. The child's attention is alerted and made ready through arousal of the cognitive system. Then, a filter that eliminates internal and external distractions is activated in order to focus his or her attention. The child's thought processes are focused on and organized using language. Language enables the child to task analyze, categorize and sort ideas, prioritize, and acknowledge cause and effect. The child's work level must be monitored for difficulty in order to be sure that lack of attention is the problem instead of tasks that are too difficult or inappropriate (Nelson, 1998).

■ FOUR AREAS OF MANAGEMENT OF ADD AND ADHD

Academic

Academically, it is important to provide structure for the child both in the classroom and at home when doing homework. Likewise, the teacher and homework helpers should individualize the interaction, working through the modalities that are the most successful for individual children. Also, structuring the environment so that the child can complete his or her assignments is critical. Fifty percent of children with ADD will fail their courses due to productivity problems. That is to say, they fail because they do not complete their work. One strategy that has been employed successfully by some teachers is to break the assignment into smaller units. For example, if the students are to complete 20 mathematics problems, the assignment could be divided into four sets of five problems for the child with **ADD** or **ADHD**. After completing the first set, the child could turn them into the teacher and pick up the next set. The same types of strategies should be employed across the academic spectrum because most children with ADD or ADHD have decreased achievement in reading, spelling, and written language.

Cantwell and Baker (1985) studied the cognitive styles of children with ADHD and noted that these children demonstrate a "cognitive impulsivity" in addition to the behavioral impulsivity commonly associated with ADHD. These children make decisions quickly without filtering through all the relevant information. Children with ADHD are often gifted, which makes one question the idea that children with ADHD may be cognitively impaired. Rather, they do not manage their knowledge in an appropriate and systematic manner. They are nonreflective about the information at hand which leads to the quick decisions that are sometimes incorrect or inappropriate (Nelson, 1993).

Memory Deficits

It is also important to focus on memory deficits when working with children with ADD or ADHD. Table 8–4 delineates the different areas of memory that are usually deficient in children with these disorders. **Selective attention** and its effects on memory are similar to focal control. When presented with a myriad of stimuli, the child cannot attend to what is important (Heyer, n.d.).

Selective attention. The ability to attend to what is important.

Focused attention requires that the child complete an activity, usually under a time constraint (Heyer, n.d.). This is important because the child may have difficulty accessing his or her memory bank to "call up" the information needed to complete a task. For example, a child who is taking a test on a story that has been read to the class may have trouble remembering the important information in the story in time to complete the test. Teachers often report that a child with ADHD seems to daydream at times when attention should be focused on a specific classroom task. The student in Figure 8-1 demonstrates this behavior.

Focused attention. The requirement that a child complete an activity, usually under a time constraint.

TABLE 8–4. Memory deficits in children with ADD or ADHD.

Selective attention	Focusing on what is important amid myriad stimuli
Focused attention	Having a specific activity that must be done, usually under a time constraint
Sustained attention	Similar to be a little less restrictive than focused attention
Divided attention	Determining how much attention can be given to each activity
Vigilance	Completing the whole task without falling behind; needed to develop a memory bank

Source: Adapted from *Programming for Children with Attention Deficit Disorders,* by J. L. Heyer, n.d., West Lafayette, IN: Purdue Research Foundation.

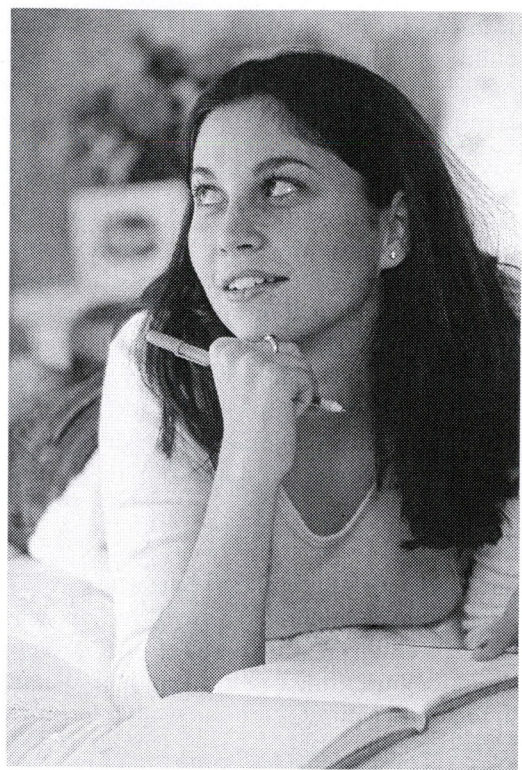

FIGURE 8–1. Students who have ADD/ADHD often find it difficult to remain focused on the task at hand, tending to daydream or be distracted by other events in the environment.

Sustained attention. The ability to remain on task, but without the time constraints of focused attention.

Sustained attention is somewhat similar to focused attention, but in this case the child does not complete the test because he or she cannot stay focused on the test, rather than having difficulty recalling the important information.

Divided attention. Determining how much attention to give to each activity.

Divided attention is a problem for the child with ADD or ADHD because he or she cannot decide how much attention to give to each activity (Heyer, n.d.). Problems with divided attention interfere with the ability to multitask. For example, most children in third grade will have homework in two or three subject areas per night. The child with ADD or ADHD will have difficulty determining how much time to allot to each subject so that all of the assignments are completed.

Vigilance. The ability to develop a memory bank.

Vigilance is important because it underlies the development of a memory bank. The child has a poor memory bank because he or she cannot stay focused enough on the information at hand in order to store it (Heyer, n.d.).

TABLE 8–5. Treatment strategies to use with children who have ADD or ADHD.

Provide a consistent routine across all environments

Break assignments down into smaller groups (e.g., 5 mathematic problems at one time instead of 20)

Simple, single instructions or directions

Prepare for changes

Strengthen the strengths as much as address the weaknesses

Maximize function and circumvent or minimize the weaknesses

For example, the young man who had difficulty with written spelling tests had trouble with vigilance. In fact, being unable to complete written spelling tests is a classic example of difficulty with vigilance. The child is busy writing word number three (for example) when the teacher calls out word number four. By the time the teacher gets to word number five, the child has fallen behind and cannot remember the words that have been called out. Consequently, these children fail to complete the spelling test because they have trouble refocusing and recalling the words that have been called out by the teacher.

As a rule, vigilance, divided attention, and sustained attention are the ones that create the biggest memory deficits in children with ADD or ADHD (Heyer, n.d.). Therefore, many children with these disorders do better on self-paced tasks cut into small units than they do on time tasks. Other treatment strategies are suggested in Table 8–5.

Behavioral

As stated previously, ADD and ADHD are not behavior management problems. However, the behavior of the children is problematic. The first step in remediation of some of the behavioral issues is to make sure the child knows that he or she is responsible for his or her own behavior. This is a time-consuming task, but it is, nonetheless, absolutely critical. It will require addressing each of the control and attention areas and developing strategies that can be used to foster their development.

Behavioral treatment can be direct **behavior modification** using a cognitive-behavioral approach, or indirect by training through parent and teacher training. Promoting communication between school and home is critical and can be accomplished through daily checklists. Setting clearly defined rules and procedures can be of benefit to the child as well, as long as the rules are consistently enforced at home and at school. Typical behavior management strategies can be adopted, including a token economy system, time out, and response cost systems (Arnold, 2002).

Behavior modification. The implementation of an intervention plan to change, modify, or correct an individual's behavior.

Medical

Drugs make the system more accessible to learning. They will help with the activity level, the impulsivity, and the attention, but they will not increase knowledge. They do increase the parent-child and teacher-child interaction time and quality, so an increase in positive responses to learning becomes a benefit of the medication.

Frequently some confusion occurs when a physician says he or she is going to treat hyperactivity by prescribing a psychostimulant. The stimulants do not stimulate behavior directly. Rather, they stimulate neurotransmitters to increase the production of dopamine which, in turn, improves the control and attention devices the child has at his or her disposal. The fact that children with ADHD respond to the psychostimulants lends support to the belief that biological factors underlie the disorder (Nelson, 1993). It is also important to note that the drugs are psychologically, not physiologically, addictive. In other words, the child may think he or she needs the drugs when they no longer are needed, but this is not a physiological craving in the way that drugs such as nicotine are.

The most common medication used for treating the hyperactivity component of ADHD is Ritalin, which has been used since 1956. Over a 16-year period between 1971–1987, the use of Ritalin among school-age children doubled every four to seven years. In an effort to curb the prescribing of Ritalin, the Drug Enforcement Agency limited production of the drug. Despite these efforts, in 1993 the production of Ritalin was three times what was allowed in 1990 and still not enough was produced to meet the demand.

Side effects of Ritalin are difficult to document owing to the fact that children taking it suffer from a wide variety of conditions and treatments. Side effects are limited primarily to loss of appetite and some trouble sleeping. These side effects frequently are dosage related, meaning they can be alleviated by adjusting the dosage. Other drugs used to treat symptoms of ADHD are Adderall®, Concerta®, and Dexedrine® Spansule. The advantages to these drugs is that they do not have to be given during school hours (Arnold, 2002).

Regardless of whether or not the physician chooses to use pharmacological agents to control hyperactivity in children with ADHD, it is important to remember that it is parents, not pills, that make children mind.

Social

The fourth area of management is the social aspect of dealing with ADD. As stated previously, many children with ADD or ADHD are perceived as rude and uncaring. They also need to be taught how to deal with their emotions appropriately. The teacher might explain ADD and ADHD to the whole class in an effort to ease some of the confusion regarding the disorder. It is also critical to monitor the social status of the child with ADD or ADHD because of the inclination to poor self-esteem and depression. Behavior therapy should be provided to help the child analyze the situations in which he or she finds himself or herself and to practice problem solving as it relates to personal and academic problems. The use of positive reinforcement is critical, and the timing is important. Remember that delayed gratification is difficult for children with ADD or ADHD, so frequent use of positive reinforcement is essential. The use of behavior management, particularly positive reinforcement, is admittedly difficult because children with ADHD tend to elicit primarily punitive responses from teachers, parents, and peers. This often results in inconsistent attempts at behavior management, with increases in depression and delinquency.

■ SUMMARY

ADD and ADHD are multifaceted disorders that can have profound effects on the academic and social growth of school-age children. The speech-language pathologist plays a key role in the diagnosis of ADD and ADHD by providing language and cognitive testing that can either rule out a learning disability or establish the possibility that the learning disability may coexist with the diagnosis of ADD. Family members and all professionals who are involved in the education and therapy process should work together to develop a consistent plan of interaction to maximize the opportunity for the child with ADD or ADHD to find success in his or her academic and social growth.

CASE STUDY

History

P is an 11-year-old boy who was referred to the University of Florida Speech and Hearing Clinic for evaluation due to poor performance in school. He lives at home with his parents, both of whom were in their late 40's. He has an older brother who was attending a technical school in another state. P is in the process of repeating 4th grade due to poor performance on a statewide assessment test, and general academic difficulties. He is receiving speech-language therapy at his school for one hour a week in a group of 5 children. According to his parents, P has always been an active child who frequently got in trouble at home and at school. He did not have any friends at school or at home. He cries with frustration almost every night when working on homework, and has difficulty organizing his assignments and remaining focused enough to be able to complete the assignments. His father is functionally illiterate.

Evaluation

On the Peabody Picture Vocabulary Test, P scored in the 83rd percentile. The Test of Language Development–Intermediate was administered with the following results:

Subtest	Raw Score	%ile	Standard Score
Sentence Combining	11	9	6
Characteristics	38	37	9
Word Ordering	9	5	5
Generals	7	2	4
Grammatic Comprehension	6	9	6

Composite scores were as follows:

	SC	CH	WO	G	GC	Sum of Std. Scores	Quotients
Spoken Language (SLQ)	6	9	5	4	6	30	73
Listening (LiQ)		9			6	15	85
Speaking (SpQ)	6		5	4		15	68
Semantics (SeQ)		9		4		13	79
Syntax (SyQ)	6		5		6	17	72

P's profile is a jagged line that is often indicative of learning disabilities. He showed relative strengths in Characteristics, and his biggest weaknesses were Generals and Word Ordering.

	Strengths	Weaknesses
Communicative	Lexicon	Written spelling
	Decoding skills	Syntax and Morphology
	General knowledge	Pragmatics
		Reading comprehension
		Poor attending skills
		Narrative writing and story development
		Short-term memory
Non-communicative	Cooperates in therapy	ADHD

Responds to behavior management techniques	Home environment not intellectually stimulating
Relative strength in mathematics	Poor handwriting
	Frustrated by school work

Therapy

When P began therapy, we initially focused on his reading comprehension and spelling skills, as well as attending skills and short-term memory. We also addressed writing narratives. His decoding skills were within normal limits, but apparently this did not translate into his spelling when taking a spelling test. His comprehension of short paragraphs was good, but broke down with longer readings.

P is in a class in school where they have a spelling test every Friday, and P typically fails these tests. It does not appear so much a matter of not being able to spell as it is not being able to keep up as the teacher goes through the spelling list. This is a source of embarrassment for him. When therapy started, P did not like to write, and his handwriting was, at times, illegible. He did not understand punctuation and thus omitted it entirely in his written assignments. He had a relative strength in mathematics, making low B/high C on most math assignments.

Over the course of therapy, it was discovered that P could spell words more accurately when he could spell them orally than when he had to write them. We contacted his teacher to see if he could take his tests orally before or after school and she agreed. His scores went from an F to a B on the spelling tests. P did not have "vigilance" that is frequently a problem area for children who have ADHD when it comes to spelling tests. P would hear the first spelling word spoken by the teacher, but by the time she had gotten to the third word he was just finishing up writing the first word and was hopelessly lost and behind. We also worked on handwriting skills and referred him to an occupational therapist for help in this area.

P loved to concoct stories, some fictional and some fabricated. For example, he frequently spoke of letters he had received from his brother. When the clinician remarked to P's mom that the letters from his brother meant a lot to P, P's mom said his brother had not written any letters to P and rarely interacted with him when he was home. P was a sports enthusiast, and this was usually the focus of his stories. An example of his written stories before intervention is depicted below. Notice the fact that there is no punctuation, several words are illegible (hence a translation is printed below the story), and there is no true introduction, elaboration, or conclusion to the story:

WRITING SAMPLE FROM AN 11-YEAR-OLD BOY WITH ADHD AND LANGUAGE-BASED LEARNING DISABILITIES

Translation (punctuation added): My Trip to the Football Game.

Me and my dad went to a football game. It was fun so much fun it took we just got there in time so we watch it was fun and it was so much fun it won and I saw a football player score a 100 touchdown. Shane Matthews his hand got hurt so he left the game. The end.

I want to be a baseball player and a football player and astronaut. I want be a catcher and I want to be on the Braves team.

After four months of intervention, P wrote the following story:

WRITING SAMPLE FROM AN 11-YEAR-OLD BOY WITH ADHD AND LANGUAGE-BASED LEARNING DISABILITIES AFTER 4 MONTHS OF INTERVENTION.

Notice the addition of periods at the end of each line (he defined a sentence as a line of words) and more cohesion within the story. There is a distinct beginning, development, and conclusion to the story, in comparison to his previous stories.

> once up a time ther woss a maney
> namd Bill ray .he had a moter.
> sikie and He hao a moter sikie
> and it was namo a
> Harley Daripson anp he cope.
> Go go fast it coun Go 295 MHP.
> qnp so he Bout a new moter.
> sikie nape Harler paripson
> anp he Gao me a ripe on heis.
> noe motrsikre he wint reil.
> Fast he ricn 300 MAP qnp .
> I wase "skoro"l
> anp I sull a squrei.
> and logt of tree's .
> Becuse he tock me on a ripe
> on a moter cikie rov rov

> the Eno

Translation (punctuation added): Once upon a time there was a man named Bill Ray. He had a motorcycle and he had a motorcycle and it was named a Harley Davidson and he could go so fast. It could go 295 miles hour per and so he bought a new motorcycle named Harley Davidson and he gave me a ride on his new motorcycle. He went real fast. He reached 300 mhp and I was "scared"! And I saw a squirrel and lots of trees. Because he took me on a ride on a motorcycle. Rev Rev. The End

Notice that this story has an introduction, an elaboration, and a conclusion. There is more elaboration and cohesion within the story. It is more legible and has fewer spelling errors. He still has not mastered the science of punctuation. When asked what a sentence is, P said it was a line of words with a dot at the end. He took this quite literally as indicated by the column of dots down the right side of the page (after each "line of words").

It should also be noted that we referred P to a local psychiatrist for evaluation of possible ADHD and consideration of medication. The psychiatrist confirmed our suspicions and prescribed Ritalin that P took each morning before school and each afternoon after school. It has been reported that sometimes the handwriting of children with ADHD improves when they are placed on Ritalin. This is because these drugs act on the frontal lobe, and this may account for the improvement we saw in the second story above.

Conclusion

P was dismissed from therapy when the family moved out of state. He was able to move on to the 5th grade and while he was not an academic star, he consistently made B's and C's. His written assignments were more organized and legible. His short-term memory improved and he made some friends which is critical for an early adolescent.

▨ REVIEW QUESTIONS

1. Which of the following groups represents behaviors/skills that are typically problematic language behaviors for children diagnosed as having ADD/ADHD?

   a. Poor problem-solving skills, good auditory skills, good sequencing skills, poor pragmatic skills
   b. Fair problem-solving skills, poor auditory skills, poor sequencing skills, poor pragmatic skills
   c. Good problem-solving skills, poor auditory skills, poor sequencing skills, fair pragmatic skills
   d. Poor problem-solving skills, poor auditory skills, poor sequencing skills, poor pragmatic skills

2. Which of the following represent the areas of management of children with ADD/ADHD?

   a. Academic, behavioral, medical
   b. Academic, behavioral, medical, social
   c. Academic, medical, social
   d. Behavioral, medical, social

3. ADD is just a learning disability.

   a. True
   b. False

4. Medications for ADHD are physiologically addictive.

   a. True
   b. False

5. Attention needed to complete a specific activity, usually under a time constraint, is

   a. Selective attention
   b. Focused attention
   c. Sustained attention
   d. Vigilance

6. Memory needed to sufficiently focus on information to develop a memory bank is

   a. Selective attention
   b. Focused attention
   c. Divided attention
   d. Vigilance

7. Difficulty with the _____ control system results in the child with ADD/ADHD having difficulty with delaying gratification.

   a. Appetite control
   b. Affective control
   c. Associative control
   d. Mental effort control

8. Inability to select what is important is due to problems with which control system?

   a. Quality control
   b. Associative control
   c. Focal control
   d. Mental effort control

9. ADHD is one of several causes of reading disabilities.

   a. True
   b. False

10. Which of the following statement(s) is/are not true?

   a. There appears to be no genetic basis for ADD/ADHD.
   b. Problems with dopamine receptors are common in ADD/ADHD.
   c. Disruptions in the development of the frontal cortex seem to occur in many children with ADD/ADHD.
   d. a and b
   e. b and c
   f. a and c

■ REFERENCES

American Psychiatric Association (1994). *Diagnostic and statistical manual of mental disorders-Revised* (4th ed.). Washington, DC: American Psychiatric Association.

Arnold, L. E. (2002). *Contemporary diagnosis and management of attention-deficit/hyperactivity disorder* (2nd ed.). Newtown, PA: Handbooks in Health Care Co.

Barkley, R. A. (2000). *Taking charge of ADHD-Revised edition.* New York: The Guilford Press.

Bass, P. M. (1988, November). Attention deficit disorder/Management in preschool, adolescent, and adult populations. Miniseminar presented at the Annual Conference of the American Speech-Language-Hearing Association, Boston, MA.

Cantwell, D. P., & Baker, L. (1985). Interrelationships of communication, learning, and psychiatric disorders in children. In C. S. Simon (Ed.), *Communication skills and classroom success: Assessment of language-learning disabled students* (pp. 43–61). Austin, TX: Pro-Ed.

Cantwell, D. P. & Baker, L. (1992). Issues in the classification of child and adolescent psychopathology. *Journal of the American Academy of Child Adolescence, 27,* 532–533.

Catts, H. W., & Kamhi, A. G. (1999). *Language and reading disabilities.* Boston: Allyn and Bacon.

Catts, H. W., & Kamhi, A. G. (2005). *Language and reading disabilities* (2nd ed.). Boston: Allyn and Bacon.

Edelbrook, C., Costello, A. J., & Kessler, M. D. (1984). Empirical collaboration of attention deficit disorder. *Journal of the American Academy of Child Psychiatry, 23,* 285–290.

Heyer, J. L. (n.d.). *Programming for children with attention deficit disorders.* Purdue University Continuing Education. West Lafayette, IN: Purdue Research Foundation.

Hynd, G. W., Lorys, A. R., Semrud-Clikeman, M., Nieves, N., Huettner, M. I. S., & Lahey, B. B. (1991). Attention deficit disorder without hyperactivity (ADD/WO): A distinct behavioral and neurocognitive syndrome. *Journal of Child Neurology, 6,* 37–43.

Lahey, B. B., Schaughency, E. A., Hynd, G. W., Carlson, C. L., & Nieves, N. (1987). Attention deficit disorder with and without hyperactivity: Comparison of behavioral characteristics of clinic-referred children. *Journal of the American Academy of Child and Adolescent Psychiatry, 26,* 718–723.

Lahey, B. B., Schaughency, E. A., Strauss, C. C., & Frame, C. L. (1984). Are attention deficit disorders with and without hyperactivity similar or dissimilar disorders? *Journal of the American Academy of Child Psychiatry, 23,* 302–309.

Morgan, A. E., Hynd, G. W., Riccio, C., & Hall, J. (1996). Validity of DSM-IV ADHD predominantly inattentive and combined types: Relationship to previous DSM diagnoses/subtype differences. *Journal of the American Academy of Child and Adolescent Psychiatry, 35*(3), 325–333.

Nelson, N. W. (1993). *Childhood language disorders in context: Infancy through adolescence.* New York: Macmillan Publishing Company.

Nelson, N. W. (1998). *Childhood language disorders in context: Infancy through adolescence.* New York: Macmillan Publishing Company.

Newhoff, M. (1986). Attentional deficit—What it is, what it is not. *The Clinical Connection* (Fall), 10–11.

Newhoff, M. (1990). Attention deficit hyperactivity disorder: Defining our role. *The Clinical Connection* (1st Quarter), 10–12.

Rutter, M., Tizard, J., & Whitmore, K. (Eds.). (1970). *Education, health, and behavior.* London: Longmans Green.

Sattler, J. M. (1988). *Assessment of children* (3rd ed.). San Diego: Author.

Shaywitz, B. A., Fletcher, J. M., Holahan, J. M., Shneider, A. E., Marchione, K. E., Stuebing, K. K., Francis, D. J., Shankweiler, D. P., Katz, L., Liberman, I. Y., & Shaywitz, S. E. (1995). Interrelationships between reading disability and attention-deficit/hyperactivity disorder. *Cognitive Neuropsychology, 1,* 170–186.

Vail, P. L. (1987). *Smart kids with school problems: Things to know and ways to help.* New York: E. P. Dutton.

Weintraub, S., & Mesulam, M. M. (1983). Developmental learning disabilities of the right hemisphere: Emotional, interpersonal, and cognitive components. *Archives of Neurology, 40,* 463–468.

Weschler, D. (1974). *Weschler Intelligence Scale for Children-Revised.* San Antonio, TX: Psychological Corporation.

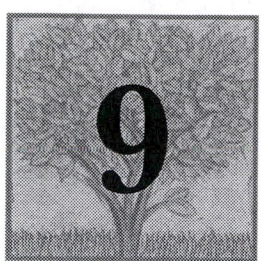

9

Language After Traumatic Brain Injury

■ LEARNING OBJECTIVES

After completion of this chapter, the reader will be able to

1. Discuss problems a clinician would expect to see in individuals who have sustained a mild TBI, a moderate TBI, and a severe TBI.

2. Discuss, list, and briefly describe the three categories of symptoms associated with TBI.

3. Discuss a minimum of five language functions within the umbrella term of executive functions.

4. Define impairment, disability, and handicap as explained by the World Health Organization.

5. Describe the language differences in diagnosis and treatment between children with TBI and adults with TBI.

6. Discuss what professionals should be involved in the multidisciplinary assessment and treatment of children with TBI and describe the roles of each.

■ INTRODUCTION

Traumatic brain injury (TBI) is defined by the National Head Injury Foundation (1985) as being damage to the brain due to an external force, not due to degenerative or congenital problems. It is estimated that 66% to 82% of all head injuries are classified as mild. The prevalence of TBI is approximately 200 persons per 100,000 people for a total of 500,000 head injuries a year. Approximately 200,000 of these injuries result in death, whereas another 200,000 persons survive with varying degrees of disability, including acquired **aphasia**. In the general population, almost twice as many males than females sustain a head injury, but in the midadolescence to early adulthood years, this ratio jumps to approximately 3–4:1. With regard to age, the highest risk categories are males aged 15 to 24 years, and males over 75 years of age (Hegde, 1996; Coelho, DeRuyter, & Stein, 1996; Murdoch & Theodoros, 2001). The prevalence of TBI in America is estimated to be a little more than 2% of the population of the United States, or 5.3 million Americans. Transportation-related accidents are the leading cause of TBIs in the age 5 to 64 population, and falls are the number one cause of TBIs in individuals age 65 and older.

In the infant and toddler age range, most head injuries are due to falls or abuse. In the older preschool population, the most common cause of injuries is falls. Elementary school-age children are most likely to acquire head injuries as a result of sports, bike accidents, skateboarding accidents, pedestrian accidents, or accidents in which they are passengers in a car. Adolescents are more likely to suffer head injuries as a result of car crashes, usually at high speeds (Reed, 2005).

Aphasia. Acquired neurological damage that results in impairment of the abilities to comprehend and express language.

Historically, research has not supported the notion of aphasia associated with TBI in children, preferring to reserve the term aphasia for use in describing adults with acquired language disorders. However, the Individuals with Disabilities Education Act (IDEA) designates TBI as a diagnostic category and defines TBI as follows:

> An acquired injury to the brain caused by an external physical force, resulting in total or partial functional disability or psychosocial impairment, or both, that adversely affect a child's educational performance. The term applies to open and closed head injuries resulting in impairments in one or more areas, such as: cognition; language; memory; attention; reasoning; abstract thinking; judgment; problem-solving; sensory, perceptual, and motor abilities; psychosocial behavior; physical functions; information processing; and speech. The term does not apply to brain injuries that are congenital or degenerative, or brain injuries induced by birth trauma. (*U.S. Federal Register,* 57[189], p. 44802, 1992)

IDEA calls for the reintegration of children with traumatic brain injury into the classrooms, and the teachers report that language disabilities are the factors that cause the greatest interference with success in school.

■ TRAUMATIC BRAIN INJURY (TBI) DEFINED

Kay and the Mild Traumatic Brain Injury Committee of the Head Injury Special Interest Group of the American Congress of Rehabilitation Medicine (1993) have defined traumatic brain injury as follows:

> Traumatically induced physiological disruption of brain function, as manifested by **at least one** of the following:
>
> 1. any period of loss of consciousness
>
> 2. any loss of memory for events immediately before or after the accident
>
> 3. any alteration in mental state at the time of the accidents (e.g., feeling dazed, disoriented, or confused)
>
> 4. focal neurological deficit(s) that may or may not be transient; but where [sic] the severity of the injury does not exceed the following:
>   - loss of consciousness for approximately 30 minutes or less;
>   - after 30 minutes, an initial Glasgow Coma Scale (GCS) of 13–15; and
>   - post-traumatic amnesia (PTA) no greater than 24 hours

Individuals with mild TBI may have a functional disability due to physical, cognitive, behavioral, or emotional symptoms that may persist after the injury. As a result of a mild head injury, the individual may have problems with memory, attention, and executive functioning. The patient may be anxious, depressed, or irritable. Language effects include mild word-retrieval deficits (Levin, Eisenberg, & Benton, 1989; Sohlberg & Mateer, 1989). Typically, three categories of symptoms are associated with TBI.

The first category consists of physical symptoms including dizziness, headaches, nausea, and vomiting. Blurred vision and sleep disturbances may also occur. Unexplained lethargy, quickness to fatigue, and other sensory losses may also occur in individuals with TBI (Green, Stevens, & Wolf, 1997).

The second category of symptoms relates to cognitive deficits. When examining and determining the cognitive deficits that have occurred as the result of a TBI, the clinician must be careful to ascertain that the cognitive deficits are not due to emotional or other causes besides the traumatic brain injury. Cognitive deficits frequently observed include poor attention skills, difficulty in concentrating, problem-solving deficits, perceptual and memory deficits, problems with speech or language, or both, and difficulty with executive functions (Green, Stevens, & Wolfe, 1997). Executive functions include goal setting, self-awareness, initiating tasks, self-directing and self-monitoring, self-evaluation, self-inhibiting, and planning (Coelho, DeRuyter, & Stein, 1996). All of these cognitive factors combine and interact with receptive and expressive language skills. Traumatic brain injury can significantly impact cognitive-communication abilities. "Cognitive-communicative impairments are those impairments of communication related to impairments of linguistic (e.g., syntax, semantics, metalinguistic skills) as well as nonlinguistic cognitive functions (e.g., attention, perception, and memory" (Coelho et al., 1996, p. S6; American Speech-Language-Hearing Association, 1987, 1990).

Behavioral changes with or without alterations in the degree of emotional responsivity constitute the third category of symptoms. Again, these symptoms must exist in the absence of other psychological, physical, or emotional stresses. Behavioral changes include emotional lability, disinhibition, irritability, and quickness to anger (Green et al., 1997).

The degree to which an individual is affected by a TBI is quite diverse, with physical deficits (as depicted in Figure 9–1), psychosocial deficits, and cognitive-communicative deficits creating varying degrees of handicap and disability.

The World Health Organization (WHO) (1987) classified injuries such as TBI in three ways: impairment, disability, and handicap. They defined impairment as the disruption or abnormality in mental or physical functioning. When an impairment limits participation in life activities, the result is a disability. In 1998, the WHO revised their terminology, substituting "activity reduction" for "disability." This terminology makes reference to a reduction in the individual's ability to effectively and successfully participate in activities that are important to a quality life such as reading comprehension,

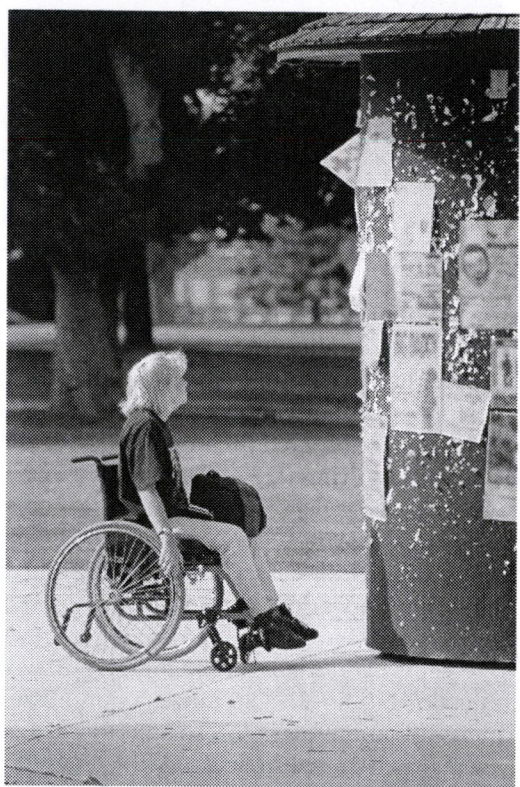

FIGURE 9–1. TBI can affect an individual's mental, social, emotional, and physical states.

conversing with others, and remaining organized and focused in work and social settings. A handicap historically referred to the social deficits that occur as a sequela to a injury or illness. In 1998, the word "participation" was substituted for "handicap." This refers to the individual's decreased ability to participate in work, school, social situations, community activities, and so on.

■ TYPES OF INJURIES

Closed head injury (CHI). A nonpenetrating brain injury in which the skull may be intact or fractured, but the meninges are intact.

It is important to differentiate among the various terms frequently used to describe head injury. A **closed head injury (CHI)** is a nonpenetrating brain injury in which the skull may be intact or fractured, but the meninges are intact (Hegde, 1996). It is possible, in these cases, to have a minor head injury without brain injury. A nonpenetrating brain injury typically results in diffuse pathological changes in the brain and are more frequent in civilian life than a penetrating head injury (Murdoch & Theodoros, 2001). The damage to the brain is usually caused by a blunt blow to the head. Shaking of the head (such as in shaken baby syndrome) is also a frequent cause of closed head injury. Closed head injuries can be due to a moving objects hitting a moving head, or due to a moving head colliding with a fixed object. Both scenarios result in the brain's moving within the skull and results in damage to the brain. These mechanisms of injury are known as acceleration/deceleration injury. This is compared to a nonacceleration injury in which a moving object collides with a stationary head which results in localized damge at the point of impact (Ylvisaker, Szekeres, & Feeney, 2001). A **penetrating head injury**, which is also known as an open head injury, results in a fracturing or perforation of the skull with the meninges becoming torn or lacerated (Hegde, 1996). An example of a penetrating head injury is a gunshot wound.

Two other terms that are frequently encountered when studying traumatic brain injury are *coup injury* and *contrecoup injury*. In a **coup injury**, the injury is at the point of impact. This type of injury occurs when a blow to the head results in the brain's moving and slamming against the point of impact. A **contrecoup injury** is a brain injury opposite from the impact. In these cases, a second injury occurs as the brain "bounces from the point of impact to the opposite side of the skull" (Blosser & DePompei, 2003, p. 17). Coup and contrecoup injuries are associated with a linear velocity mechanism that frequently is the result of trauma in the front or the back of the head (Ylvisaker et al., 2001).

It is also important to know if the child has a focal lesion or a diffuse lesion. In a **focal lesion**, the damage is limited to a small area of the brain. This is in contrast to a **diffuse lesion**, which causes widespread damage. In diffuse lesions, frequently a twisting movement of the brain occurs, which can force tissues together, pull tissues apart, or create a tearing of axonal fibers as the injury occurs (Blosser & DePompei, 2003). Depending on the site of the damage, a diffuse lesion would be expected to be much more devastating to the child's cognition and language than a focal lesion. The majority of injuries are consistent with frontolimbic damage and the deficits can be grouped into three categories: cognitive, executive functions, and psychosocial/behavioral (Ylvisaker et al., 2001).

Nelson (1993) advocates dividing brain injury into four etiological categories: "(1) focal acquired lesions, (2) diffuse lesions associated with traumatic brain injury, (3) acquired childhood aphasia secondary to convulsive disorder, and (4) other kinds of brain injury or encephalopathy" (p. 116). Focal acquired lesions are frequently caused by strokes in children. These strokes are commonly the result of embolisms associated with congenital heart disease. They may also be associated with vascular disorders due to sickle cell anemia. The strokes often result in left hemisphere lesions, from which recovery usually is fairly complete. Nelson (1993) does warn of possible enduring effects on language development and learning, however. Diffuse lesions associated with TBI resulting from falls, vehicular accidents, or abuse are the primary focus of this chapter. In these cases, it is not unusual to see relatively good language recovery in young children; however,

Penetrating head injury. An open head injury resulting in a fracturing or perforation of the skull with the meninges being torn or lacerated.

Coup injury. Injury at the point of impact, occurring when a blow to the head results in the brain's moving and slamming against the point of impact.

Contrecoup injury. A brain injury opposite from the impact as the brain bounces from the point of impact to the opposite side of the skull.

Focal lesion. A lesion in which the impact is concentrated in one small area of the brain.

Diffuse lesion. A lesion in which the damage is spread throughout a large area of the brain or over several small areas, resulting in comprehensive deficits.

long-term sequelae in terms of linguistic processing and cognition are common (Ewing-Cobbs, Fletcher, & Levin, 1985; Satz & Bullard-Bates, 1981).

Acquired aphasia secondary to convulsive disorders often includes unknown etiological factors. The problems can be either sudden or gradual in onset. Landau-Kleffner syndrome is a convulsive disorder characterized by epileptic discharges and severe language comprehension deficits (Nelson, 1993). Finally, Nelson refers to encephalopathies that are secondary to infection or irradiation. These include disorders due to tumors, encephalitis, meningitis, and cancer treatments. The extent of the damage in the last two categories varies with the extent and location of tissues involved, the age of the child, and the general health of the child.

Aphasias in the pediatric population due to deficits in categories one, three, and four are relatively uncommon. In 1989, the death rate for children under 15 years of age from cerebrovascular disease (which contributes to stroke) was 4 per 100,000, compared to 2296 per 100,000 in adults. Over one-third of strokes in children occur in the first two years of life. Usual etiological factors are sickle cell anemia, cardiac disease, vascular occlusions or malformations, and hemorrhage (Reed, 1994). Reed summarized much of the research in this area as outlined in Table 9–1.

TABLE 9–1. Associated physical, cognitive, perceptual motor, behavioral, and social problems in children with acquired aphasia due to traumatic brain injury.

Area	Effect of Traumatic Brain Injury
Gross and fine motor	• Severe TBI: spasticity, delayed motor milestones • Mild TBI: fine motor and visuomotor deficits, reduction in age-appropriate play and physical activity
Cognitive	• Problems with long- and short-term memory, conceptual skills, problem solving • Reduced speed of information processing • Reduced attending skills
Perceptual motor	• Visual neglect, visual field cuts • Motor apraxia, reduced motor speed, poor motor sequencing
Behavioral	• Impulsivity, poor judgment, disinhibition, dependency, anger outbursts, denial, depression, emotional lability, apathy, lethargy, poor motivation
Social	• Does not learn from peers, does not generalize from social situations • Behaves like a much younger child, withdraws • Becomes distracted in noisy surroundings and becomes lost even in familiar surroundings

Source: Adapted from *An Introduction to Children with Language Disorders* (2nd ed.), by V. A. Reed, 1994, p. 368. Copyright 1994, Macmillan College Publishing Company.

In the pediatric population, lesions causing language deficits initially may be limited to the surface structure of the brain. However, as the learning demands increase, as they do in grades three and four, the deficits become more apparent. Clinicians must understand the relationship between cognition and language because impaired cognitive processes (i.e., perception, memory, reasoning, and problem solving) interfere with language processes (Russell, 1993). A summarization of the primary and secondary mechanisms associated with the different types of brain trauma is found in Figures 9–2 and 9–3.

Underlying Complications

Cognitive and language deficits due to TBI are rarely related to a single factor. Many secondary mechanisms exist that can create complications after the immediate injury. For example, the patient may have seizure activity. In fact, many head injury patients are placed on seizure medications as a prophylactic measure to minimize or prevent the occurrence of seizures. Swelling of the brain tissues also may be present. In closed head injuries (CHI), when tissue swells, a tight cavity is created between the brain and the cranium, leaving no place for the excess fluid. Therefore, the intracranial pressure increases and results in a decline in the patient's status. Hypoxia (lack of oxygen), hemorrhage, and the development of blood clots can also contribute to increased damage following the actual accident.

Secondary damage may occur after a TBI, and it may also affect the degree of impairment experienced by the patient. One example of secondary damage is cerebral edema which can contribute to increased intracranial pressure. Cerebral edema is the "accumulation of fluid between the brain and skull, within the ventricles, or within the brain lesion" (Ylvisaker et al., 2001, p. 748). The edema may be limited to the area of the brain around the injury site, or throughout the brain. Intracranial pressure is due to accumulation of cerebrospinal fluid, water, or blood within the skull. The fluid accumulation can compress or displace brain tissue.

Another type of secondary damage is hemorrhage. There are two types of hemorrhage: intracerebral, in which blood is in the brain tissue causing diffuse axonal injury, and extracerebral in which there is bleeding into the meninges.

Seizures, a fourth type of secondary damage, may occur within one week post injury (early-onset), or after the first week (late-onset). Finally, hypoxic-ischemic damage may occur as a result of reduced oxygen and blood supply to the brain. This can be due to cardiopulmonary deficits, an increase in intracranial pressure, or cerebral vasospasms. In addition, critical areas of the brain such as the hippocampus may suffer further damage from pathological neurotransmitter surges that may occur (Ylvisaker et al., 2001).

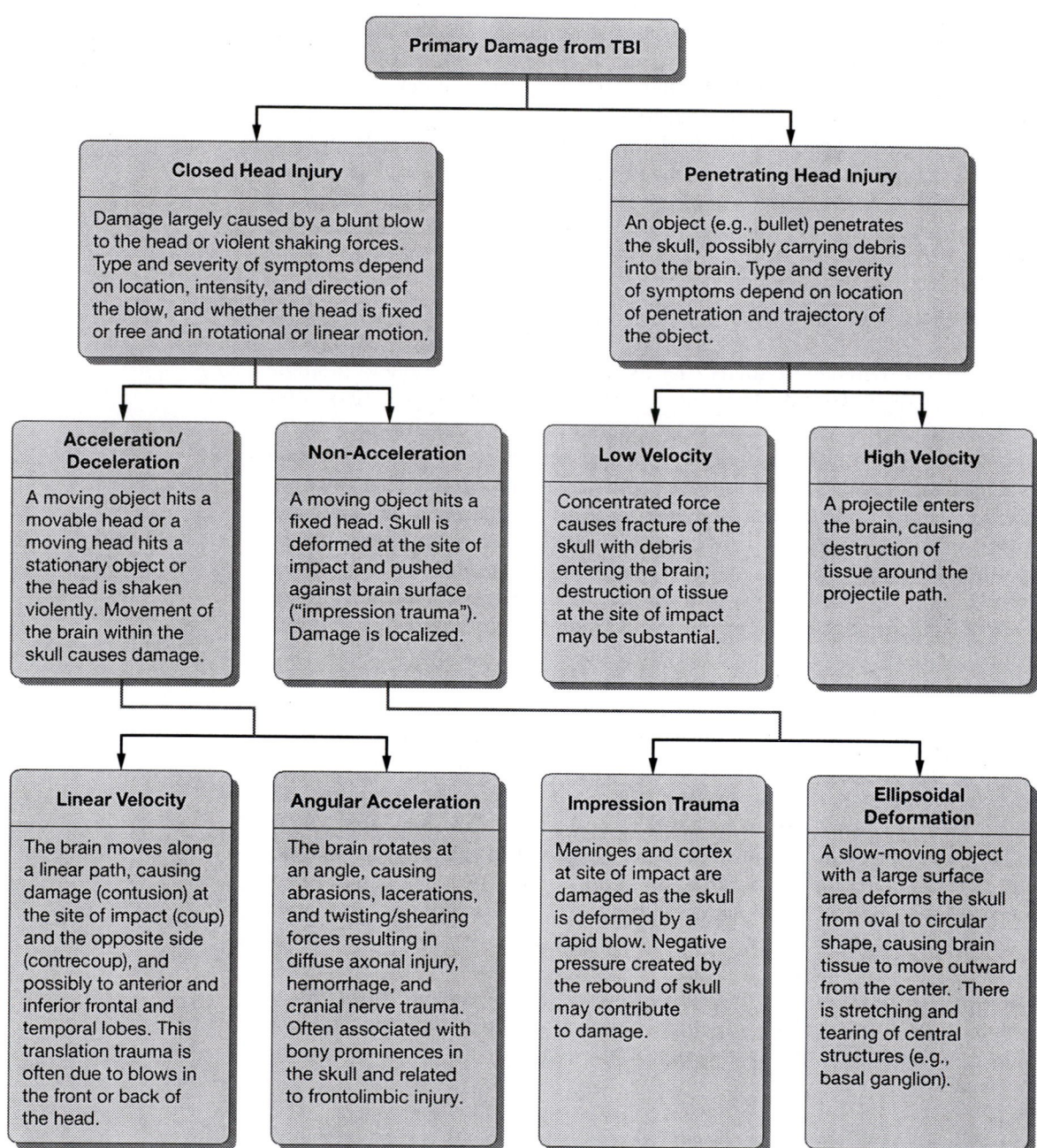

FIGURE 9–2. Mechanisms of immediate injury in closed and open traumatic brain injury. *Source:* From Communication Disorders Associated with Traumatic Brain Injury, by M. Ylvisaker, S. Szkeres, and T. Feeney. In *Language Intervention Strategies in Aphasia and Related Neurogenic Communication Disorders,* 4th ed. R. Chapey, Ed. Philadelphia: Lippincott Williams & Wilkins. Copyright 2001 by Lippincott Willias & Wilins. Reprinted with permission.

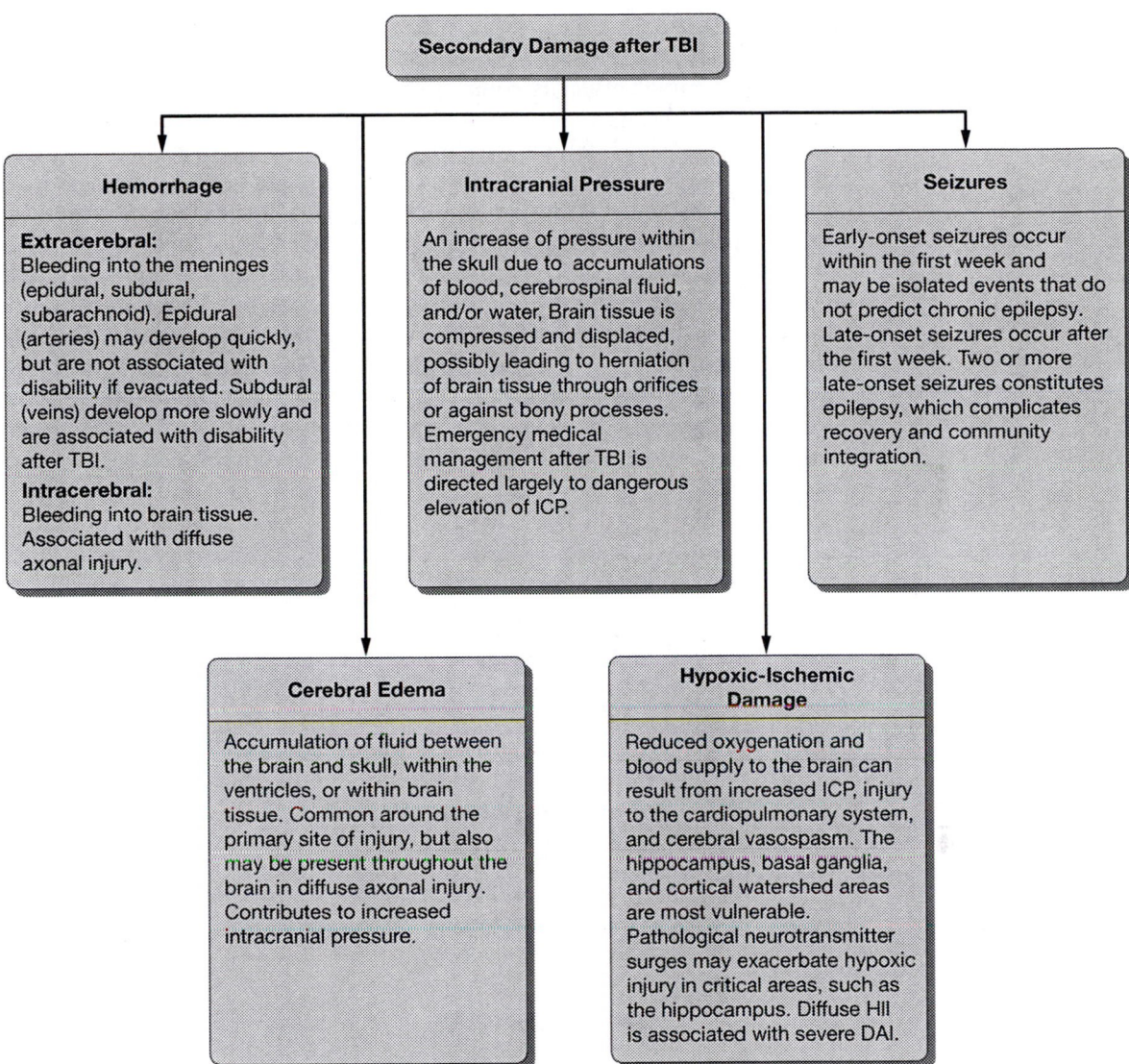

FIGURE 9–3. Pathologic events that often follow severe TBI and contribute to impairment. *Source:* From Communication Disorders Associated with Traumatic Brain Injury, by M. Ylvisaker, S. Szkeres, and T. Feeney. In *Language Intervention Strategies in Aphasia and Related Neurogenic Communication Disorders,* 4th ed. R. Chapey, Ed. Philadelphia: Lippincott Williams & Wilkins. Copyright 2001 by Lippincott Williams & Wilkins. Reprinted with permission.

■ EFFECTS OF CLOSED HEAD INJURY (CHI) AND TBI

The resultant sequelae of TBI should be evaluated in terms of the effects that occur immediately after the injury, those that are observed during the acute recovery period, and those that are long-term, or residual, effects.

Initial Effects

A frequent initial effect is coma. Confusion and posttraumatic amnesia are also observed frequently immediately after the injury. In mild injuries commonly associated with a *concussion,* a loss of consciousness occurs that lasts less than 30 minutes, and posttraumatic amnesia (PTA) lasts less than 1 hour. An injury is regarded as moderate if a loss of consciousness or posttraumatic amnesia is present for more than 30 minutes, but less than 24 hours. In severe cases, the coma lasts for more than 6 hours, and the PTA lasts for one to seven days. In very severe cases, the PTA lasts for more than seven days (Russell, 1993). The status of the patient on the Glasgow Coma Scale (Table 9–2) and the length of the PTA can be predictors of how the patient will do with regard to recovering language and cognitive functions. However, in the pediatric population, this needs to be interpreted with much caution as the Glasgow Coma Scale was developed for use with adults.

TABLE 9–2. Glasgow Coma Scale.

Eye opening (E)	
spontaneous	4
to speech	3
to pain	2
nil	1
Best motor response (M)	
obeys	6
localizes	5
withdraws	4
abnormal flexion	3
extensor response	2
nil	1
Verbal response (V)	
oriented	5
confused conversation	4
inappropriate words	3
incomprehensible sounds	2
nil	1

Coma score (E + M + V) = 3 – 15

13–15	Mild brain injury
9–12	Moderate brain injury
3–08	Severe brain injury

Source: From *Management of Head Injuries,* by B. Jennett and G. Teasdale, 1981, p. 78. Philadelphia: F. A. Davis. Copyright 1981 by F. A. Davis Company. Reprinted with permission.

The patient may also have **retrograde amnesia**, which is difficulty remembering events leading up to the accident. Abnormal behaviors such as irritability, aggression, anxiety, hyperactivity, lethargy, and withdrawal may also be observed in the immediate period after the injury. Motor dysfunctions such as rigidity, tremor, spasticity, ataxia, and apraxia may also be observed.

Retrograde amnesia. A common sequela of traumatic brain injury that creates difficulty in remembering events that led up to the accident.

Acute Recovery Period

During the acute recovery period, speech production deficits may occur such as difficulty with the production of consonants and possible mutism. The patient also may have speech comprehension problems and word retrieval deficits during the acute recovery stages. When shown common objects, the child may have difficulty describing them. Syntactic problems including a limited mean length of utterance, difficulty in constructing sentences, and fewer utterances, may be observed. In children old enough to write, deficits in this area may be noted.

Long-term (Residual) Effects

Possible long-term effects include persistent word retrieval problems and a reduction in spontaneous speech. When speech does occur, it may be characterized by reduced fluency, in part due to the word retrieval difficulties. Pragmatic problems are common. Subtle comprehension problems that result in reading problems, poor mathematic reasoning skills, and, in general, poor academic performance may be present. Memory problems may persist. Behaviorally, hyperactivity and impulsivity are frequently observed in post-TBI patients. An additional problem may involve residual confusion, in which the child is unable to recognize his or her own deficits.

Language characteristics occurring after closed head injury are outlined in Table 9–3. In addition to the language characteristics, psychological difficulties, which include depression, anger, and behaviors inappropriate for the situation, are frequently noted.

The child who sustains a TBI will have deficits in specific language areas, as well as in metacognitive and metalinguistic skills. These deficits also impact the child's ability to organize narratives (Reed, 2005). Ylvisaker and Szekeres (1989) identified seven problem areas in the academic arena for children who have sustained a TBI:

1. Limited self-awareness with regard to their communication problems

2. Poor planning, impacting the quality and organization of narratives

3. Difficulty initiating conversation with teachers and peers

TABLE 9–3. Language deficits in children with TBI.

Concentration
Sustained attention
Memory
Nonverbal problem solving
Part or whole analysis and synthesis
Conceptual organization and abstraction
Processing
Reasoning
Executive functioning (formulating goals, planning to achieve goals, carrying out plans)

Source: Adapted from *Mild Traumatic Brain Injury: A Therapy and Resource Manual,* by B. S. Green, K. M. Stevens, and T. D. W. Wolfe, 1997, San Diego: Singular Publishing Group. Copyright 1997 by Singular Publishing Group. Adapted with permission.

4. Problems with inhibition, leading to the use of inappropriate statements

5. Failure to self-monitor, affecting behavior and comprehension

6. General self-evaluations that do not lead to constructive responses

7. Lack of flexibility in problem solving

It is helpful for intervention purposes to work with the child in his natural settings to facilitate the development of language skills that can be used to combat these problem areas.

According to National Institutes of Health criteria (1984), three types of personality changes exist following a TBI. The first is apathy, in which the child does not care about what happens. He or she has reduced interest in the usual activities and challenges, which is often misinterpreted as compliance or absence of a behavior problem. However, that misinterpretation often reinforces the apathy. In other words, the caregivers treat the child as if he or she has a behavior problem, and, since the child may have trouble making them understand otherwise, the apathy is reinforced. The second personality change occurs when the child is overly optimistic regarding the extent of the disability. Although positive thinking can be a good trait, caution should be taken to ensure that the child has realistic expectations regarding the rate and degree of recovery. The third change entails a loss of social restraint and judgment. In these cases, the patient often becomes tactless and talkative. He or she can become hurtful, which frequently damages his or her relationships with family members. He or she may also have rage outbursts of abnormal intensity in response to trivial frustration.

■ PEDIATRIC VERSUS ADULT APHASIA

Pediatric patients usually exhibit nonfluent aphasia with mutism, effortful speech, and impaired repetition skills. Syntactic problems, auditory comprehension deficits, anomia, and reading and writing difficulties also may be present. Children are less likely than adults to show **paraphasia**, jargon, and fluent aphasia.

Paraphasia. The unintentional substitution of an incorrect word for an intended word.

In fluent aphasia, the patient does not have difficulty initiating speech, but he or she typically uses few, if any, content words. Syntax and prosody frequently remain intact, so the person appears to be speaking in sentences, but the sentences cannot be understood with regard to content.

Associated deficits in pediatric acquired aphasia include attentional disturbances and language impairments. As already mentioned, these language impairments include **anomia**. Also included are trouble with figurative and abstract language, difficulty in organizing the production of language, and problems in comprehending language. Cognitive and communication deficits result in academic underachievement. In her examination of the long-term residual effects of pediatric aphasia, Lees (1997) observed that, with adequate treatment, some children may achieve a relatively normal language profile based on testing used to measure progress after intensive therapy. However, Lees cautioned that, for some children, these normal language profiles masked persistent high-level difficulties, such as auditory verbal processing and lexical recall, which interfered with successful progress in school. Organically based behavioral and emotional deficits interfere with social interactions and impede the social-emotional growth that normally occurs during the school-age years. The child also may have perceptual-motor deficits that results in visual-field cuts, motor apraxia, or both.

Anomia. Lack of the ability to recall names of people, common objects, and places.

The individual who has sustained a TBI initially may demonstrate an aphasia-like set of symptoms. However, much of the research indicates that the traditional aphasic syndromes are uncommon following TBI in children and adults. A patient who has a diffuse injury is more likely to demonstrate impairment in receptive and expressive language accompanied by persistent cognitive deficits. Ylvisaker and colleagues (2001) write that "communication challenges following TBI are most often 'nonaphasic' in nature, that is, they co-exist with intelligible speech, reasonably fluent and grammatical language, and comprehension adequate to support everyday interaction" (p. 754).

Patients who do not present with aphasia in its classical terms still are likely to have language deficits that are not evident in routine interactions. Specifically, these deficits include problems with following complex oral directions, confrontational naming, and word fluency (Sarno, 1984). Ylvisaker and colleagues (2001) reflect the findings of many clinicians and caregivers in noting that patients with TBI often have deficits in interactive competence as the cognitive and social demands increase. Taken together, the array of communication deficits exhibited by patients with TBI are labeled by the American Speech-Language-Hearing Association (ASHA) as cognitive-communicative impairment (Ylvisaker, Hanks, & Johnson-Green, 2003), A listing of impairments with frontolimbic damage can be found in Table 9–4.

As a rule, recovery from mild TBI in children is usually excellent, while recovery from severe TBI is less certain. However, generally speaking, recovery in children is more complete than in adults regardless of the severity of the TBI (Bijur, Haslum, & Gloning, 1990). Murdoch and Theodoros (2001) suggest three reasons why recovery is more complete in children than in adults:

> First, it may be due to the different nature of the impacts causing TBI in children versus adults, childhood TBI generally being associated with lower-speed impacts; second, it may be related to differences in the basic mechanisms of brain damage following head injury in the two groups, which in turn are related to differences in the physical characteristics of children's heads and adult's heads; third, it may be the result of greater plasticity in the child's brain. (p. 248)

Even though their recovery is more complete, children with severe TBI frequently have residual and persistent language deficits as one would find in aphasia. These deficits include word-finding and naming problems, difficulty with expressive language (verbal, gestural, and written output) (Alajouanine & Lhermitte, 1965), and deficient repetition of words and sentences (Murdoch & Theodoros, 2001). In a study by Levin and Eisenberg (1979), the Neurosensory Center Comprehensive Examination for Aphasia (NCCEA; Spreen & Benton, 1969) was administered to a group of children and teenagers who had sustained a closed head injury. Eleven percent of their subjects had deficits in auditory comprehension; 4% had impaired verbal repetition; 12% had dysnomia. The same test and a similar age grouping was used in a study by Ewing-Cobbs and colleagues (1985) who found linguistic impairments (especially naming problems, dysgraphia, and reduced verbal production) in a significant portion of their subjects when they were less than six months post event. Ewing-Cobbs and colleagues concluded that their subjects demonstrated a "subclinical aphasia" due to the stages of language acquisition their subjects were in when they incurred their injury. In a later study by Ewing-Cobbs and colleagues (1987), they administered the NCCEA to 23 children and 33 adolescents who had TBI. In this study, they found significant language impairment in most of their subjects, with graphic and expressive functions being the most affected.

In a series of studies by Jordan and colleagues (Jordan, Ozanne, & Murdoch, 1988), 20 children between the ages of 8 and 16 years who had sustained a TBI were tested using the Test of Language Development series and the

TABLE 9–4. Vulnerable frontolimbic structures and frequently associated impairments.

Frontolimbic Injury and Executive System Impairment
- reduced awareness of personal strengths and weaknesses
- difficulty setting realistic goals
- difficulty planning and organizing behavior to achieve the goals
- impaired ability to initiate action needed to achieve the goals
- difficulty inhibiting behavior incompatible with achieving the goals
- difficulty self-monitoring and self-evaluating
- difficulty thinking and acting strategically, and solving real-world problems in a flexible and efficient manner
- general inflexibility and concreteness in thinking, talking, and acting

Frontolimbic Injury and Cognitive-Communication Impairment
- disorganized, poorly controlled discourse or paucity of discourse (spoken and written)
- inefficient comprehension of language related to increasing amounts of information to be processed (spoken or written) and to rate of speech
- imprecise language and word-retrieval problems
- difficulty understanding and expressing abstract and indirect language
- difficulty reading social cues, interpreting speaker intent, and flexibly adjusting interactive styles to meet situational demands in varied social contexts
- awkward or inappropriate communication in stressful social contexts
- impaired verbal learning

Frontolimbic Injury and Cognitive Impairment
- reduced internal control over all cognitive functions (e.g., attentional, perceptual, memory, organizational, and reasoning processes)
- impaired working memory
- impaired declarative and explicit memory (encoding and retrieval)
- disorganized behavior related to impaired organizing schemes (managerial knowledge frames, such as scripts, themes, schemas, mental models)
- impaired reasoning
- concrete thinking
- difficulty generalizing

Frontolimbic Injury and Psychosocial/Behavioral Impairment
- disinhibited, socially inappropriate, and possibly aggressive behavior
- impaired initiation or paucity of behavior
- inefficient learning from consequences
- perseverative behavior; rigid, inflexible behavior
- impaired social perception and interpretation

Source: From "Communication Disorders Associated with Traumatic Brain Injury," by M. Ylvisaker, S. F. Szekeres, and T. Feeney. In *Language Intervention Strategies in Aphasia and Related Neurogenic Disorders* (4th ed.), R. Chapey (Ed.), pp. 745–808. Copyright 2001 by Lippincott Williams & Wilkins.

Dysnomia. Loss of ability to name people, places, or things; may also be referred to as anomia.

NCCEA. When compared to a control group matched for age and sex, the children with TBI were mildly language-impaired 12 months after the injury. The language impairment was similar to that found in adults, creating the impression of a "subclinical aphasia" with **dysnomia**. At 24 months post injury, Jordan and Murdoch (1990) found that the naming deficit had persisted and verbal fluency had declined. This further solidifies the argument that children who sustain a moderate to severe TBI will have residual language deficits (Murdoch & Theodoros, 2001).

■ ASSESSMENT

Neuropsychological testing of an individual who has sustained a TBI should be completed by a multidisciplinary team that includes professionals from medicine, nursing, social work, psychology, physical therapy, occupational therapy, psychiatry, audiology, and speech-language pathology.

Mood and behavior changes can be due to the injury or an emotional reaction to the injuries. Testing of cognitive abilities includes assessment of auditory and visual processing skills and a determination of attention abilities, similar to those assessed in attention deficit disorder. Of particular interest are the child's abilities to sustain attention and to use selective attention, divided attention, and **alternating attention** (Mateer & Moore-Sohlberg, 1992).

Alternating attention. The ability to shift attention between tasks that have different cognitive demands.

Testing of language abilities should concentrate on the comprehension of single words and sentences, auditory discrimination skills, and expressive language abilities. Assessment of memory and learning should be done in conjunction with language testing and should focus on auditory and visual memory, immediate and delayed recall, and the ability to learn new information. Intelligence testing should analyze verbal intelligence, nonverbal intelligence, and general knowledge.

Communication should be assessed and analyzed in a variety of contexts. This involves observing the individual with TBI interacting in a multiplicity of settings with different individuals. It will be necessary to evaluate how they interact with each other and to eventually modify the communication behavior of the injured individual as well as his or her communication partners. Blosser and DePompei (2003) present a diagram that illustrates the interrelated aspects of communication. This is depicted in Figure 9–4.

Executive functioning refers to setting and executing goals and the ability to self-evaluate. Many individuals who have suffered a TBI have trouble with motivation and personal drive. Accident-induced lethargy contributes to this problem, which may occur even in individuals who were highly motivated and self-directed prior to the accident. Tests of dissimulation that assess the patient's effort and motivation also should be completed (Green et al., 1997).

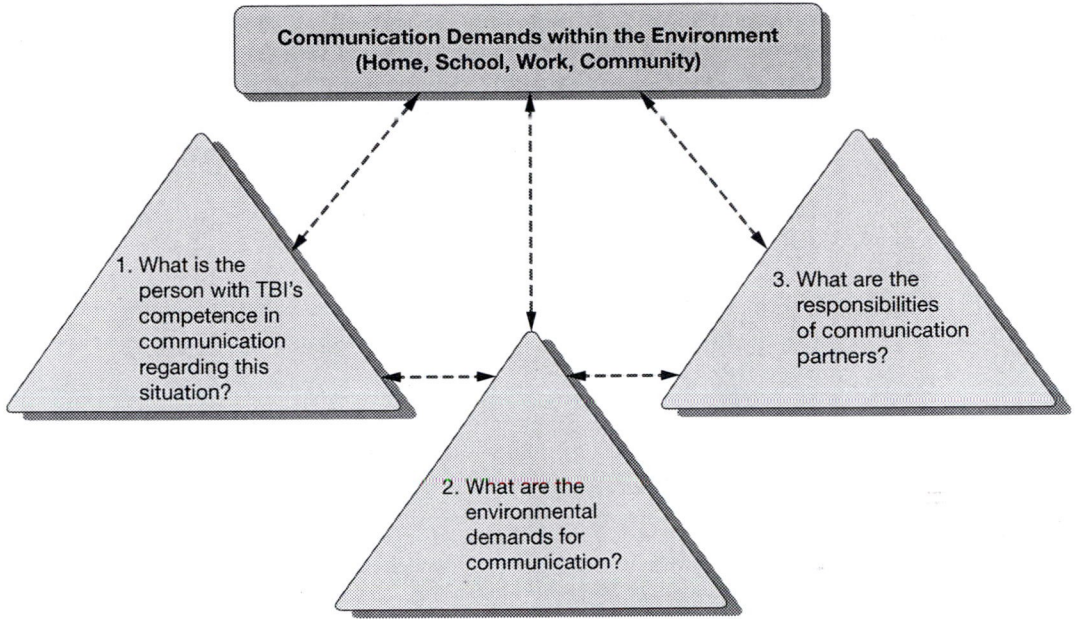

FIGURE 9–4. Interrelated aspects of communication. *Source:* From Pediatric Traumatic Brain Injury: Proactive Intervention, by J. Blosser & R. DePompei. Clifton Park, NY: Delmar Thomson Learning. Copyright 2003 by Delmar Thomson Learning. Reprinted with permission.

Problems with executive functioning may be manifested as reduced deficit awareness, poor goal-setting skills, lack of initiation of tasks, poor self-monitoring, difficulty in making and keeping a schedule, and poor time efficiency.

Testing of academic skills and achievement should include subject-specific testing. This includes mathematics, vocabulary, reading, and spelling. Abstract reasoning and concept formation should address problem-solving skills and the ability to make appropriate judgments. Motor strength, coordination, and manual dexterity should be part of the assessment of fine motor control and speed. Orientation in space and time, visual and tactile perceptual abilities, and responses to varying sensations may have a negative effect on the testing of sensory and perceptual skills.

Finally, a complete personality inventory and psychosocial examination should be done. Many patients who have suffered a TBI are reported to undergo personality changes after the accident, so this should be assessed by a competent psychologist or psychiatrist, or both (Green et al., 1997).

When assessing the strengths and weaknesses of an individual who has suffered a TBI, the professionals involved must communicate frequently and regularly in order to follow the changes that occur as the patient's physical injuries resolve. It is important to remember that the patient may fatigue easily, so testing should be done in several short sessions, as opposed to one long session. Sensitivity to the patient's emotional state is also important so that the individual does not become overly frustrated or depressed by his or her performance on the varying tasks that are presented.

A list of assessment tools that are appropriate for use with children who have sustained a TBI is found in Table 9–5.

There are many tests and scales that can be used to determine the severity of a brain injury and to measure associated disability. These tests are listed in Table 9–6.

TABLE 9–5. Language tests suitable for use with children with TBI.

Test	Authors
Preschool Language Scale-3 (PLS-3)	Zimmerman et al. (1992)
Receptive-Expressive Emergent Language Test—Second Edition (REEL-2)	Bzoch and League (1991)
Clinical Evaluation of Language Fundamentals—Third Edition (CELF-3)	Semel, Wiig, and Secord (1995)
Clinical Evaluation of Language Fundamentals—Preschool (CELF-P)	Wiig, Secord, and Semel (1992)
Peabody Picture Vocabulary Test-Third Edition (PPVT-III)	Dunn and Dunn (1997)
Hundred Pictures Naming Test (HPNT)	Fisher and Glenister (1992)
Boston Naming Test (BNT)	Kaplan et al. (1983)
Test of Language Competence-Expanded Edition (TLC)	Wiig and Secord (1989)
Test of Word Knowledge (TOWK)	Wiig and Secord (1992)
Test of Problem Solving-Elementary (TOPS-Elementary)	Bowers et al. (1994)
Test of Problem Solving-Adolescent (TOPS-Adolescent)	Bowers et al. (1991)
Queensland University Inventory of Literacy (QUIL)	Dodd et al. (1996)
Test of Phonological Awareness (TOPA)	Torgesen and Bryant (1994)
School Age Oral Language Assessment (SAOLA)	Allen et al. (1993)

Source: Reprinted from *Traumatic Brain Injury: Associated Speech, Language, and Swallowing Disorders.* By B. B. Murdoch and D. G. Theodoros, p. 265. Copyright 2001 by Delmar.

TABLE 9–6. Assessments commonly used to measure injury severity and associated disability.

Assessment Procedure	Description
Glasgow Coma Scale (Teasdale and Jennett, 1974)	A 3-category (eye opening, motor response, verbal response), 15-point scale commonly used to measure the initial severity of TBI. Scores of 8 or lower within the first several hours after injury typically classified as severe injuries, 11–12 as moderate, and 13–15 as mild.
Duration of Coma	Generally based on time from injury to eye opening and resumption of normal sleep-wake cycles. Measured in minutes or hours for mild to moderate injuries and in days, weeks, or months for severe injuries. Sometimes used more informally to refer to the period of significantly altered consciousness.
Duration of Post-Traumatic Amnesia	Based on time from injury to resumption of orientation and integration of day-to-day memories. Very hard to establish with precision in severe cases.
Galveston Orientation and Amnesia Test (GOAT) (Levin et al., 1979)	A 10-question test of orientation to person, place, and time and of memory for recent, post-injury events as well as for most recent preinjury events.
Glasgow Outcome Scale (Jennett and Bond, 1975)	A 5-category global outcome scale: death, persistent vegetative state, severe disability (conscious, but disabled and dependent), moderate disability (disabled but independent), and good recovery (relatively normal life, but possibly with ongoing minor impairment).
Rancho Los Amigos Levels of Cognitive Functioning (Hagen, 1981)	An 8-level scale of cognitive recovery, based on observations of responsiveness, purposeful activity, orientation, memory, self-regulation, spontaneity, independence. Levels: no response, generalized response, localized response, confused-agitated, confused-nonagitated, confused-appropriate, automatic-appropriate, and purposeful-appropriate.
Disability Rating Scale (Rappaport et al., 1982)	A rating scale developed to track improvement of people with TBI from coma to community. Includes subscales for impairment (similar to GCS), disability (cognitive ability for feeding, toileting, and grooming), and handicap (level of community functioning and employability).

(continued)

TABLE 9–6. (*continued*)

Assessment Procedure	Description
Functional Assessment Measure (FIM + FAM) (Hall, 1992)	A rating scale that adds 12 domains for disability to the 12 domains of the older Functional Independence Measure (FIM). The additional items, added specifically for individuals with brain injury, include swallowing, reading, writing, orientation, attention, safety judgment, emotional status, and adjustment to limitations.
ASHA-FACS (Frattali et al., 1995)	A rating scale designed to assess functional communication with greater precision than is possible with most general disability rating tools.
Communication Effectiveness Survey (Beukelman, 1998)	A survey designed to assess functional communication in natural contexts.
Community Integration Questionnaire (Willer et al., 1994)	A 15-item questionnaire designed to assess home and social integration and productivity in the following domains: household activities, shopping, errands, and leisure activities.

Source: From "Communication Disorders Associated with Traumatic Brain Injury," by M. Ylvisaker, S. F. Szekeres, and T. Feeney. In *Language Intervention Strategies in Aphasia and Related Neurogenic Disorders* (4th ed.), R. Chapey (Ed.), pp. 745–808. Copyright 2001 by Lippincott Williams & Wilkins.

■ STAGES OF RECOVERY/IMPROVEMENT

Szekeres, Ylvisaker, and Holland (1985) have defined three stages of improvement that are based on the Rancho Los Amigos Levels of Cognitive Functioning (Hagen, 1981). As described by Szerkeres colleagues, the early stage is compatible with the Ranchos Los Amigos (RLA) levels 2 to 3. The behaviors at this stage range from the initial generalized responses to environmental stimuli to external stimulus-specific responses. These stimulus-specific responses would include localizing to sound, visual tracking, appropriately using common objects, and following simple commands. This stage is frequently referred to as the sensory or coma stimulation stage of treatment, with the patient needing intensive support from others.

During the middle stage (RLA levels 4–6), the patient may initially be disoriented, confused, and agitated but will be more active and alert than in the early stage. Typically, these patients experience improvement slowly. They may become more goal-directed but will still have difficulty in planning a course of action to achieve the goals, Memory continues to be impaired, although some improvement in episodic memory and focused attention may occur. They will continue to need support from others in their environment although simplifying and structuring the environment may facilitate eventual independence.

The last stage is equivalent to the RLA levels 7, 8, and beyond. The goal at this stage is to help the patient achieve his or her ultimate level of independence through the fading of environmental supports. The patient may have residual communication and cognitive deficits, with therapy focusing on the development of compensatory strategies and functional skills that can be used in the patient's natural settings (Ylvisaker et al., 2001).

■ TREATMENT

Whether the patient is an adult or a child, his or her treatment must consist of a team approach. Rehabilitation specialists functioning as a multidisciplinary team must be involved in order to work toward a positive resolution of any residual deficits. Family counseling in which family members are assigned their own roles in the rehabilitation process also is critical. The speech-language pathologist will "help to identify effective and functional supports to enable cognitively disabled individuals to be as independent and successful as possible. Such supports may include cognitive prosthetic devices (e.g., memory logs)" and changes to expectations and environments to facilitate re-introduction into the child's natural settings (Coelho et al., 1996, p. S7).

Factors affecting treatment include the stage of recovery, etiological factors, and age at the time of injury. Age is important because the younger the child, the greater the plasticity of the brain. Plasticity refers to the ability of the undamaged areas of the brain to compensate for the damaged areas of the brain. It is believed that the more plasticity the brain has, the better the chances for natural recovery of some function. Regardless, therapy is needed to help manipulate the plasticity to ensure that the child recovers his or her maximum abilities (Rose, Johnson, & Attree, 1997):

> Environmental enrichment is a key to recovery. A common consequence of traumatic brain injury in humans is a reduction in cerebral arousal-activation. In combination with other common neuropsychological impairments, for example, inattention, memory, and motivation, this can result in significantly reduced levels of interaction between the patient and his environment. Coexisting sensory and motor impairments can restrict interaction still further. Clinicians agree that to increase levels of interaction between brain damaged patients and their environments is a vital part of any rehabilitation process. (p. 4)

Rose and colleagues advocate the use of computerized virtual reality therapy to create real-life and imaginary situations as a method of facilitating environmental interaction in a safe environment. Since most children have access to computer games, this method of bringing a variety of environments into a safe therapeutic setting holds great promise in therapy with the pediatric population (Rose et al., 1997). However, there has not been sufficient research in this form of intervention to make any conclusive statements.

Because many patients suffering from residual effects of TBI fatigue easily, it is usually recommended that initial therapy sessions be brief and frequent. In other words, four 15-minute sessions per day may be more productive than a single 1-hour session. Functional communication goals should be targeted in individual and group therapy. Determining readiness to return to school or work should be a prime consideration. Thus, it is important to focus not only on functional goals but also compensatory strategies that can be used to minimize the deficits. The rehabilitation team, including the family members, will also need to work closely with the patient's school/work personnel to facilitate the transition back into the patient's natural settings. Initially, an appropriate classroom setting may be a class specifically designed for children recovering from TBI or a classroom for students with learning disabilities (Iskowitz, 1997).

During the acute phase, therapy is likely to focus on sensory stimulation and working closely with the family to encourage responses from the child. Although speech and language abilities are a concern, during this stage issues related to self-care, swallowing, and feeding may be paramount. However, as the child progresses, more attention can be focused on speech and language goals and preparing the child to return to his or her home and school environment. This includes focusing on prospective memory, which is the ability to remember to do things at the appropriate time (such as taking prescribed medications) and functional memory. Functional memory includes the skills needed to learn new information, recall old information, remember situational details, and to function independently (Green et al., 1997). It will also be important to address pragmatic issues with the client with emphasis on social skills such as carrying on a conversation, sharing, greeting, and cooperating in order to facilitate interaction with others in the client's natural environments (Ylvisaker et al., 1992).

Cognition will also be a focus in therapy. This will include addressing memory, attention, reasoning ability, organization, efficient information processing, perceptual skills, and learning. However, there are impediments inherent in TBI that make therapy more challenging. For example, people with TBI frequently have difficulty taking previous consequences into consideration when making decisions. They also frequently have reduced initiation which can also impede executive functions such as decision making. Deficits in working and strategic memory, poor organizational skills, and impaired memory of previous consequences to decisions impede improvement in cognition. There is also difficulty with maintenance and generalization of skills beyond the therapy setting to the patient's natural environments. Patients with TBI frequently exhibit oppositional behavior and this, combined with poor ability to learn from previous consequences impede behavior management in patients with TBI (Ylvisaker et al., 2001).

Regardless of the age of the individual with TBI, treatment needs to be focused on having the patient be an active participant in the therapy process. Therapy should address the development of skills that will enable the patient to succeed

TABLE 9–7. Individual skills necessary for effective communication in various environments.

School	Employment
maintain adequate vocabulary	attend regularly
request information	communicate effectively
respond to questions	follow directions
follow directions	organize day and job routines
comprehend lectures	adapt to changes
read for functional comprehension	recognize mistakes
write for functional expression	correct mistakes
organize for planning and sequencing	care for work area
store and recall information for later use	ask for help
Social	use socially acceptable manners
monitor actions	use non-aggressive socially correct language
manage time	demonstrate initiative
understand cultural diversity	cope with constructive criticism
respect others	**Independent Living**
use correct pragmatics	plan daily routine
demonstrate socially acceptable	carry out daily routine
manners and language	use public transportation
	know community resources and how to access
	advocate for self without offending others
	manage finances

Source: From *Pediatric Traumatic Brain Injury: Proactive Intervention* (2nd ed.), by J. L. Blosser and R. DePompei, p. 172. Copyright 2003 by Delmar Learning.

in school, independent living, working environments, and social activities. Blosser and DePompei (2003) have delineated the skills needed to effectively communicate in each of these settings. These skills are outlined in Table 9–7.

■ SUMMARY

Based on studies conducted over the last 20 years, Murdoch and Theodoros (2001) have concluded that while children who suffer a mild TBI usually fully recover, those who have moderate to severe TBI events do not fully recover. Receptive language is not as impaired as expressive language, and the children have compromised "expressive oral language skills, including verbal fluency and naming to confrontation" (p. 251). In the initial stages, the child typically has reduced verbal output (even to the point of mutism in some cases). Long term, they have subtle high-language deficits characterized by poor verbal fluency, word-finding difficulties, and dysnomia. Generally speaking, the language impairments following moderate to severe TBI in children is similar to those found in adults. Speech-language pathologists will be seeing these children in therapy as they are integrated back into their home and school setting following the TBI.

Over the last several years, speech-language pathologists have held discussions regarding the need to establish medical tracks and school-based tracks in speech-language pathology coursework. However, the population of students with TBI helps point out the need to have both types of education, regardless of the professional's primary employment site. Those who work with a child in the medical setting need to understand the educational setting to which the child will return as soon as possible. Likewise, those in the educational setting need to be familiar with the long-term sequelae of TBI and to understand the nature of the injury and recovery process. These children also need to be followed closely throughout their academic careers to monitor possible residual deficits that may play a role in a child's educational and social progress.

Adults returning to their work settings, like children returning to their school settings following a TBI, need to be monitored to gauge the effect the TBI and its residual deficits have on the individual. Careful attention needs to be paid to his or her ability to adapt to the old surroundings and to be sure the patient does not become depressed and/or frustrated to the point that it is not possible for him or her to continue in that setting. This may involve providing therapy in the community-based settings, with the clinician going to the client instead of having the client come to a therapy setting. Functional goals should be established that relate to the needs and interests of the client (Blosser & DePompei, 1989; DePompei & Blosser, 1987, Coehlo et al., 1996).

CASE STUDY

History

L, a 19-year-old left-handed male was seen on July 23, 2004 for an initial speech and language evaluation. He had suffered a gun shot wound to the left frontal lobe in a drive-by shooting when he was 17 years old and, consequently, had aphasia. During the first six months following the trauma, L received speech-language therapy, physical therapy, and occupational therapy five times a week in a residential rehabilitation center.

During this time, he also worked with a homebound teacher on his schooling. He has continued with out patient speech-language therapy two times a week since he was discharged from the residential rehabilitation center. L and his family recently moved to Gainesville and have been referred to the University of Florida Speech and Hearing Clinic for continued therapy. L had difficulty with the subject matter at the ninth grade level and did not return to school following discharge from the rehabilitation center. He did continue to work with a homebound teacher for three months until he was 18 but did not graduate.

L wears glasses, has a brace on his right leg, and has a moderate hearing (40 dB) loss in his right ear. L has taken 100 mg of Dilantin three times a day since the shooting to control seizures.

Assessment

L's speech, language, and cognitive functions were assessed using the Western Aphasia Battery during his initial visit to our clinic. The results of the subtests were as follows.

Spontaneous Speech	Information Content	9/10
	Fluency, grammatical competence, paraphasias	5/10
	Total	14/20
Auditory Comprehension	Yes/No questions	60/60
	Auditory word recognition	51/60
	Sequential commands	47/80
	Total	158/200
Repetition		84/100
Naming	Object Naming	44/60
	Word fluency	10/20
	Sentence completion	10./10
	Responsive speech	8/10
	Total	72/100
Reading	Comprehension of sentences	34/40
	Reading commands	14/20
	Written word stimulus—object choice matching	6/6
	Written word stimulus—picture word matching	6/6
	Written word stimulus—written word choice matching	6/6

	Spoken word stimulus—written word choice matching	3/4
	Letter discrimination	4/6
	Spelled word recognition	1/6
	Spelling	2/6
	Total	76/100
Writing	Not assessed due to L's fatigue	
Apraxia		60/60
Constructional, Visuospatial & Calculation Tasks	Drawing	26/30
	Block design	9/9
	Calculation	18/24
	Raven's Progressive Matrixes	31/37
	Total	84/100
Aphasia Quotient		75

In the spontaneous speech test, L's speech was characterized as often being telegraphic; however, some grammatical organization was evident. Certain paraphasias were noted. On the auditory comprehension subtest, L answered yes/no questions with 100% accuracy. On the auditory word recognition section, he achieved 85% accuracy and did not demonstrate difficulty with any particular category. L scored 59% on sequential commands, which demonstrates his difficulty when commands are increased in length and complexity (two or more steps).

On the repetition subtest, L performed with 84% accuracy. The longer sentences and phrases proved to be the most difficult for the client to repeat.

L was able to name objects with 73% accuracy. On the word fluency section, he was able to name 10 animals in one minute, indicating decreased word fluency. One paraphasia was noted ("canteloupe" for "antelope"). He was 100% accurate on the sentence completion section, and his responsive speech was 80% accurate.

On reading comprehension of sentences, L was 85% accurate. It took him a long time (average 3 to 5 minutes) to complete the task. The additional time appeared to help him answer items correctly. On the reading commands section, L was 70% accurate. He had difficulty reading each command aloud and received only partial points on the more complex commands. On choice matching of written and spoken words, L was 75% to 100% accurate. He had more difficulty identifying the written word from an orally presented target, as opposed to pointing to a picture or object that matched the written word, or pointing to the written word that matched the picture.

On the letter discrimination section, L was 67% accurate. He performed with 17% accuracy on spelled word recognition and 33% accuracy on spelling words. It was noted that L finger spelled the letters on the table, but he was unable to process what individual letters together would spell.

The client was able to perform upper limb, facial, instrumental, and complex gestures upon command with 100% accuracy. His responses were quick and appropriate.

L showed little difficulty with constructional tasks. He was able to free-handedly draw the figures required with 87% accuracy. All but one of his drawings were appropriate; he drew a square when asked to draw a circle. On the Block Design subtest, which tests visuospatial skills, he was able to quickly put four blocks together in the desired pattern with 100% accuracy.

Calculation tasks were 75% accurate. He showed no difficulty with addition and multiplication but had some errors in subtraction and division. This may have been partially due to the examiner's presentation of the cards; combined oral and visual stimulation was not provided.

The Cinderella story was used to assess L's expressive narrative speech and language ability. His speech was characterized as nonfluent with an abundance of fillers such as "ya know," "and all this," and "and everything," and contained many pauses. He had much difficulty initiating sentences, and produced false starts throughout the story.

Summary

L presents with mild auditory and reading comprehension problems, even though his scores were relatively high for these subtests. This was evidenced by his frequent delay of response, and/or request for a repetition. His speech is nonfluent and is characterized by a short mean length of utterance, frequent pauses, false starts, and fillers. His speech, at times, was also telegraphic. L demonstrated letter-processing problems visually and auditorily. He also showed problems spontaneously naming functional objects, and performing sequential commands.

Impression

L presents with Broca's aphasia, characterized by his nonfluent speech, a greater production of nouns and verbs compared to other grammatical forms, agrammatic speech, and an abundance of pauses and fillers.

Recommendations

It was recommended that L receive individual therapy two times a week for one hour sessions. Therapy concentrated on sentence production of "Wh" interrogatives and object relatives. It was also recommended that he receive a full audiological evaluation.

■ REVIEW QUESTIONS

1. A contrecoup injury is one in which the injury to the brain is at the point of impact only.
   a. True
   b. False

2. Severe TBIs are characterized by a loss of consciousness lasting 1 to 24 hours.
   a. True
   b. False

3. Individuals who have sustained a closed head injury are likely to demonstrate attention disorders, impulsivity, and fluctuating moods.
   a. True
   b. False

4. Falls are the leading cause of TBIs in the age 5 to 64 population.
   a. True
   b. False

5. According to IDEA, TBI includes brain injuries that are congenital.
   a. True
   b. False

6. As defined by the WHO, which of the following defines an impairment?
   a. A decreased ability to participate in work, school, social situations, and so on
   b. A reduction in the individual's ability to effectively and successfully participate in activities of life
   c. A disruption or abnormality in mental or physical functioning

7. Cerebral edema is an example of primary damage resulting from a TBI.
   a. True
   b. False

8. Children who have sustained a TBI usually exhibit nonfluent aphasia as opposed to a fluent aphasia.
   a. True
   b. False

9. Which of the following should be included in an assessment battery for children with a TBI?

   a. Tests of academic skills and achievement

   b. Tests of executive functioning

   c. Language tests

   d. Personality inventory and psychosocial examination

   e. All of the above

   f. a, b, and c

   g. a, c, and d

10. Usually receptive language is not as impaired as expressive language in individuals who have sustained a moderate to severe TBI.

   a. True

   b. False

■ REFERENCES

Alajouanine, T. & Lhermitte, F. (1965). Acquired aphasia in children. *Brain, 88,* 653–662.

Allen, L., Leitao, S., & Donovan, M. (1993). *School Age Oral Language Assessment.* South Fremantle, Western Australia: Language-Learning Materials, Research and Development.

American Speech-Language-Hearing Association (ASHA). (1987). The role of speech-language pathologists in the rehabilitation of cognitively impaired individuals: A report of the subcommittee on language and cognition, *Asha, 29,* 53–55.

American Speech-Language-Hearing Association (ASHA). (1990). Guidelines for speech-language pathologists serving persons with language, socio-communicative, and/or cognitive communicative impairments. *Asha, 32,* 85–92.

Beukelman, D. R. (1998). Communication effectiveness survey. In D. R. Beukelman, P. Mathy, & K. Yorkston, Outcomes measurement in motor speech disorders. In C. M. Frattali (ed.), *Measuring outcomes in speech-language pathology* (pp. 334–353). New York: Thieme.

Bijur, P. E., Haslum, M., & Gloning, J. (1990). Cognitive and behavioral sequelae of mild head injury in children. *Pediatrics, 86,* 337–344.

Blosser, J. L., & DePompei, R. (1989). The head injured student returns to school: Recognizing and treating deficits. *Topics in Language Disorders, 9,* 19–32.

Blosser, J. L., & DePompei, R. (1994). *Pediatric traumatic brain injury: Proactive intervention.* San Diego: Singular Publishing Group.

Blosser, J. L., & DePompei, R. (2003). *Pediatric traumatic brain injury: Proactive Intervention,* 2nd ed. Clifton Park, NY: Delmar Learning.

Bowers, L., Huisingh, R., Barrett, M., Orman, J., & LoGuidice, C. (1991). *Test of problem solving-elementary.* Nerang East, Queensland, Australia: Pro-Ed.

Bowers, L., Huisingh, R., Barrett, M., Orman, J., & LoGuidice, C. (1994). *Test of problem solving-elementary.* Nerang East, Queensland, Australia: Pro-Ed.

Bzoch, K. R., & League, R. (1991). *Receptive-expressive emergent language test, second edition.* Austin, TX: Pro-Ed.

Coelho, C. A., DeRuyter, F., & Stein, M. (1996, October). Treatment efficacy: Cognitive-communicative disorders resulting from traumatic brain injury in adults. *Journal of Speech and Hearing Research, 39*(5), S5–S17.

DePompei, R., & Blosser, J. (1987). Strategies for helping head-injured children successfully return to school. *Language, Speech, and Hearing Services in the Schools, 18,* 292–300.

Dodd, B., Holm, A., Qerlemans, M., & McCormack, M. (1996). *Queensland University Inventory of Literacy.* Nerang East, Queensland, Australia: The University of Queensland.

Dunn, L. M., & Dunn, L. M. (1997). *Peabody picture vocabulary test-third edition.* Circle Pines, MN: American Guidance Service.

Ewing-Cobbs, L., Fletcher, J. M., & Levin, H. S. (1985). In M. Ylvisaker (Ed.), *Head injury rehabilitation: Children and adolescents* (pp. 71–89). Austin, TX: Pro-Ed.

Ewing-Cobbs, L., Fletcher, J. M., Levin, H. S., & Landry, S. H. (1985). Language disorders after pediatric head injury. In J. K. Darby (Ed.), *Speech and language evaluation in neurology: Childhood disorders* (pp. 97–112). Orlando, FL: Grune & Stratton.

Ewing-Cobbs, L., Levin, H. S., Eisenberg, H. M., & Fletcher, J. M. (1987). Language functions following closed head injury in children and adolescents. *Journal of Clinical and Experimental Neuropsychology, 9,* 575–592.

Fisher, J. P., & Glenister, J. M. (1992). *The Hundred Pictures Naming Test.* Victoria: ACER.

Frattali, C. M., Thompson, C. K., Holland, A. L., Wohl, C. B., & Ferketic, M. M. (1995). *The American Speech-Language-Hearing Association functional assessment of communication skills for adults (ASHA FACS).* Rockville, MD: ASHA.

Green, B. S., Stevens, K. M., & Wolfe, T. D. W. (1997). *Mild traumatic brain injury: A therapy and resource manual.* San Diego: Singular Publishing Group.

Hagen, C. (1981). Language disorders secondary to closed head injury. *Topics in Language Disorders, 1,* 73–87.

Hall, K. M. (1992). Overview of functional assessment scales in brain injury rehabilitation, *NeuroRehabilitation, 2,* 98–113.

Hegde, M. N. (1996). *Pocketguide to assessment in speech-language pathology.* San Diego: Singular Publishing Group.

Iskowitz, M. (1997, June 16). Overcoming obstacles of pediatric TBI. *Advance for Speech Language Pathologists, 7*(24), 5.

Jennett, B., & Bond, M. (1975). Assessment of outcome after severe brain damage: A practical scale. *Lancet, 1,* 480–484.

Jennett, B., & Teasdale, G. (1981). *Management of head injuries.* Philadelphia: F. A. Cavis Company.

Jordan, F. M., & Murdoch, B. E. (1990). Linguistic status following closed head injury: A follow-up study. *Brain Injury, 4,* 147–154.

Jordan, F. M., Ozanne, A. E., & Murdoch, B. E. (1988). Long-term speech and language disorders subsequent to closed head injury in children. *Brain Injury, 2,* 179–185.

Jorgenson, C., Barrett, M., Huisingh, R., & Zachman, L. (1981). *The word test.* East Moline, IL: Linguisystems.

Kaplan, E., Goodglass, H., & Weintraub, S. (1983). *Boston naming test.* Philadelphia: Lea & Febiger.

Kay, T., & the Mild Traumatic Brain Injury Committee of the Head Injury Special Interest Group of the American Congress of Rehabilitation Medicine. (1993). Definition of mild traumatic brain injury. *Journal of Head Trauma Rehabilitation, 8*(3), 86–87.

Kertesz, A. (1982). *Western aphasia battery.* Orlando, FL: Grune and Stratton.

Lees, J. (1993). *Children with acquired aphasias.* London: Whurr Publishers.

Lees, J. (1997). Long-term effects of acquired aphasias in childhood. *Pediatric Rehabilitation, 1*(1), 45–49.

Levin, H. S., & Eisenberg, H. M. (1979). Neuropsychological impairment after closed head injury in children and adolescents. *Journal of Pediatric Psychology, 4,* 389–402.

Levin, H. S., Eisenberg, H. M., & Benton, A. L. (1989). *Mild head injury.* New York: Oxford University Press.

Levin, H. S., O'Donnell, V. M., & Grossman, R. G. (1979). The Galveston orientation and amnesia test: A practical scale to assess cognition after head injury. *Journal of Nervous and Mental Diseases, 167,* 675–684.

Mateer, C., & Moore-Sohlberg, M. (1992, September). Current perspectives in cognitive rehabilitation. Presented at a conference entitled Speaking of Cognition . . . Assessment and Intervention Strategies. Sponsored by Rehabilitation Services Midwest Medical Center, Indianapolis, IN.

Murdoch, B. E., & Theodoros, D. G. (2001). *Traumatic brain injury: Associated speech, language, and swallowing disorders.* Clifton Park, NY: Delmar.

National Head Injury Foundation (1985). *An educator's manual: What educators need to know about students with traumatic brain injury.* Framingham, MA: Author.

National Institutes of Health. (1984). *Head injury: Hope through research.* NIH Publication No. 84–2478, pp. 1–37. Bethesda, MD: Author.

Nelson, N. W. (1993). *Childhood language disorders in context: Infancy through adolescence.* New York: Macmillan Publishing Company.

Rappaport, M., Hall, K. M., Hopkins, H. K., Belleza, T., & Cope, D. N. (1982). Disability rating scale for severe head trauma: Coma to community. *Archives of Physical Medicine and Rehabilitation, 63,* 118–123.

Reed, V. A. (1994). *An introduction to children with language disorders* (2nd ed.). New York: Macmillan Publishing Company.

Reed, V. A. (2005). *An introduction to children with language disorders* (3rd ed.). New York: Macmillan Publishing Company.

Rose, F. D., Johnson, D. A., & Attree, E. A. (1997). Rehabilitation of the head-injured child: Basic research and new technology. *Pediatric Rehabilitation, 1*(1), 3–7.

Russell, N. K. (1993, April). Educational considerations in traumatic brain injury: The role of the speech-language pathologist. *Language, Speech, and Hearing Services in the Schools, 24,* 67–75.

Sarno, M. T. (1984). Verbal impairment after closed head injury: Report of a replication study. *Journal of Nervous and Mental Disease, 172,* 475–479.

Satz, P., & Bullard-Bates, C. (1981). Acquired aphasia in children. In M. T. Sarno (Ed.), *Acquired aphasia* (pp. 399–426). New York: Academic Press.

Semel, E., Wiig, E. H., & Secord, W. A. (1995). *Clinical evaluation of language fundamentals-third edition.* San Antonio, TX: Pro-Ed.

Sohlberg, M. M., & Mateer, C. A. (1989). *Introduction to cognitive rehabilitation theory and practice.* New York: Guilford Press.

Spreen, O., & Benton, A. L. (1969). Neurosensory centre comprehensive examination for aphaisa. Victoria, British Columbia, Canada: University of Victoria.

Szekeres, S., Ylvisaker, M., & Holland, A. (1985). Cognitive rehabilitation therapy: A framework for intervention. In M. Ylvisaker (Ed.), *Head injury rehabilitation: Children and adolescents.* Boston: College-Hill Press/Little, Brown.

Teasdale, G. M., & Jennett, B. (1974). Assessment of coma and impaired consciousness: A practical scale. *Lancet, 2,* 81–84.

Torgensen, J. K., & Bryant, B. R. (1994). *Test of phonological awareness.* Nerang East, Queensland, Australia: Pro-Ed.

Wiig, E. H., & Secord, W. A. (1989). *Test of language competence-expanded edition.* San Antonio, TX: The Psychological Corporation.

Wiig, E. H., & Secord, W. A. (1992). *Test of word knowledge.* San Antonio, TX: The Psychological Corporation.

Wiig, E. H., Secord, W. A., & Semel, E. (1992). *Clinical evaluation of language fundamentals-preschool.* San Antonio, TX: The Psychological Corporation.

Willer, B., Ottenbacher, K. J., & Coad, M. L. (1994). The community integration questionnaire. *American Journal of Physical and Medical Rehabilitation, 73,* 103–107.

World Health Organization (1987). *International classification of impairments, disabilities, and handicaps.* Geneva, Switzerland: Author.

Ylvisaker, M., Hanks, R., & Johnson-Green, D. (2003). Rehabilitation of children and adults with cognitive-communication disorders after brain injury. *Asha Supplement, 23,* 59–72.

Ylvisaker, M., & Szekeres, S. (1989). Metacognitive and executive impairments in head-injured children and adults. *Topics in Language Disorders, 9,* 34–49.

Ylvisaker, M., Szekeres, S., & Feeney, T. (2001). Communication disorders associated with traumatic brain injury. In R. Chapey (Ed.), *Language intervention strategies in aphasia and related neurogenic communication disorders* (4th ed.). Philadelphia: Lippincott Williams & Wilkins.

Ylvisaker, M., Szekeres, S., Haarbauer-Krupa, J., Urbanczyk, B., & Feeney, T. (1992). Speech and language intervention. In G. Wolcott & R. Savage (Eds.), *Educational programming for children and young adults with acquired brain injury.* Austin, TX: Pro-Ed.

Zimmerman, I. L., Steiner, V. G., & Pond, R. E. (1992). *Preschool language scale-3.* San Antonio, TX: The Psychological Corporation.

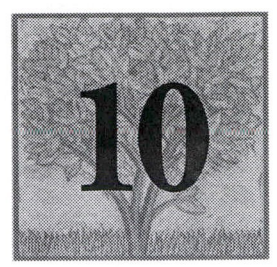

Assessment of Language Disorders in School-Age Children

■ LEARNING OBJECTIVES

After completion of this chapter, the reader will be able to

1. Describe three goals that guide the evaluation process.

2. Cite four key questions that should be asked when analyzing a language sample of a school-age child.

3. Explain why IQ/achievement discrepancy is not a good tool for diagnosing a child as dyslexic.

4. Discuss three constructs that should be noted through the analysis of a language sample.

5. Discuss why it is better to assess narrative discourse and expository discourse than straightforward discourse analysis when testing adolescents.

6. Discuss why it is difficult to differentially diagnose auditory processing disorders, language problems associated with ADD/ADHD, and language-based learning disabilities.

■ INTRODUCTION

When discussing the assessment of language disorders in preschool children, consideration must be given to lexicon, semantics, syntax, morphology, and pragmatics, and analyzing the presence and absence of these areas of language against normal development. In the school-age population, however, the clinician needs to be concerned about the impact of the features of language on learning, and, particularly, the impact of language deficits on reading, spelling, writing, and socialization. The population of school-age children with language delays and disorders is quite diverse. One faction of this population is made up of children whose preschool delays evolve into disorders during the school years as greater language demands are placed on the child. These children were discussed in Chapter 5. However, the bulk of the children seen for assessment and treatment during the school years have problems that affect their reading, spelling, and writing. These children have a language-based learning disability that has a negative impact on their academic, social, and vocational progress. These children are the focus of Chapters 10 and 11.

■ COMPONENTS OF THE EVALUATION

The evaluation process is guided by three goals. The first objective is to determine the reality of the problem. The child's communication behavior needs to be described with particular emphasis on the areas of greatest deviation from expected behaviors. Is the child's language within normal limits, delayed, or disordered? Because few norms are available against which to compare diagnostic data in the school-age population, it is important to compare the information gained through the diagnostic process with acceptable criteria for the mental and chronological ages of the student. It is also necessary to make a severity statement, including a notation as to how much of a problem the disorder is for the child. This includes evaluating the impact that the language or learning disability has on the child's academic and social progress.

A second goal of the diagnostic process is to determine the etiology of the problem. What causal factors may be related to the presenting problem? Emerick and Haynes (1986) differentiate predisposing, precipitating, and perpetuating etiologic factors, and this distinction is particularly important when talking about the school-age population. **Predisposing factors** are defined as "agents that dispose or incline an individual toward communication impairment" (Emerick & Haynes, 1986, p. 9).

In children with language delays in the preschool years, a persistence of the delay may occur as a disorder. Thus, the language delay could be a predisposing factor in the child's language disorder. **Precipitating factors** "actually bring about the onset of the problem" (Emerick & Haynes, 1986, p. 9) and may not always be identifiable.

Perpetuating factors are "responsible for the persistence of the abnormality" (Emerick & Haynes, 1986, p. 9). These may include such factors as lack of early identification and treatment, unreasonable demands in the classroom when the disorder is taken into account, and the student's own lack of understanding about his or her language deficits.

The third goal of the evaluative process with school-age children is to provide a clinical focus. When all of the information is gathered, what can be done to help the child improve with regard to language, academic progress, and social goals needs to be addressed. Effectively obtained diagnostic information is the basis for clinician accountability when determining therapy goals. To this end, when evaluating adolescents, it is particularly important to make sure they understand the importance of what you are doing. The clinician should be straightforward with the child and acknowledge the pressure the child may feel in the evaluation process. Alternatives could be discussed, as well as the socioeconomic repercussions of language disorders that affect the child's learning in school and carry over into adulthood. Adolescents need to feel that they have some control, so it is a good idea to let the adolescent be the focus during the interviews. Questions should be directed to the adolescent during the history-gathering process, and the results should be discussed directly with the adolescent.

Predisposing factors. Factors that dispose or incline an individual toward an impairment related to his or her language and communication skills.

Precipitating factors. Factors that result in the onset of the language or communication problem, or both.

Perpetuating factors. Factors that result in the persistence of the language or communication problem, or both.

Screening

In most school settings, a child's speech and language skills can be screened without getting permission from the parents. A screening serves to identify children who are not using speech and language as expected based on the child's chronological age and academic abilities. A screening simply provides information that, based on the test used to provide a preliminary evaluation of the child's speech and language skills, there is or is not reason to suspect a possible speech or language deficit. Screenings can be administered individually using instruments that take 5 to 15 minutes to determine if a child is at risk. Some screening tools can be administered as paper-and-pencil tasks to an entire classroom at one time. Regardless of the type of screening done, the only conclusion that can be drawn is that the child apparently is within normal limits with regard to speech and language skills, or the child is at risk for speech and language problems and should be evaluated further. A screening does not result in a diagnosis.

Case History

As with any evaluation, the history is a critical component in the assessment of an individual with a language-based learning disability. It may be gathered through a written history form and through a preassessment interview with the student and his or her family. When evaluating the effect of language on a child's academic and social development, it is critical to analyze carefully the child's daily environment and the impact that his or her family and peers have on the child's language. It is also important to look at the child's educational history. What academic subjects are particularly challenging for the child? What are his or her grades? Does the child actively participate in the educational process? The answers to these questions can provide important guidance to the clinician in planning the assessment and treatment processes. The passage of the Individuals with Disabilities Education Act (IDEA) reinforced the educational expectations outlined in Public Laws 94-142 and 99-457 but added an educational focus on the child's transition from school to work. Transition is a required focus for all children receiving special education services who are 16 years old and older. However, for children with severe deficits or multiple problems, educators are encouraged to introduce vocational training prior to age 16 years. Thus, the case history of a school-age child should also reflect information related to vocational (previous, current, and future) education.

A detailed medical history also should be taken. The presence of seizure disorders should be carefully noted, as well as any medications that the child takes on a regular basis. The presence of allergies or autoimmune disorders in the child or family members should be documented carefully because some studies show a history of these types of disorders in the families of children with language-based learning disabilities. Also, any history of drug abuse by the child should be documented.

Previous testing should be reviewed carefully, although usually there is no need to go back to developmental milestones for children with language-based learning disabilities. For children who have severe delays that are carrying over into the school-age years, the milestones may be of interest, particularly those relating to the development of the features of language.

Student Interview

An interview is a directed conversation that proceeds in an orderly fashion to obtain data, to convey certain information, and to provide release and support for the sharing of information. For older elementary, middle school, and high school students, it is particularly important to make the student feel that he or she has some control over what happens in the assessment process. Time should be given to the student to vent any concerns, problems, or feelings with regard to the disorder and its diagnosis and treatment. When assessing a student who has a language-based learning disability, it is important to get the student's perspective on the problem (Larson and McKinley, 1995). This is particularly important when assessing students who are in middle or high school. Larson and McKinley (1995) suggest that the clinician determine the student's feelings and attitudes about thinking, listening, and speaking. Negative attitudes can adversely affect the logical thought processes needed to survive in academic and social situations. As stated earlier, many students with language-based learning disabilities develop a sense of learned helplessness in which they come to believe that outcomes cannot be controlled. They become passive participants in the academic world and develop an inability to be persistent in their approach to learning. These students are likely to become ineffective problem-solvers; they believe they cannot think, so they do not think. They believe that educators, family members, and clinicians have low expectations, and this influences their desire to set and achieve higher goals. All of these factors are compounded into a negative self-image and an increased prevalence of depression in the learning-disabled population when compared to their nondisabled classmates.

Larson and McKinley (1995) also point out the importance of knowing the student's feelings and attitudes toward listening. Many students with language-based learning disabilities will express listening barriers that are excuses for their poor academic achievement. For example, frequent comments include statements such as, "The teacher is boring" and "The teacher does not like me." The students may criticize the speaker's looks, actions, and speaking style. They may also listen for isolated facts without taking in the whole picture. Some students may get overly stimulated or emotionally involved with the topic, sometimes allowing their own personal prejudices to interfere with listening to the speaker and with their comprehension of the subject. They may listen as long as the topic is easy, but shut down when the content becomes more complicated.

Feelings and attitudes toward speaking also are important to ascertain (Larson & McKinley, 1995). The first step is to determine if poor communication is due to a poor attitude about speaking or to a disordered communication system, or to both. Does the student believe he or she has nothing to say, in which case the root of the problem may be language-based, or does he or she have a speech disorder (voice, fluency, articulation) that interferes with his or her desire to communicate with others? Does his or her attitude vary from setting to setting or speaker to speaker? Many adolescents will not admit to a communication disorder unless it affects communication with their peers.

Auditory learner. A person who learns primarily by listening.

Assessing the student's learning environment also is important. What is the child's learning style? Is he or she an **auditory learner** or a **visual learner**? Does he or she do better on oral or written examinations? Are there environmental factors or social-emotional factors that affect the student's ability to learn?

Visual learner. A person who learns primarily and most effectively through a visual modality.

All of the above information should be obtained prior to proceeding with the testing portion of the diagnostic process.

Language Sample

A predominant part of any evaluation of a school-age child is the language sample, in which the clinician gathers approximately 50 to 100 utterances (depending on the analysis system to be used) and carefully analyzes the child's spontaneous language use. In younger elementary school-age children, a language sample should be obtained in the assessment situation. Usually, toys and books can be presented to encourage the child to engage in dialogue with the assessing clinician. To thoroughly assess the speech and language of an adolescent (middle and high school students), it is beneficial to get one language sample of the child talking with a peer, one talking to a teacher, and one talking with a family member (Hegde, 1996).

A language sample is a critical part of the evaluation of any individual with a communication impairment. In Table 10–1, Weiss, Tomplin, and Robin list activities that can be used to elicit a language sample for different age groups as well as ideas as to what to look for when analyzing the language sample. The sample should be analyzed from several perspectives and can be one of the most valuable pieces of diagnostic data that the clinician has. First, just as with preschoolers and younger school-age children, the sample should be analyzed in terms of the features of language. Does the child have appropriate semantics, syntax, and prosody? The presence of word-retrieval problems should also be documented. Differentiations between speech dysfluencies and dysfluency due to language-based problems should be noted. Does the child use false starts, verbal mazes, circumlocution, imprecise language, excessive pauses,

TABLE 10–1. Language sampling across the life span.

Age Range	Suggested Sampling Activities	Look for:	Helpful References
Infants and Toddlers (Preverbal to Emerging Language: approximately 0 to 2 years of age)	• Observation of the child with the primary caregiver(s). • Use a variety of familiar and unfamiliar toys; place some just out of reach or make them otherwise inaccessible without assistance from an adult. • Coggins & Carpenter (1981) suggest a sample of 45 minutes duration.	• Evidence of responsiveness on the part of the caregiver(s) to the child's initiated bids. Compare styles of interactions. Does the infant provide clear signals of interest in interaction? • Evidence of developing communicative interactions, e.g., protoimperatives and protodeclaratives. • Evidence of nonlinguistic comprehension strategies, e.g., "imitation of on-going actions," versus evidence of true word comprehension. • Evidence of the child's repertoire of volitional vocalizations and speech sounds; precursors to word use. • Evidence of real word use: (1) resemblance to an adult word, (2) consistent phonetic form, (3) used in consistent context. • Analysis of early words in terms of pragmatic function and semantic categorization.	Rossetti (1990) Coggins & Carpenter (1981) Bates (1976) Chapman (1978) Proctor (1989) Owens (1996) Dore (1974); Bloom (1973); Nelson (1973)
Preschoolers (approximately 2 to 5 years of age)	• Collect several language samples with different coconversationalists in different settings and with different degrees of structure. 50–200 utterances are usually recommended. • Use materials that lend themselves to the creation of scenarios, e.g., dollhouse, toy farm.	• Evidence of assertiveness and responsiveness in conversations and their different proportions relative to the different samples collected. • Evidence of age-appropriate syntactic structure and use of grammatical morphemes as per mean length of utterance and Developmental Sentence Scoring, for example.	Fey (1986) Brown (1973) and Miller (1981) for MLU analysis; Lee (1974) for DSS, and Retherford (1993)

(continued)

TABLE 10–1. *(continued)*

Age Range	Suggested Sampling Activities	Look for:	Helpful References
Preschoolers	• Use open-ended requests for information that do not constrain response length and complexity, e.g., "Tell me about . . ." • Use a variety of familiar and unfamiliar materials and follow the child's lead. • Although conversation samples are most often used, you can also use prompts for personal narratives, scripts, and story retelling. Be sure to use a lot of visual support materials.	• Evidence of a variety of vocabulary words in the sample, e.g., Type–Token Ratio, as per Templin (1957). • Evidence that the child is accommodating language to his/her listeners via responses to or requests for clarification, presuppositional skills; question comprehension is evident by appropriate responses made to questions asked. • Evidence of observation of turn taking rules; little if any "simultalk" occurs. • Child can maintain a topic for several turns.	Brinton & Fujiki (1989)
School-age children (approximately 6 to 12 years of age)	• Provide prompts for personal narratives, fictional stories, and scripts with visual support, e.g., "Make up a story about something that's not real." • Use of interview questions as per Evans & Craig (1992): (1) What can you tell me about your family? (2) Tell me about school. (3) Tell me about what you like to do when you are not in school. • For older children, collect both written and oral samples. • Collect samples of classroom discourse from both ends of the formal-informal continuum.	• Evidence of a cohesive discourse structure: What is the overall structure of the discourse and how adequate is it? • Use of later-developing syntax forms: postmodification of nouns, coordinate conjunctions, adverbial clauses, infinitives, complements, and subjunctive modals. • Evidence of more sophisticated sentence repair strategies or use of alternation rules when faced with communication breakdowns.	Hughes, McGillvray, & Schmidek (1997); Roth & Spekman (1986) Scott (1988); Nippold (1998); Weiss & Johnson (1993) Damico (1991); Westby (1994)

Age group			
Adolescents (junior high school and high school age)	• Use activities that require story creation or retelling either with or without visual support. • Collect a sample of expository discourse. • Elicit samples of both oral and written discourse. • Use written materials to prompt conversations, e.g., a provocative newspaper article.	• Evidence of perspective taking and acknowledgment of others' perspectives and opinions. • Greater finesse should be expected in terms of discourse cohesion and structure. • Comparison of cohesion in samples where information is shared versus not shared with the audience.	Hughes, McGillvray, & Schmidek (1997)
Adults	• Story generation and story retelling without visual stimuli; context not shared. • Fable retelling, proverb interpretation, picture descriptions; use of picture sequences, cartoon stimuli.	• Sentence complexity, completeness of episode structure, proportion of core information presented (in recall); proportion of revisions, words per minute.	Nicholas & Brookshire (1993), Chapman (1997); Chapman, Ulatowska, Franklin, Shobe, Thompson, & McIntire (1997); Chapman, Levin, & Culhane (1995); Ulatowska, Chapman, Highley, & Prince (1998)

Source: From "Language Disorders" by A. L. Weiss, J. B. Tomlin, and D. A. Robin. In J. B. Tomlin, H. L. Morris, and D. C. Spriesterbach (Eds.), *Diagnosis in Speech-Language Pathology* (2nd ed.). Copyright, 2000, Singular Publishing Group, San Diego, pp. 153–155. Reprinted with permission.

repetitions, and other devices that interfere with his or her expressive language skills? The mean length of utterance also should be determined.

Second, the language sample should be analyzed with regard to the child's use of language for various functions. For example, using the Damico (1985) analyses of conversational language, it can be determined if a student is an active or passive communicator by comparing the number of times the student initiates conversation with the number of times he or she responds to the initiations of his or her conversation partner. It can also be used to determine if a child uses language for a variety of functions, such as sharing information, receiving information, greeting, and negotiating.

The language sample should be analyzed in terms of the quality and the quantity of information. Is the student able to generate a sample of 50 to 100 semantically and syntactically acceptable utterances? It not, what factors interfered with the student's production of an adequate sample? With regard to the quality of information, the clinician should look at the accuracy of the message. Are the topics discussed relevant and coherent? Is the message full of verbal mazes, or is it fluent with appropriate pragmatics? These issues should be considered carefully when analyzing the quality of a language sample (Larson & McKinley, 1995).

Metalinguistics

Children must make a transition from acquiring functional use of language during the preschool years and developing the ability to think and talk about language as a tool during the school-age years. They learn that language can be used to think, learn, problem solve, and communicate. As a child's language matures, he or she becomes more able to attend not only to the context of a message, but also to how the message is transmitted (Brown, 1978; Flavell, 1977; Flavell & Wellman, 1977). This is due, in part, to an increase in metalinguistic skills. Metalinguistic skills allow a child to think about language in a critical manner and to make judgments with regard to the accuracy and appropriate use of language skills and functions. These skills appear to be related to environmental stimulation, play, cognitive development, academic achievement, and reading ability (Saywitz & Cherry-Wilkinson, 1982).

The development of metalinguistic skills also leads to the formation of metacognitive skills. Metacognitive skills refer to an increasing ability to think about and analyze how a problem can be solved. In other words, metacognition is a skill that underlies a child's ability to become a logical thinker and problem solver.

Discourse Parameters

The child's language should be analyzed in terms of his or her use of cohesion devices to maintain conversational continuity. These devices include repetitions of key words in the conversation and following a logical progression of thought as the dialogue progresses. Critical listening is a primary component of comprehension of a conversation. To be a critical listener, one must be a critical thinker. This implies that, to be a mature conversationalist, a child must have well-developed metalinguistic and metapragmatic skills. Critical listening includes the ability to engage in inductive and deductive thinking, to distinguish between facts and opinions, and to make inferences (Larson & McKinley, 1995).

Narrations

The role of narratives in the assessment of language in school-age children must not be overlooked. At age 5 to 7 years, children can produce true narratives. This is a good age to begin narrative journals to track the child's development in writing as he or she progresses through the elementary years. Children aged 7 to 11 years can summarize and categorize stories. By age 11 to 12 years, they can produce more complex stories; between the ages of 13 to 15 years, children learn to analyze stories. By the time a child is 16 years old, he or she should be able to formulate abstract statements about the themes and messages of books (Larson and McKinley, 1995).

In addition to knowing what kind of information a child can glean from a story, it is important to assess a child's knowledge of story structure. Can he or she identify the common elements of a story? Does the child understand the rules that dictate the construction of a story? (Mandler & Johnson, 1977; Rumelhart, 1975; Stein & Glenn, 1979; Thorndyke, 1977).

Thus, with regard to language in school-age children, it is important to assess the child's ability to comprehend and produce narratives. A child's abilities with regard to narration can provide a window of observation into how well he or she integrates information conveyed through language (Larson & McKinley, 1995).

General Testing

Clinicians who provide services for school-age children must be adept at analyzing the language skills of students from preschool age through late adolescence. Language-based learning disabilities are multifaceted disorders that need specialized assessment using modality-specific testing instruments. The assessment battery should consist of tests that assess language and cognition using instruments, such as the Woodcock-Johnson III (2001) Psychoeducational Battery (Woodcock & Johnson, 1977) and the Detroit Test of Learning Aptitude (Hammill, 1998). Tests should be used that enable the clinician to compare the child's overall verbal skills with his or her nonverbal (frequently referred to as performance) skills. Many schools use a discrepancy score between verbal and nonverbal IQ as an eligibility criterion for placement in special education or related services in the schools.

■ TESTING CHILDREN WITH AUDITORY PROCESSING DISORDERS

It is estimated that some degree of auditory processing difficulty is present in 3% to 5% of the school-age population. In addition, a much higher percentage of auditory processing disorders occurs in children with learning disabilities than in the general population (Holston, 1992). These prevalence figures may be low because many children with learning disabilities are not referred for auditory processing assessment.

Hearing starts at the outer ear and ends at the auditory nerve, which transports the auditory information to the brain. The auditory signal is then separated from nonessential background sound and translated into a meaningful, clarified message. The skills needed for this translation develop mostly in the first 5 years of a child's life.

Auditory acuity. The sharpness and clarity with which sound is perceived by the ear.

Although auditory perception and auditory processing frequently are used interchangeably, there are distinct differences in the meanings of this terminology. **Auditory acuity** refers to the sharpness and clarity with which sound is perceived by the ear. Auditory perception is the identification, interpretation, or organization of sensory data received through the ear (Holston, 1992). A central auditory processing disorder refers to "auditory processing that begins at the level of the cochlear nuclei in the brain stem, ascending ultimately to the cortex" (Wallach & Butler, 1994, p. 383). Auditory processing refers to the processing of auditory information throughout the auditory system, including the outer and middle ear. Sometimes, *auditory processing* and *central auditory processing* are used interchangeably. Young (1985) defines processing as the neuropsychological transmission of the stimuli from one point in the brain to another. He refers to the comprehension of the stimuli as perception.

Individuals with auditory processing problems have normal hearing acuity and intelligence but are unable to process auditory information effectively. Most authorities report that auditory processing disorders cause difficulties in detection, interpretation, and categorization of sounds and that these problems may be due to some type of dysfunction in lower or higher level cortical processes (Schow & Nerbonne, 1996).

On the basis of several different profiles, children are frequently referred for auditory processing testing. Children who are believed to have reading problems or language-based learning disabilities are often referred to an audiologist for testing to rule out auditory processing as a causative factor in their learning problems. Children who have poor academic achievement, ADD, ADHD, behavior problems, phonological deficits, and problems with oral language also should be referred for further evaluation of their auditory processing abilities (Wallach & Butler, 1994).

It is sometimes difficult to separate an auditory processing disorder from a language deficit, owing to the underlying role of language in processing and learning. Young (1985) proposed that two types of auditory processing disorders may be present in children. The first is related to attentional deficits, whereas the second includes both attentional problems and language deficits.

At times, it is difficult not only to separate language disorders from auditory processing disorders but also to differentiate between children with ADHD and children with auditory processing disorders. This is because many of the symptoms of ADHD are also reported as symptoms for auditory processing problems. These symptoms include hyperactivity, impulsivity, distractibility, and difficulty in staying on task (Holston, 1992). In Table 10–2 there is a list of typical behaviors associated with auditory processing disorders in childhood that classroom teachers can use as a guide.

Auditory processing disorders often are diagnosed through a team approach involving the speech-language pathologist and the audiologist. The speech-language pathologist typically uses tests based on information processing,

TABLE 10–2. Typical behaviors for teachers to look for when referring children for auditory processing assessment.

Says "huh" or "what" frequently

Gives inconsistent responses to auditory stimuli

Often misunderstands what is said

Has poor auditory attention

Is easily distracted

Has difficulty following oral directions

Has difficulty listening in the presence of background noise

Has difficulty with phonics and speech sound discrimination

Has poor auditory memory

Constantly requests that information be repeated

Has poor receptive and expressive language skills

Gives slow or delayed responses to verbal stimuli

Has reading, spelling, and other academic problems

Learns poorly through the auditory channel

Exhibits behavior problems

Source: Adapted from *Fisher Auditory Problems Checklist,* by L. T. Fisher, n. d. Cedar Rapids, IA: Grant Wood Area Education Agency.

task analysis, and multimodality comparisons of information processing. The role of the speech-language pathologist on many teams is to determine, through comprehensive testing, why the child is having academic difficulties (Dempsey, 1993). The audiologist's role is to determine the site of the lesion within the auditory pathway and to assess the child's ability to understand speech in a variety of conditions (Wallach & Butler, 1994).

Testing for auditory processing disorders is based on three important assumptions. The first is that testing auditory processing requires a conglomeration of tests that assess auditory memory, auditory closure, auditory discrimination, and auditory figure-ground perception (Keith, 1988). A second assumption is that the auditory system is redundant; therefore, it is necessary to reduce and manipulate the redundancies by filtering, alternating between the right and left ears, compressing the message, lowering the signal-to-noise ratio, and presenting competing noise in the opposite or same ear. The neuroanatomical and language redundancies challenge the mechanism, so the testing should also address the redundancies (Keith 1988).

The third assumption had to do with cause and effect. If a child tests positive for auditory processing disorders, it is difficult to determine if the auditory processing problems are the cause or the result of the language problem (Northern & Downs, 1991). It is almost certain that, since language has a strong auditory component, the auditory processing disorder contributes to the language difficulties. However, until a definitive relationship can be forged between language disorders and auditory processing disorders, the reader should take care when considering the diagnostic information for purposes of labeling a child's disorder and determining eligibility for services. It is possible that some children do not perform well on auditory processing tests owing to metalinguistic and metacognitive disorders that affect the outcome of the testing (van Kleeck, 1984).

A sample battery of tests for auditory processing disorders is found in Table 10–3.

TABLE 10–3. Sample APD battery used at the University of Florida.

Synthetic Sentence Identification (SSI)	Jerger and Jerger (1974)
Dichotic Digits	Musiek (1983)
Staggered Spondaic Words (SSW)	Katz (1962)
Pitch Pattern Sequence (PPS)	Pinheiro (1977)
Duration Pattern Sequence (DPS)	Baran, Musick, Gollegly et al. (1987)
Random Gap Detection Test (RGDT)	Keith (2000)
Test for Auditory Processing Disorders in Children (SCAN-C) or Adults (SCAN-A)	Keith (1986)

■ TESTING LANGUAGE SKILLS IN CHILDREN WITH SPECIFIC LANGUAGE IMPAIRMENT (SLI)

Early identification of children with SLI is particularly important since communication functions and academic development are frequently at risk in this population. Children with SLI frequently have reading disorders in addition to more global impairment in academic subjects (Aram, Ekelman, & Nation, 1984; Catts, 1991, 1993; Stark et al., 1984). Not only is early identification important, but it is also advantageous to reassess the children over time (even if they are receiving intervention) in order to monitor linguistic variables that are typically associated with long-term deficits in children with SLI.

The child's use of morphosyntactic structures should be followed, as well as more general measures such as mean length of utterance and quantitative and qualitative growth in lexicon. The best way to measure these constructs is through a spontaneous language sample (in addition to more formalized measures) (Goffman & Leonard, 2000). The assessment of language in children who have specific language impairment should include comparisons both across and within language domains. This would involve comparing the child's performance on tasks assessing form (phonology, morphology, and syntax), content (semantics), and use (pragmatics). Bliss (2002) writes, "At more specific levels, comparisons should be made within grammatical categories for noun and verb phrase expansion (e.g., articles versus demonstrative pronouns or auxiliaries versus copulas) and between grammatical categories and grammatical structures (e.g., auxiliaries versus simple and complex sentence use)" (p. 35).

It is also important to assess the child's usage of verbs because this is language form that is typically problematic for children with SLI (Goffman & Leonard, 2000; Grela & Leonard, 2000; Bliss, 2002).

In addition, adolescents who have language-based learning disabilities should be assessed and provided with intervention as early as is feasible. This is due to the impact that language-based learning disabilities have, not only on language, but on academic, social, and subsequent vocational activities. Bliss (2002) advocates the use of discourse analysis but cautions the reader that basic conversation is not necessarily problematic for these adolescents, so it may not reflect the extent of the language/learning deficits. Narrative discourse is useful for the assessment of topic maintenance, referencing, and event sequencing. Likewise, expository discourse, which is commonly encountered in the classroom, can provide insight into the child's ability to describe and explain different phenomena, persuasion, and argumentation (Larson & McKinley, 1995; Nelson, 1998; Paul, 2001). Metalinguistic skills, metapragmatic skills, and metacognitive skills should also be assessed in adolescents with language-based learning disabilities, as well as social skills and word-retrieval skills (Bliss, 2002).

Ultimately, the best test of the abilities child with SLI will be to assess his or her functional communication ability in a wide variety of settings. How well does he or she exchange information with others? Are his or her pragmatics appropriate? Damico (1993) notes that effective communication is based on three criteria: "the effectiveness of meaning transmission, the fluency of meaning transmission, and the appropriateness of meaning transmission" (p. 29). Larson and McKinley (1995) advocate that a descriptive assessment that includes a descriptive analysis and an explanatory analysis be done.

> A descriptive analysis would focus on directly observing and recording behaviors that (1) have been found to be necessary for successful communication in selected contexts in which the student is likely to communicate and in selected modalities that the student is likely to use, and (2) are believed to be valid indices of communicative difficulty, An explanatory analysis would determine the causal factors for the communication disorder that was observed during the descriptive analysis. (p. 83)

It is important that when assessing a school-age child or adolescent with a specific language impairment that an evaluation of the student's environment, including curriculum variables, teachers' attitudes and philosophies, and social demands be conducted (Larson & McKinley, 1995). All of these factors can greatly affect the student's ability to learn and use language, and to succeed socially and academically.

■ TESTING LANGUAGE SKILLS IN SCHOOL-AGE CHILDREN WITH COGNITIVE CHALLENGES

Testing the school-age child with cognitive challenges poses a different set of problems than testing most school-age children. They are likely to have attention and motivation problems, lack of conventional verbal output, poor motor skills, and cognitive skill deficits. It may be necessary to divide the testing into several short periods of time instead of one long session. In addition, it may be helpful to increase the amount of reinforcement that is offered to the child in order to help keep him or her motivated to complete the tasks. If the child is nonverbal and/or has physical problems that negate pointing as a response mode, it may be necessary to use an alternative response mode such as eye gaze or head wands for pointing. It also may be necessary to give the child extended time in which to respond. Multiply handicapped children may need time not only to formulate the correct response but also to motor plan how to make that response.

Other test adaptations may be necessary such as modifying the test items, but this would result in an invalid administration. At times, one may have to use a standardized test to gain specific information about the child's language. However, if the test does not include handicapped children in its normative sample, the test would not be valid for the handicapped child. It could be used to gain information about some of the child's language constructs, but the test could not be scored. A clinician can employ "out-of-level testing" (Berk, 1984) which involves using a test for a child whose age is not included in the normative sample. Again, this would enable the clinician to gain information about the child, but no score can be obtained. For lower functioning school-age children, it may be beneficial to use developmental checklists and tests such as the Communication and Symbolic Behavior Scales—Developmental Profile (CSBS-DP) (Wetherby & Prizant, 2002). The CSBS is normed for developmental ages 8 to 24 months, and chronological age 9 months to 6.0 years. The results of the CSBS and similar tests (see Chapter 3) can be used to guide further assessment, plan intervention, and document change over time.

In 1988, Sattler proposed a *testing of limits* as a method of adaptations for following up on standardized test administrations. These modifications include providing extra time to respond, providing supplemental cues to the child, changing the response modality (for example, using gestural output instead of verbal output), and asking questions that can help the child clarify and prepare his response. Testing of limits can provide information as to how the child approaches a task, and the impact of his disabilities on his test performance (McCauley, 2001).

Another type of testing that can be done is discrepancy testing. McCauley (2001) defines discrepancy testing as "the comparison of performances in two different behavioral or skill areas (e.g., between ability and achievement) to determine whether a discrepancy exists" (p. 158). Some school districts use discrepancy testing as a means of justifying educational assistance for a child.

Generally speaking, the child with cognitively challenged should be tested in a variety of settings in order to get a true picture of his or her communicative abilities. Behavioral observations and language samples can be helpful in providing an adequate assessment of their functional communication skills (Bliss, 2002).

■ TESTING LANGUAGE SKILLS IN CHILDREN WITH ADHD

Children with ADHD frequently are restless and fidgety, unable to sit still for the duration of a test, and excessively talkative. All of these behavioral manifestations of ADHD can contribute to making it difficult to assess a child with ADHD. According to Barkley (2000), lack of behavioral inhibition is at the root of the impulsivity, inattention, and hyperactivity seen in children who have ADHD. Behavioral inhibition is a cognitive deficit that significantly interfere with executive functioning skills as described in Chapter 7. This, in turn, has the potential to affect assessment results in these children. This is particularly important when one considers that there may be overlap of language impairments and ADHD, with estimates that co-morbidity of these two problems ranges from 20% to 60% (Oram et al., 1999).

Oram and colleagues (1999) propose three hypotheses related to language assessment of children who have ADHD. The first hypothesis is that the children's behavioral manifestations of ADHD do not interfere with formal testing. This may be due in part to the nondistracting environment and one-on-one interaction that typically characterize language assessments. Contrary to this first hypothesis, the second hypothesis is that the ADHD does interfere with testing which may lead to an underestimation of the child's true ability on language tasks. The third hypothesis is that the ADHD will interfere with the child's performance on specific tasks, namely, those "that require a greater degree of sustained attention, inhibition, and/or organization" (p. 73). Oram and colleagues designed a study to test the third hypothesis through the language testing of three groups of children: controls (24 private school children), children with ADHD and language impairment, and children with ADHD only. Fifty-three children aged 7 to 11 years old who were diagnosed with ADHD were tested using the three language tests. These tests were the Test of Word Finding (TWF; German, 1986), the Clinical Evaluation of Language Fundamentals-Revised (CELF-R; Semel, Wiig, & Secord, 1987), and the Auditory Analysis Test (Rosner & Simon, 1971). "Language impairment was defined by performance: (a) at least 1.5 SD below the mean for age on at least one of TWF Accuracy Score, Rosner raw score, CELF-R Receptive Language Score, or CELF-R Expressive Language Score; or (b) at least 1 SD below the mean for age on two or more of these scores" (Oram et al., 1999, p. 74). As a result of the testing, the 53 children with ADHD were divided into two groups: those with ADHD only (25 children) and those with ADHD and Language Impairment (28 children). This particular study was actually part of a larger study conducted by Tannock and colleagues (1998) in which children referred for medical treatment of ADHD (but not referred due to concerns about language) were given several standardized language tests in addition to assessment of auditory processing, conversational and narrative language, cognitive functioning, and academic skills. Oram and colleagues further hypothesized as to which tasks would be most problematic for the children with ADHD. These included tasks "requiring high levels of sustained attention, inhibition, working memory, or planning/organization" (p. 73). A list of the tasks and their nonlinguistic demands is found in Table 10–4.

TABLE 10–4. Nonlinguistic demands of standardized language tasks on systems impaired in ADHD.

Nonlinguistic Demand	Subtest	Description
Sustained attention	CELF-R Listening to Paragraphs	Listen to narrative paragraphs
	TWF Description Naming	Listen to three-part word definitions
	CELF-R Oral Directions	Listen to multipart directions
Inhibition	CELF-R Oral Directions	Do not point until examiner says "Go"
Working memory	CELF-R Oral Directions	Remember all parts of direction while executing each step
	CELF-R Word Classes	Remember four words while selecting two related in meaning
	CELF-R Formulated Sentences	Remember target word while formulating a sentence using it
	Rosner Level VII	Remember target syllable to delete while segmenting multisyllabic word
Planning/Organization	CELF-R Sentence Assembly	Avoid making same arrangements of word groups that already were unsuccessful

Source: From "Assessing the Language of Children with Attention Deficit Hyperactivity Disorder," by J. Oram, J. Fine, C Okamoto, and R. Tannock. In *American Journal of Speech-Language Pathology.* Copyright, February 1999, American Speech-Language-Hearing Association.

Results were as follows.

1. On most subtests, the ADHD-only and control groups did not differ in their performance, with both groups doing significantly better than the group of children with ADHD and Language Impairment (LI).

2. On the CELF-R subtests, the ADHD-only children and the controls performed within normal limits, but the children with ADHD and LI scored more than one SD below the mean on two subtests and borderline for two other subtests.

3. On the three CELF-R expressive language subtests, the controls and ADHD-only children did better than the ADHD-LI group.

4. On the three CELF-R expressive language subtests, those children with ADHD-only did significantly worse than the controls on Formulated Sentences, Word Structure, and Sentence Assembly.

5. On the Sentence Assembly subtest, "only the mean score for the group with ADHD+LI approached clinical levels" (p. 76).

6. Mean scores for all three groups were within the normal range on the Word Structure subtest.

7. The differences in performance by the ADHD-only and control groups on Word Structure and Sentence Assembly are not clinically relevant.

8. Both ADHD groups scored at least within the borderline range on the Formulated Sentences subtest, making this subtest "more challenging in children with ADHD relative to their unaffected peers, even in the absence of LI" (p. 77).

On the Formulated Sentences subtest, there were three patterns of errors by the children with ADHD-only: no response, missing clause, and responses with the target at the beginning. Since these three responses occurred more frequently by the ADHD-only group than by the controls, it is possible that they were a factor in the lower scores achieved by the ADHD-only group. The ADHD-LI group scored even lower than the ADHD-only group, indicating that their language weaknesses also contributed to poor performance on the Formulated Sentences subtest. Another factor that may have contributed to the lower performance on the Formulated Sentences subtest is pragmatics. All the children with ADHD exhibited pragmatic deficits such as poor turn-taking skills, providing insufficient and ambiguous information, talking excessively and inappropriately, and difficulty initiating and maintaining a topic. All of these findings have implications for the assessment of language disorders in children with ADHD.

■ MULTICULTURAL ISSUES IN ASSESSMENT OF SCHOOL-AGE CHILDREN

Demographic Issues

As of 1994, approximately 7 million children and 42 million Americans of all ages spoke English as a second language, (Owens, 1995). In the next 10 years, it is estimated that one-third of the speech-language pathology caseload in the schools will be from Black, Hispanic, Asian, and Native American cultures (Larson & McKinley, 1995). Furthermore, it was estimated that by the year 2004 (Owens, 2004), 7 million members of minority populations would have a communication disorder that requires intervention (Larson & McKinley, 1995). Over 33% of today's clinicians have at least one bilingual client on their caseloads, yet over 80% of these clinicians do not feel confident in their abilities to treat bilingual clients (Owens, 1995).

If the clinician conducting the evaluation is not fluent in the child's language, it will be necessary to find a colleague who is. If another clinician cannot be located, it is acceptable to use an interpreter. Taking the time to train the translator in test administration, paying particular attention to the use of inadvertent nonlinguistic cues is critical. It is strongly recommended that one interpreter be used consistently with a client (ASHA, 1989). It is also important to remember that a word-for-word translation of English into any other language is not possible. Thus, the validity and reliability of any test that is translated by an interpreter will be affected.

Interpreters can also be of benefit when analyzing language samples when the clinician and client speak different languages or dialects of the same language. The clinician should collect language samples in several different contexts to check for code-switching and dialect use. Monologue and dialogue settings should be analyzed, as well as static tasks such as describing objects, dynamic tasks such as narration, and abstract tasks such as expressing opinions (Owens, 1995).

In cases in which a dialectal difference occurs, but not English as a second language, it is important to compare the presence of dialectal variations in oral language and written language. In any vernacular, differences occur in the functional and structural properties of language used for writing and spoken language (Rubin, 1987). Rubin also points out that research shows that African Americans show fewer instances of Black English vernacular in the written language than in the spoken language.

Differences Are Linguistic and Cultural

Difficulty with English is the primary reason for referral for determination of eligibility for special education placement. Minority children are also known to have a greater drop-out rate, frequently are less successful in school, and are, in fact, overrepresented in special education classes and underrepresented in classes for gifted students (Polakow, 1993). Until 1983, ASHA recognized several minority groups based on physical, mental, or hearing handicaps. At that time, it adopted the federal government's designation of minority groups as consisting of Blacks, Hispanics, Asians, and Native American Indians (including native Alaskans). One of the complicating issues is that what constitutes a difference or a disorder in one culture may not be one in another setting. For example, Native American children are taught that it is disrespectful to establish eye contact with their elders. This lack of eye contact could be interpreted as a pragmatic deficit by a clinician who is not familiar with the culture of the Native Americans. Unfortunately, very few data exist, particularly from Third World countries, to define a communication disorder. According to a sociocultural perspective, the clinician must keep in mind that a difference or disorder would exist on a continuum related to culturally based norms for that speech community. Nonetheless, clinicians must be prepared to assess and treat individuals from different cultural and linguistic backgrounds. In fact, not only is it logical and ethical but also it is federally mandated that the assessment and remediation of communication disorders in minority language speakers require specific skills and background knowledge. These skills are discussed more thoroughly in Chapter 11.

When one is assessing children who are linguistically and culturally different, there are many factors that require attention from the speech-language pathologist. Some of these considerations are diagrammed in Figure 10–1. As depicted in the model, the first thing that should be done is to screen language of standard American English (SAE) speaking students. If the child fails, he should then be screened using a test standardized on the child's linguistic-cultural group, if available. Based on the child's performance, he or she continues for further testing and intervention, or is determined to be competent in his or her native language. It is important to remember that children may demonstrate a language deficit in English but be competent in their native language.

Legal Mandates Related to Multicultural Issues

Several federal and case laws address the assessment and treatment of individuals from multicultural backgrounds.

PL 95-561 (The Bilingual Education Act of 1978; Title VII of the Elementary and Secondary Education Act of 1968). Reauthorized in 1978, PL 95-561 provided federal assistance for programs to aid children speaking limited English.

Equal Education Opportunity Act (EEOA) of 1974. The EEOA stated that education opportunities could not be denied to an individual because of the failure by an educational agency to take appropriate action to overcome language barriers that impede equal participation by its students.

Diana vs. Board of Education (1970). This case addressed the overidentification of children of Mexican migrant workers for placement in special education classes. Upon investigation, it was ascertained that the children were being tested in English, even though, for the majority of the children, Spanish was their first language and their English was extremely limited. The ruling in this case mandated that children should be tested in their native language.

Lau vs. Nichols (1974). "No equality of treatment" was the issue in San Francisco, where more than half of the students of Chinese descent received no instruction to overcome English-language deficiencies. A Supreme Court decision led to a resolve to give special instruction to teach English to the students of Chinese descent.

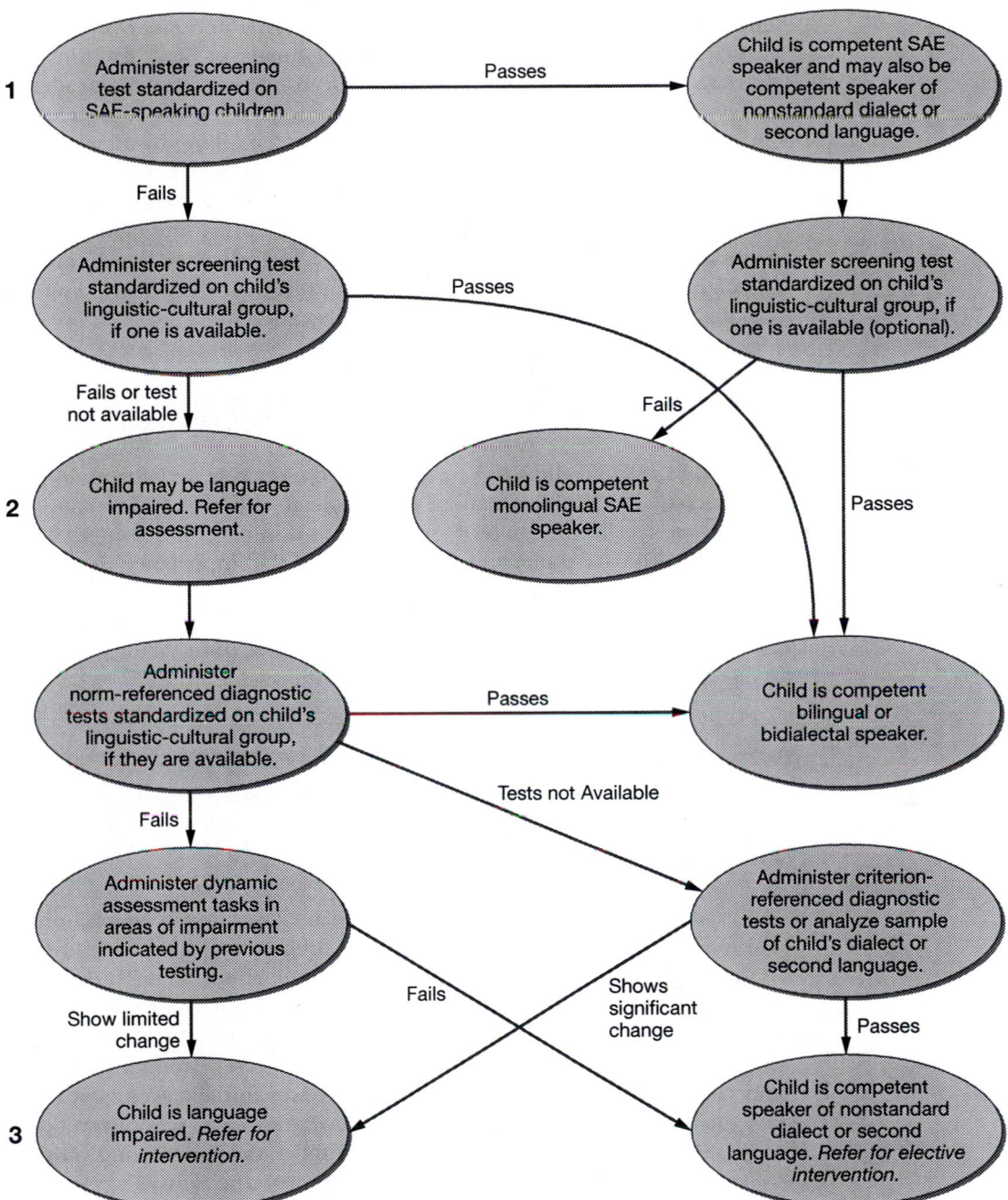

FIGURE 10–1. Model of differential diagnosis for linguistically-culturally diverse children. (From: S. Long, "Language and Linguistically-Culturally Diverse Children," in V.A. Reed (Ed.), *An Introduction to Children with Language Disorders*, 3rd ed., Figure 9.1, p. 326. Copyright Pearson Education, Inc., 2005.)

Martin Luther King, Jr., Elementary School vs. Ann Arbor School District Board (1979). This is a case that addressed the legitimacy of Black English. The parents of several African-American children believed that the academic progress of their children was being hindered and impeded, particularly in language-based classes, such as reading and spelling, by a lack of understanding and appreciation of Black English. Speech-language pathologists were designated by the courts to take an active role in assisting teachers to be sensitive to cultural dialects while providing instruction in standard English. This case is often referred to as the case that found the Black English dialect to be a legitimate and distinct dialect with cultural origins that deserved recognition and acceptance.

■ SUMMARY

PL 94-142, PL 99-457, and IDEA have all played a key role in determining the importance of adequate evaluations of school-age children. IDEA mandates increased services in the areas of assessment and intervention and serves to heighten health care professionals' awareness of the importance of early intervention. The final determination of a child's disorder and eligibility for therapy should be a synthesis of the clinician's knowledge of norms, adequate testing procedures and techniques, test results, observations, effective and empathetic relationships, and creative intuition.

CASE STUDY

History

MW is an 11-year-old girl in the fifth grade at Clark Elementary School. The developmental history and Mrs. W's pregnancy with M are unremarkable. Mr. W has reported that he struggled with reading and was a "slightly below average student" when he was in school, but he was never tested or diagnosed with a reading problem. M's learning problems were first apparent toward the end of second grade. M is repeating fifth grade and continues to struggle academically. She was initially evaluated two and one-half years ago when she was in third grade by a school psychologist and was found to have low average intellectual functioning with a full-scale IQ of 85. She was further tested by the school's speech-language pathologist who determined that M has a moderately severe language disorder with apparent deficits in auditory processing. After more than two years of group therapy at Clark, M has demonstrated little progress. M's parents have brought her to the Communicative Disorders Diagnostic Clinic (CDCC) at Memorial Hospital for further assessment.

Evaluation

On September 9, 2003, M was tested for language-based learning disabilities at the CDDC at Memorial Hospital. Tests administered included the Token Test-Revised, the Woodcock-Johnson Psychoeducational Battery, the Test of Language Development-Intermediate, and the Word Test. Additional nonstandardized diagnostic procedures were also done.

On the Token Test-Revised, M's overall age standard score of 496 and overall grade standard score of 495 were within the average performance range. On each subtest of the TOLD-I, she scored more than one standard deviation below the mean. A summation of her scores on the TOLD-I is as follows.

Subtest	Raw Score	Percentile	Standard Score
Sentence Combining	11	9	6
Characteristics	38	37	9
Word Ordering	9	5	5
Generals	7	2	4
Grammatic Comprehension	6	9	6

On the Word Test, M achieved a raw score of 21 with an age equivalent of 7:9. Results of the Woodcock-Johnson Psychoeducational Battery Tests of Cognitive Ability are as follows.

Cluster	Grade Score	Age Score	Percentile
Verbal Ability	5:6	10:8	50
Reasoning	1:0	3:10	<1
Perceptual Speed	2:8	8:4	9
Memory	2:8	8:0	17

On the Broad Cognitive Ability Scale, M achieved an age score of 7:4 and a grade score of 1:8. This is equivalent to a moderately deficient functioning level. On the Tests of Achievement, M performed as follows.

Cluster	Grade Score	Age Score	Functioning Level
Reading	2:3	7:6	Severely Deficient
Mathematics	1:7	6:11	Severely Deficient
Written	1:8	7:4	Severely Deficient
Knowledge	4:7	10:0	Average

On the Calculation subtest, M added all problems including the subtraction and multiplication problems, only completing 4/13 correctly. M's strongest performance was on Blending, and her lowest performances were on the Analysis and Synthesis subtest and the Concept Formation subtest. She was also weak on the Dictation subtest.

M was asked to write a brief narrative about her best friend. On this narrative that consisted of six sentences, M wrote two incomplete sentences (e.g., "Go to school twogather."), and used simple sentence structure for the remaining four sentences (e.g., "April is nice. she is my friend sins preskool."). She used two adjectives and used capital letters inconsistently.

M was able to complete two-step commands in order (10/10), but completed only 6/10 three-step commands in the proper sequence.

Behavioral Observations

M is a pleasant young lady who put forth excellent effort during the testing session. She would occasionally get frustrated on the tasks presented and frequently inquired as to how she was doing on the tests. M professes that she does not like school and wishes her mom would arrange for home schooling.

Summary

This evaluation found that M has difficulties in math, reading, spelling, and verbal expression skills in addition to the previously determined deficits in auditory processing.

Recommendations

Recommendations given to the parents and sent to the school include the following:

1. It would be beneficial for M to be tested by a reading specialist to determine her level of phonemic awareness and phonological memory prior to initiating a therapy program that targets reading and spelling skills. Participation in a multisensory, phonetics-based reading therapy program such as the Barton program, the LiPS program, or the Orton-Gillingham method is recommended.

2. Address auditory discrimination, auditory memory, and visual memory skills. M possibly may benefit from the use of an FM system in her classroom.

3. Incorporate problem-solving activities into the academic and therapy settings.

4. Minimize visual and auditory distractions in the school room and home study area.

The clinician shared M's thoughts about attending school and suggested that the parents consider an alternative school setting. There is a Montessori school in town that goes from kindergarten to eighth grade, and all children who attend the school have reading, spelling, and other language-based academic difficulties. There is a full-time speech-language pathologist on staff who works collaboratively with the teachers to facilitate development of language skills that impact on academic ability. M expressed an interest in visiting this school, and the parents were given the principal's name and phone number. Perhaps this would be a happy compromise between mainstreamed public school and home schooling.

■ REVIEW QUESTIONS

1. Language screening identifies a child's strengths and weaknesses in language tasks and results in a specific diagnosis.

    a. True
    b. False

2. When comparing the assessment of preschoolers and school-age children, typically more cognitive assessment is included in the testing of preschoolers than in the testing of school-age children.

    a. True
    b. False

3. Factors that result in the onset of a language or communication problem, or both, are _____ factors.

    a. Precipitating factors
    b. Perpetuating factors
    c. Predisposing factors

4. A set of auditory skills that integrates what is heard with language at the cortical level is

    a. Auditory perception
    b. Auditory acuity
    c. Auditory processing

5. The first objective of the assessment process with school-age children is to determine the etiology of the problem.

    a. True
    b. False

6. Assessment batteries for language-based learning disabilities should include
   a. Modality-specific testing
   b. Tests of language and cognition
   c. Comparison of verbal and nonverbal skills
   d. All of the above.

7. Which of the following can be tested through the analysis of a spontaneous language sample?
   a. Mean length of utterance
   b. Use of morphosyntactic structures
   c. Lexicon
   d. Pragmatics
   e. All of the above
   f. a, c, d
   g. a, b, d
   h. a, b, c

8. Which of the following cases address overidentification of minority children as having speech and/or language deficits?
   a. *Diana* vs. *Board of Education*
   b. *Lau* vs. *Nicols*
   c. The Bilingual Education Act
   d. *Martin Luther King, Jr. Elementary School* vs. *Ann Arbor School District*
   e. All of the above
   f. a, c, d
   g. a, b, c
   h. a. b. d

9. Some schools use discrepancy testing as a means of justifying educational assistance for a child.
   a. True
   b. False

10. Auditory perception and auditory processing can be used interchangeably.
   a. True
   b. False

■ REFERENCES

American Speech-Language-Hearing Association (ASHA). (1989). Clinical management of communicatively handicapped minority language populations. *ASHA Desk Reference, 4,* IV-2–IV-6.

Aram, D., Ekelman, B., & Nation, J. (1984). Preschoolers with language disorders: Ten years later. *Journal of Speech and Hearing Research, 27,* 232–244.

Baran, J., Musiek, F., Gollegly, K., et al. (1987). Auditory duration pattern sequences in the assessment of CANS pathology. Paper presented at the American Speech-Language-Hearing Association annual meeting, New Orleans, November 15.

Barkley, R. A. (2000). *Taking charge of ADHD: The complete authoritative guide for parents.* New York: Guildford Press.

Bates, E. (1976). *Language in context.* New York: Academic Press.

Berk, R. A. (1984). *Screening and diagnosis of children with learning disabilities.* Springfield, IL: Thomas.

Bliss, L. S. (2002). *Discourse impairments: Assessment and intervention applications.* Boston: Allyn and Bacon.

Bloom, L. (1973). *One word at a time: The use of single-word utterances before syntax.* The Hague Mouton.

Brinton, B., & Fujiki, M. (1989). *Conversational management with language-impaired children: Pragmatic assessment and intervention.* Rockville, MD: Aspen Publishers.

Brown, R. (1973). *A first language.* Cambridge, MA: Harvard University Press.

Brown, A. (1978). Knowing when, where, and how to remember: A problem in metacognition. In R. Glaser (Ed.), *Advances in instructional psychology.* Hillsdale, NJ: Lawrence Erlbaum.

Catts, H. (1991). Early identification of dyslexia: Evidence from a follow-up study of speech-language impaired children. *Annals of Dyslexia, 41,* 163–177.

Catts, H. (1993). The relationship between speech-language impairments and reading disabilities. *Journal of Speech and Hearing Research, 36,* 948–958.

Chapman, R. (1978). Comprehension strategies in young children. In J. Kavanaugh & W. Strange (Eds.), *Speech and language in the laboratory, school, and clinic* (pp. 308–327). Cambridge, MA: MIT Press.

Chapman, S. (1997). Cognitive-communication abilities in children with closed head injury. *American Journal of Speech-Language Pathology, 6,* 50–58.

Chapman, S., Levin, H., & Culhane, K. (1995). Language impairment in closed head injury. In H. Kirschner (Ed.), *Handbook of neurological speech and language disorders* (pp. 387–414). New York: Marcel-Dekker.

Chapman, S. B., Ulatowska, H. K., Franklin, L. R., Shobe, J. L., Thompson, J. L., & McIntire, D. D. (1997). Proverb interpretation in fluent aphasia and Alzheimer's disease: Implications beyond abstract thinking. *Aphasiology,* 11, 337–350.

Coggins, T., & Carpenter, R. (1981). The communicative intention inventory: A system for coding children's early intentional communication. *Applied Psycholinguistics, 2,* 235–251.

Damico, J. (1991). Clinical discourse analysis: A functional approach to language assessment. In C. Simon (Ed.), *Communication skills and classroom success: Assessment and therapy methodologies for language and learning disabled students* (pp. 165–206). Eau Claire, WI: Thinking Publications.

Damico, J. S. (1985). Clinical discourse analysis: A functional approach to language assessment. In C. S. Simon (Ed.). *Communication skills and classroom success:* Assessment of language-learning disabled students. San Diego: College-Hill Press.

Damico J. (1993). Language assessment in adolescents: Addressing critical issues. *Language, Speech, and Hearing Services in Schools,* 24, 29–35.

Dempsey, D. (1983). Selecting tests of auditory function in children. In E. Z. Lasky & J. Katz (Eds.), *Central auditory processing disorders: Problems of speech, language, and learning* (pp. 203–221). Austin, TX: Pro-Ed.

Dore, J. (1974). A pragmatic description of early language development. *Journal of Psycholinguistic Research, 4,* 343–350.

Emerick, L. L., & Haynes, W. O. (1986). *Diagnosis and evaluation in speech pathology.* Englewood Cliffs, NJ: Prentice Hall.

Fey, M. C. (1986). *Language intervention with young children.* Needham Heights, MA: Allyn and Bacon.

Fisher, L. I. (n. d.). *Pisher auditory problems checklist.* Cedar Rapids, IA: Grant Wood Area Education Agency.

Flavell, J. H. (1977). *Cognitive development.* Englewood Cliffs, NJ: Prentice Hall.

Flavell, J. H., & Wellman, H. (1977). Metamemory. In R. Kail & J. Hagen (Eds.), *Perspectives on the development of memory and cognition.* Hillsdale, NJ: Lawrence Erlbaum.

German, D. J. (1986). *Test of word finding.* Allen, TX: DLM Teaching Resources.

Goffman, L., & Leonard, J. (2000). Growth of language skills in preschool children with specific language impairment: Implications for assessment and intervention. *American Journal of Speech-Language Pathology, 9,* 151–61.

Grela, B. G., & Leonard, L. B. (2000). The influence of argument-structure complexity on the use of auxiliary verbs by children with SLI. *Journal of Speech, Language, and Hearing Research, 43,* 1115–1125.

Hammill, D. D. (1998). *Detroit test of learning aptitude-4.* Austin, TX: Pro-Ed.

Hegde, M. N. (1996). *PocketGuide to assessment in speech-language pathology.* San Diego: Singular Publishing Group.

Holston, J. T. (1992, February). *Assessment and management of auditory processing problems in children.* Paper presented at the Winter Conference of the Florida Speech-Language-Hearing Association, Gainesville, FL.

Hughes, D., McGillvray, L., & Schmidek, M. (1997). *Guide to narrative language: Procedures for assessment.* Eau Claire, WI: Thinking Publications.

Jerger, J., & Jerger, S. (1974). Auditory findings in brainstem disorders. *Archives of Otolaryngology, 99,* 342–349.

Katz, J. (1962). The use of staggered spondaic words for assessing the integrity of the central auditory system. *Journal of Audiology Research, 2,* 327–337.

Keith, R. W. (1986). *SCAN: A screening test for auditory processing disorders.* San Antonio, TX: Psychological Corporation.

Keith, R. W. (1988). Central auditory tests. In N. J. Lass, L. V. McReynolds, J. L. Northern, & D. E. Yoder (Eds), *Speech, language, and hearing: Vol. 3, Hearing disorders,* (pp. 1215–1236). Philadelphia: W. B. Saunders.

Keith, R. W. (2000). Diagnosing central auditory processing disorders in children. In K. Roeser, H. Hosford-Dunn, & M. Valente (Eds.). *Audiology: Diagnosis, treatment, strategies, and practice management* (pp. 337–355). New York: Thieme.

Keith, R. W. (2000). *Randon gap defection test.* St. Louis, MO: Auditec.

Larson, V. L., & McKinley, N. (1995). *Language disorders in older students: Preadolescents and adolescents.* Eau Claire, WI: Thinking Publications.

Lee, L. (1974). *Developmental sentence analysis.* Evanston, IL: Northwestern University Press.

Mandler, J., & Johnson, N. (1977). Remembrance of things passed: Story structure and recall. *Cognitive Psychology, 9,* 111–151.

McCauley, R. J. (2001). *Assessment of language disorders in children.* Mahwah, NJ: Lawrence Erlbaum Assocates, Publishers.

Miller, J. (1981). *Assessing lanuage production in children: Experimental procedures.* Baltimore, MD: University Park Press.

Musiek, F. (1983). Assessment of central auditory dysfunction: The dichotic digits test revisited. *Ear and Hearing, 4,* 79–83.

Nelson, K. (1973). Structure and strategy in learning to talk. *Monographs of the Society for Research in Child Development, 38* (1–2, Serial No. 149).

Nelson, N. W. (1998). Childhood language disorders in context: Infancy through adolescence (2nd ed.). Boston: Allyn and Bacon.

Nicholas, L., & Brookshire, R. (1993). A system for quantifying the informativeness and efficiency of the connected speech of adults with aphasia. *Journal of Speech and Hearing Research, 36*, 338–350.

Nippold, M. (1998). *Later language development: The school-age and adolescent years* (2nd ed.). Austin, TX: Pro-Ed.

Northern, J. L., & Downs, M. P. (1991). *Hearing in children* (4th ed.). Baltimore, MD: Williams & Wilkins.

Oram, J., Fine, J., Okamoto, C., & Tannock, R. (1999). Assessing the language of children with hyperactivity disorder. *Journal of Speech-Language Pathology, 8*(1), 72–80.

Owens, R. (1995). *Language disorders: A functional approach to assessment and intervention* (2nd ed.). Boston: Allyn and Bacon.

Owens, R. (1996). *Language development: An introduction* (4th ed.). Boston: Allyn and Bacon.

Owens, R. E. (2004). *Language disorders: A functional approach to assessment and intervention* (4th ed.). Boston: Pearson/Allyn and Bacon.

Paul, R. (2001). *Childhood language disorders in context: Infancy through adolescence* (2nd ed.). Boston: Allyn and Bacon.

Pinheiro, M. (1977). Test of central auditory function in children with learning disabilities. In Keith, R. (Ed.). *Central auditory dysfunction.* New York: Grune & Stratton.

Polakow, V. (1993). *Lives on the edge: Single mothers and their children in the other America.* Chicago: University of Chicago Press.

Proctor, A. (1989). Stages of normal noncry vocal development in infancy: A protocol for assessment. *Topics in Language Disorders, 10*(1), 43–56.

Retherford, K. (1993). *Guide to analysis of language transcripts* (2nd ed.). Eau Claire, WI: Thinking Publications.

Rosner, J., & Simon, D. P. (1971). The auditory analysis test: An initial report. *Journal of Learning Disabilities, 4*, 384–392.

Rossetti, L. (1990). *Infant-toddler assessment: An interdisciplinary approach.* Boston: Little, Brown & Co.

Roth, F., & Spekman, N. (1986). Narrative discourse: Spontaneously generated stories of learning disabled and normally achieving students. *Journal of Speech and Hearing Disorders, 51*, 8–23.

Rubin, D. L. (1987). Divergence and convergence between oral and written communication. *Topics in Language Disorders, 7*(4), 1–18.

Rumelhart, D. (1975). Notes on a schema for stories. In D. Bobrow & A. Collins (Eds.), *Representation and understanding: Studies in cognitive science* (pp. 211–236). New York: Academic Press.

Sattler, J. M. (1988). *Assessment of children.* San Diego: Author.

Saywitz, K., & Cherry-Wilkinson, L. (1982). Age-related differences in metalinguistic awareness. In S. Kaczaj (Ed.), *Language development: Vol. 2, Language, thought, and culture.* Hillsdale, NJ: Lawrence Erlbaum.

Schow, R. L., & Nerbonne, M. A. (1996). *Introduction to audiologic rehabilitation.* Needham Heights, MA: Simon & Schuster Company.

Scott, C. (1988). Spoken and Written syntax. In M. Nippold (Ed.), *Later language development: Ages nine through nineteen* (pp. 49–55). Austin, TV: Pro-Ed.

Semel, E., Wiig, E. H., & Secord, W. (1987). *Clinical evaluation of language fundamentals-revised.* New York: The Psychological Corporation, Harcourt Brace Jovanovich.

Semel, E., Wiig, E., & Secord, W. (1997). *Clinical evaluation of language fundamentals-III.* San Antonio, TX: The Psychological Corporation.

Stark, R. E., Bernstein, L., Condino, R., Bender, M., Tallal, P., & Catts, H. (1984). Four-year follow-up study of language impaired children. *Annals of Dyslexia, 34,* 49–68.

Stein, N., & Glenn, C. (1979). An analysis of story comprehension in elementary school children. In R. Freedle (Ed.), *New directions in discourse processing, 2* (pp. 53–120). Norwood, NJ: Ablex.

Tannock, R., Fine, J., & Ickowicz, A. (1998). Language abilities of children with attention deficit hyperactivity disorder. *Journal of Child Psychology, 21,* 103–117.

Thorndyke, P. (1977). Cognitive structures in comprehension and memory of narrative discourse. *Cognitive Psychology, 9,* 77–110.

Ulatowska, H., Chapman, S., Highley, A., & Prince, J. (1998). Discourse in health old-elderly adults: A longitudinal study. *Aphasiology, 12,* 619–633.

van Kleeck, A. (1984). Metalinguistic skills: Cutting across spoken and written language and problem solving abilities. In G. Wallach & K. Butler (Eds.), *Language learning disabilities in school-age children* (pp. 53–89). Baltimore, MD: Williams & Wilkins.

Wallach, G. P., & Butler, K. G. (1994). *Language learning disabilities in school-age children and adolescents:* Some principles and applications. New York: Macmillan.

Weiss, A., & Johnson, C. (1993). Relationships between narrative and syntactic competencies in school-age hearing-impaired children. *Applied Psycholinguistics, 14,* 35–59.

Westby, C. (1994). The effects of culture on genre, structure, and style of oral and written texts. In G. Wallach & K. Butler (Eds.), *Language learning disabilities in school-age children and adolescents* (pp. 180–218). New York: Merrill-Macmillan College Publishing Company.

Wetherby, A., & Prizant, B. M. (1993). *Communication and symbolic behavior scales.* Itasca, IL: Riverside Publishing.

Wetherby, A., & Prizant, B. (2002). *Communication and Symbolic Behavior Scales—Developmental Profile (CSBS-DP).* Baltimore, MD: Brookes Publishing.

Wilkinson, G. (1993). *The wide range achievement test,* 3rd ed. Wilmington, DE: Jastak.

Woodcock, R. W. (1987). *Woodcock reading mastery tests-revised.* Circle Pines, MN: American Guidance Service.

Woodcock, R. W., & Johnson, M. B. (1977). *Woodcock-Johnson psycho-educational battery.* Allen, TX: DLM Teaching Resource.

Woodcock, R. W., McGrew, K. S., & Mather, N. (2001). *Woodcock-Johnson III tests of achievement.* Itasca, IL: Riverside.

Woodcock, R. W., McGrew, K. S., & Mather, N. (2001). *Woodcock-Johnson III tests of cognition.* Itasca, IL: Riverside.

Young, M. (1985). Central auditory processing through the looking glass: A critical look at diagnosis and management. *Journal of Childhood Communication Disorder, 9,* 31–42.

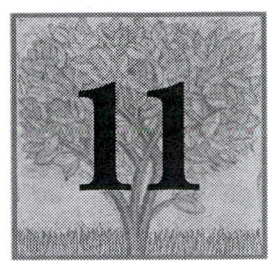

Treatment in the School-Age Population

■ LEARNING OBJECTIVES

After completion of this chapter, the reader will be able to

1. Discuss some factors that could negatively impact accomplishing therapy goals for school-age children.

2. Discuss some special issues that need to be considered when planning and implementing language therapy for adolescents.

3. Compare and contrast the three primary models of intervention in the schools.

4. Discuss the four steps of Merritt and Culatta's view of collaboration in the problem-solving process.

5. Discuss the steps involved in planning and implementing the therapy process.

6. Discuss some of the academic changes and demands that occur beginning in third grade.

7. Discuss the importance of developing metalinguistic skills and their impact on academic success.

8. Discuss the focus of language therapy for adolescents, including critical thinking, listening, and writing.

9. Differentiate between and discuss the three philosophies regarding provision of therapy services to individuals from minority cultural groups.

■ INTRODUCTION

Language-impaired children are students who are unable to use language to fulfill the academic and social demands of school (Naremore, Densmore, & Harman, 1995). One of the first steps in the therapeutic process is to set the goals, objectives, and procedures that will guide the therapy for the school-age child. According to Van Hattum (1985), three questions should guide the determination of goals, objectives, and procedures for therapy. The first question is, "What does the child need to communicate successfully in his or her environment?" This question is particularly important to address in terms of the several environments (i.e., home, school, social settings) in which school-age children function. A second question that should be addressed is, "What skills is the child currently demonstrating?" Using the four-box system (see Chapter 3), this question should be answered in terms of the communicative and noncommunicative strengths that the child exhibits in the different environments. The third question has its impact after the new skills have been learned in the therapy setting. At that time, the major question facing the clinician is, "How do I facilitate the child's use of the newly learned skills in his or her natural environment?"

TABLE 11–1. Deciding if goals and objectives are appropriate.

1. Do the goals and objectives take the student's environmental demands into consideration?
2. Are the goals and objectives useful and relevant?
3. Can the goals and objectives be transferred and maintained?
4. Do the goals and objectives provide a foundation for response generalization?
5. Can the objectives be broken down into smaller steps?
6. Are the goals achievable?

It is also important to be sure that the goals and objectives are appropriate for the child's age and overall cognitive abilities. Table 11–1 delineates six questions that can be used as guidelines for determining the appropriateness of the goals and objectives that the clinician has developed for therapy.

With regard to question 1 in Table 11–1, the environments of a school-age child are greatly expanded in comparison to those of a preschool child. Therefore, the issue of environmental demands is much more critical when setting goals and objectives for school-age children. The usefulness and relevance of the goals, as expressed in question 2, can be determined only in light of the different environments in which the child functions on a daily basis. The use of the skills in the child's daily environment leads to the issue expressed in questions 3 and 4 in Table 11–1 with regard to the maintenance and generalization of the skills. The fifth question brings forth a critical concern. Perhaps one of the hardest jobs in determining goals and objectives is to be sure that the steps are appropriate in their demands. If steps are too big, the student will not make efficient progress and will become discouraged. If the steps are too small, critical therapy time is wasted on reviewing what is already known. This also ties in with question 6 in that it is important that the objectives be achievable. Many times emotional, physical, or mental capacity problems may exist that affect the achievability of the goals and objectives. Given the potential for emotional distress due to unmet goals, particularly in older elementary and middle school-age children, the answers to questions 5 and 6 are critical for success with school-age children in speech-language therapy.

When planning therapy for adolescents, it is first important to look at the educational commitment of the student. Does this student value education, or does he or she resent being in school (Larson & McKinley, 1995)? Does the child complete homework assignments, is he or she motivated to achieve, and what are his or her educational aspirations? A student who does not value the education he or she is receiving is going to be negative about most attempts at therapy. Therefore, extra time will need to be spent developing a rapport with the student and making him or her understand the importance of achieving the therapy goals that have been set. Children with language-based learning disabilities often have a negative attitude toward school because of a feeling of failure that is based on poor academic performance due to the learning disability. In these cases, it is important to gain the trust of the student and help him or her see the educational relevance of the objectives in speech-language therapy (Larson & McKinley, 1995). A high school student recently started therapy for dyslexia at the University of Florida Speech and Hearing Clinic. After several sessions, the clinician asked her whether she thought the therapy was helping. The student replied that she understood her history lessons for the first time and had even volunteered to read aloud in class. Clearly, this student made the connection between what was happening in therapy and the changes it could create in the classroom.

Second, tied in with the student's educational commitment are his or her values. Does the student value the educational process? Does the student care about the feelings of other people? Does the student value helping other people? The student should be asked these questions as part of the history-gathering process so that the values can be taken into account when developing the goals and objectives for therapy (Larson & McKinley, 1995).

Third, a special issue with adolescents is social competence, which taps into issues related to self-esteem, assertiveness, decision-making skills, friend-making abilities, planning skills, and the student's personal view of his or her own future. As seen in Chapter 5, self-esteem and depression are major concerns when working with adolescents with language-based learning disabilities.

Providing therapy for students with language-based learning disabilities is a multidimensional issue. Careful consideration needs to be given to establishing rapport with the student, particularly students beyond the elementary school years. For the therapy to be successful, the student must see the value of the therapy and have a sense of trust in the clinician.

■ ELIGIBILITY FOR THERAPY

Children who are considered language impaired as preschoolers may have their condition variously labeled as a reading disability or learning disability in elementary schools (Bashir et al., 1983; Snyder, 1984; Wallach & Liebergott, 1984). Thus, it is important to understand the school environment, the curriculum, the child's language abilities, interactive learning styles, and the child's language problems when planning intervention for school-age children with language-based learning disabilities.

When determining eligibility for therapy, the clinician can look toward exclusionary criteria or discrepancy criteria, or both (Naremor, Densmore, &

Harman, 1995). Using exclusionary criteria, the therapist would diagnose the language-based learning disability based on the fact that the child has language or learning problems that are not related to mental handicaps, sensory impairments, or physical conditions. If the clinician uses discrepancy criteria, he or she is typically referring to a gap between the child's expected level of language achievement based on his or her overall intellectual functioning and sociocultural opportunities and his or her language abilities. The discrepancy can be in any or all of the components of language and can affect both receptive and expressive language (Naremore et al., 1995).

The American Speech-Language-Hearing Association (ASHA) published a paper in 1989 in which the association took issue with using discrepancy definitions to determine eligibility for therapy. Specifically, one of the concerns was the possible use of a single aspect of language to validate the presence of a discrepancy. The association also was concerned about poor availability of age-appropriate and psychometrically valid testing instruments for the school-age population. This is not as much as problem today as it was in 1989, but that concern is still valid if a clinician applies labels could be applied using inadequate standardized testing. Related to the lack of age-appropriate and valid testing instruments is the fact that tests are developed on the basis of different theoretical constructs and standardized on different populations. Thus, it can be psychometrically incorrect to compare test scores from different tests. Many tests also fail to provide important qualitative information regarding the nature of the learning or language deficits (ASHA, 1989). These are certainly critical concerns when determining a label for a child's disorder that may be needed to qualify for services in the schools. In fact, ASHA went so far as to say that "the exclusive use of a discrepancy formula as a required procedure for determining eligibility for language intervention should be viewed with extreme caution and avoided whenever possible" (ASHA, 1989, p. 115).

■ MODELS OF INTERVENTION

Historically, school-based clinicians primarily have employed the "pull-out" method for therapy. Using this model, students were assigned to specific times for therapy, and the clinician would take the children to the "speech room" where he or she would provide therapy before taking the child back to the classroom. The pull-out model places an extra demand on the classroom teacher because the clinician relies on the teacher to provide feedback as to how well the child is generalizing his or her therapy skills into the classroom.

The **collaborative model** of intervention, as illustrated in Figure 11–1, a partnership between the teacher and the speech-language pathologist, is becoming increasingly popular among school-based speech-language pathologists. In the collaborative model, each professional has a view of the "whole child," not myriad professional viewpoints (Naremore et al., 1995).

Collaborative model. Classroom-based or curriculum-based intervention that focuses on learning strategies and using them in materials related to the curriculum.

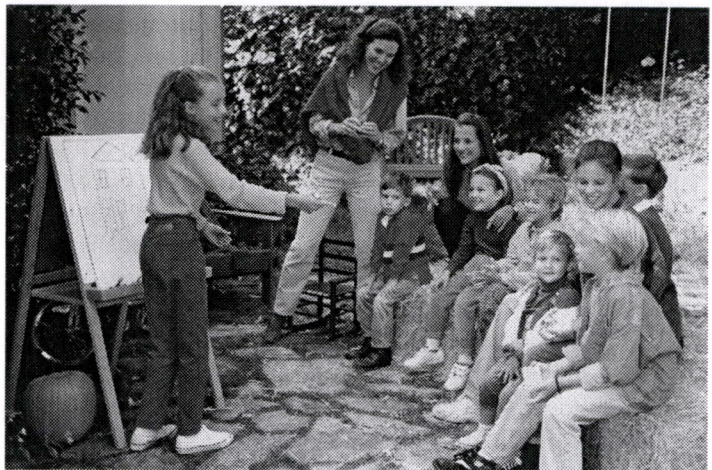

FIGURE 11–1. In the collaborative model, the speech-language pathologist and teacher work together in the classroom to facilitate generalization of skills in the academic setting.

TABLE 11–2. Samples of behavioral objectives.

Andrew will independently match the phonemes /b/, /p/, /s/, and /t/ with the corresponding grapheme with 90% accuracy on 20 trials.

With no more than 2 verbal prompts from the clinician, Nicole will place 5 story strips in the proper sequence for 3 different stories.

Sam will list 2 synonyms for each of the 10 words on a vocabulary list with 80% accuracy.

The collaborative model, also known as classroom-based intervention or curriculum-based intervention, focuses on learning strategies and using them in materials related to the curriculum. The underlying philosophy of the collaborative model is that "language learning is intrinsic to literary development" (Naremore et al., 1995).

In 1991, ASHA supported the collaborative model as the most efficient and effective model of intervention for students with language-based learning disabilities in public schools (ASHA, 1991). Merritt and Culatta (1998) view collaboration as a "problem-solving process" consisting of four steps: identification of the problem, planning of intervention, implementation, and evaluation. During the identification phase, the teachers and clinicians work together to write behavioral objectives consisting of a description of the behavior that needs to be changed, the conditions under which the behavior will occur, and the criteria for measuring progress. Examples of behavioral objectives for speech-language pathology are in Table 11–2.

During the identification stage, the clinician also presents any baseline data against which progress will be measured and identifies the most problematic behaviors to determine the priority in which multiple goals will be addressed.

During the stage in which the intervention is planned, the involved personnel brainstorm ideas and do the equivalent of a feasibility study to develop a realistic action plan and timeline. The implementation stage consists of putting the plan into action, following the timeline, and collecting the data. In the final stage, evaluation of the program, the teachers and clinicians compare the pre- and post-intervention data and make a decision as to whether to continue with the intervention, revise the goals, or terminate the intervention (Merritt & Culatta, 1998).

In spite of ASHA's strong support of the collaborative model, there has been some hesitancy on the part of educators to adopt this service delivery model. General educators were found to be less favorable of within-class services (the foundation of the collaborative model) but did agree that it was less detrimental academically, as the children remain in the classroom. Furthermore, both regular and special education teachers have questioned the teacher's need to be in class when the speech-language pathologist is present (Sanger, Hux, & Griess, 1995). Clinicians adopting the collaborative model must stress that it is based on collaboration between the classroom teacher and the clinician. It is not intended that the speech-language pathologist be a temporary substitute for the teacher. Rather, both professionals should work as a team in coordinating language therapy goals, objectives, and procedures with curricular demands in the classroom.

In the **consultative model**, the speech-language pathologist provides indirect therapy through workshops and individualized input to classroom teachers on appropriate methods for encouraging effective speech and language skills. In this model, the clinician provides preventive and direct intervention information. Other indirect methods of therapy include counseling, tutoring, and adapting education materials to intermingle communication and language into the standard classroom curriculum. A comparison of all three models is in Table 11–3.

Consultative model. A service delivery model in which the speech-language pathologist provides indirect therapy through inservice and input to classroom teachers on appropriate methods for encouraging effective speech and language skills.

TABLE 11–3. Direct service and consultation models.

Model Type	Options	Description
Direct service models	Pull-out	The SLP provides services in individual or small group sessions in a setting separate from the regular education classroom; goals and objectives typically are unrelated to curricular demands; teacher may or may not reinforce approaches.

(continued)

TABLE 11–3. (*continued*)

Model Type	Options	Description
Direct service models	Pull-in (parallel instruction)	The SLP conducts individual or small group sessions in the classroom; incorporates specific speech and language objectives within a curricular focus; teacher assists in generalizing skills.
Consultation models	Instructional consultation	The SLP is a consultant to the classroom teacher, assisting in interpreting formal and informal assessment data, developing intervention approaches, and monitoring progress.
	Monitoring	The SLP observes the student in the classroom context and collects data relative to established language goals and objectives.
	Prereferral teacher assistance	The SLP participates in a problem-solving team that attempts to meet the educational needs of children in the classroom by varying instructional approaches and strategies.

SLP: Speech-language pathologist

Source: From "Collaborative Partnerships and Decision-Making," by J. DiMeo, D. D. Merritt, and B. Culatta in *Language Intervention in the Classroom,* edited by D. D. Merritt, & B. Culatta, 1998, p. 74. San Diego: Singular Publishing Group. Copyright 1998 by Singular Publishing Group. Reprinted with permission.

■ INDIVIDUALIZED EDUCATION PLANS (IEPS)

Individualized education plan (IEP). Required by IDEA, the academic plan required for all students who are in special education or related services in the public schools.

Individualized education plans (IEPs) are supposed to address four domains: curriculum and learning environment, independent functioning, social and personal concerns, and communication. The curriculum and learning environment incorporate the academic subjects, including reading, writing, listening, speaking, mathematics, and problem solving. With the passage of IDEA, *transition* became a major focus of the IEP to encourage educators to consider what skills a student will need to make the transition from school to work. Thus, the curriculum portion of the IEP includes job preparation, use of tools and technology, and employability skills.

Independent functioning includes personal care (daily living skills) and self-management, which addresses personal planning, decision making, and appropriate conduct in daily living and work roles. The social and personal domains concentrate on working with others, focusing on group and interpersonal relationships. With regard to communication, the IEP needs to address the student's ability to participate effectively in communication exchanges.

The IEP should also specify the level of functioning the child is expected to achieve. At the "independent level" of functioning, the student is capable of working and living independently, even though occasional assistance may be needed. To achieve independent functioning, the IEP needs to address functional academics and functional daily living and working skills. The "supported level" of functioning means that the student is expected to be capable of living and working in a supported setting. This student will need skills that address daily living tasks and activities and skills that can maximize independence and personal effectiveness. Finally, a level of functioning may be specified as "participatory." This means that the student is capable of participating in major life activities but will require extensive support systems. The student will need opportunities for participation in tasks and activities of daily living. Regardless of the level of expected functioning, it is critical that the curriculum focus on functional goals and objectives. In other words, subjects need to provide "real-life" applications to facilitate the generalization of the academic preparation to the work place. "A Case for Teaching Functional Skills" (Lewis, 1987) is provided in Appendix 5A. It is an eloquent story that highlights the importance of providing therapy that is based on functional goals for school-age children with language delays and disorders.

■ TREATMENT SEQUENCE

Regardless of the student's age and the type of language-based learning disability, a general sequence of events is part of planning and implementing the therapy process. The first step is to select the target behavior. This ties in very closely with the evaluative-planning process because an appropriate assessment protocol that is properly administered can provide the necessary baseline data from which to select the language skills to be targeted in therapy.

A second step is to plan the sequence in which the targets will be addressed in therapy. Most children who have a language-based learning disability will have difficulty with a number of aspects of language. Thus, it is the job of the clinician to prioritize the objectives. The ability to task analyze a goal is absolutely critical at the planning stage of therapy. Task analysis is important because many of the language and communication objectives people use incorporate a chained sequence of behaviors. The clinician must know the components of the skill in order to plan effective and efficient therapy. Objectives and procedures need to be small enough to be readily achievable, yet not so small that the student does not progress at a satisfactory rate in therapy. Using the four-box system, a clinician can ascertain the strengths and weaknesses that were identified in the assessment process to help prioritize the skills to be addressed in therapy. The information and data gathered from the assessment process also are critical in the documentation of baselines. Baselines reflect the student's level of performance prior to intervention. Baselines help document the need for therapy, serve as a basis for documenting improvement, and establish the clinician's accountability (Hegde, 1996).

The third step involves writing the therapy plan. This includes the selection of stimulus materials and the determination of which procedures will be used. At this point, the clinician defines the expected cause and effect considerations by selecting stimuli to facilitate the accuracy and rate of responses from the student. Materials should be age-appropriate and in accordance with the child's level of functioning. For example, when teaching reading to a middle school-age child, it is important to use literature that is not significantly beyond the child's level of ability yet is appropriate for the student in terms of the content and interest level. Complexity of the responses should be graded on a continuum from words to phrases, then to simple shorter sentences. As the child progresses, longer and more complex sentences should be used, followed by establishing maintenance of the skills from each level (Hegde, 1996).

Maintenance. The independent use of therapy skills in a person's natural settings.

Another consideration when writing the therapy plan is the development of a **maintenance** and **generalization** plan. It does not do any good for a child to be able to develop and use new language skills in a controlled setting if there is no plan to incorporate the skills into the child's daily settings and activities.

Generalization. The addition of new stimuli or environmental factors to elicit the same response obtained in a controlled setting.

The fourth step in the therapy process is putting the plans for therapy, maintenance, and generalization into action. The goal is to establish the new skills in a controlled setting, then to practice the skills to ensure that they will be generalized and maintained when stimuli and reinforcement schedules are changed. The clinician should always be moving toward effective communication. Strategies to facilitate the movement toward conversation include the ability to initiate and maintain a topic. Turn-taking and eye contact should also be addressed. The child should also be taught "conversational repair" strategies, such as requesting verification when a message is not understood (Hegde, 1996). Once the child can maintain a skill in a controlled setting, the emphasis shifts to the generalization of the skills into the child's daily environments and routines.

The final step in the treatment process is the reviewing of the data and making any needed modifications. This evaluative process leads to a decision on whether to modify current goals, objectives, or procedures, and whether to continue or dismiss the child from therapy.

■ INTERVENTION WITH ELEMENTARY SCHOOL-AGE CHILDREN

During the elementary school years, the development of literacy skills predominates the academic curriculum. As mentioned previously, the transition in third grade from "learning to read" to "reading to learn" (Roth & Worthington, 2001, p. 146) represents a major milestone in the academic world. Other academic demands include increasingly complex written and oral language and the use of narratives as part of the instructional protocol for teaching more advanced language forms. It is assumed that, by the time the child enters third grade he or she will have mastered skills needed to succeed academically and socially. Some of these skills are the development of good work habits, the ability to work independently, self-organization skills, and "rapid and automatic application of knowledge" (Roth & Worthington, 2001, p. 146). Children with a history of language and/or phonological deficits may experience difficulty with these aspects of his or her schooling.

Development of Metalinguistic Skills

Metalinguistic skills are needed for a child to be able to analyze his or her language and its functions. They are critical in order for the child to manipulate the components of language so that he or she can appreciate humor, understand idioms, provide definitions of words, and use phonemic awareness tasks including segmentation of words and blending of sounds to create words (Roth & Worthington, 2001).

Three Language Teaching Methods

Olswang and Bain (1991) described three intervention methods based on the amount of structure used in the therapy process. The first one, milieu teaching, involves providing therapy in the child's natural environments. Goals and activities are based on the interest and attention of the child, and the natural reinforcements in the environment promote language growth. Procedures include incidental teaching, mand-model teaching, and delay (Warren & Yoder, 1994). In incidental teaching the therapist, teacher, and caregivers build language into the child's daily activities and routines. A variety of techniques can be used, and it is highly dependent on the interests of the child. Mand-model intervention is the more typical therapy approach in that it is adult-directed, with the adult presenting a stimulus, asking for a particular response, and, if necessary, providing a prompt to elicit the response. If the child responds correctly, he or she is reinforced by the clinician. If the child responds incorrectly, the clinician uses a variety of techniques to elicit the desired response. Using delay as a teaching technique must be done carefully in order not to frustrate the child. In using delay, the adult looks expectantly at the child for about 15 seconds while waiting for an appropriate request for an action or object. Lack of response from the child can be met with modeling the desired behavior, then waiting again (Reed, 2005).

The second model is joint action routines, or, as it is sometimes called, script therapy. In joint action routines, the adult sets up "interactive, systematic repetitions of events in which each partner has predictable language and behavioral patterns to complete" (Reed, 2005, p. 476). The routines set up the need to communicate in a contrived, social situation. As the child's involvement in the routines increases, language demands become more complex. It is hoped that the child will generalize the routines to his or her natural environment, but this is sometimes problematic.

The most structured teaching method, inductive teaching, is the third model proposed by Olwsang and Bain (1991). The child looks for patterns in communicative exchanges that are developed and manipulated by the adult. This procedures assumes that the induction process is an innate process, and that if the communicative exchanges are arranged correctly, the child will hypothesize, or induct, the rule governing the pattern of the exchanges.

Most therapists will use a combination of the three models, with the child's abilities and interests guiding which one is implemented at any given time.

■ INTERVENTION WITH ADOLESCENTS

Roth and Worthington (2001) delineate three main stages of adolescence as explained in Table 11–4. The development of metalinguistic skills continues in this age period, with increased ability to use and appreciate humor, proverbs, metaphors, and idioms. The use of figurative language enhances oral and written language as the child learns to "go beyond the conventional meaning of language for correct interpretation or use" (Roth & Worthington, 2001, p. 158). Other advances in language include increased mean length of utterance and increased complexity of sentences, the use of linguistic cohesion devices, expository writing, and continued development of lexicon and word knowledge. Metalinguistic skills are a major target of intervention with adolescents with language-based learning disabilities. They play a role in both oral and written language, and they facilitate the acquisition and use of independent problem-solving strategies (van Kleeck, 1994).

TABLE 11–4. Stages of adolescence and corresponding therapeutic emphasis.

Stage	Age	Therapeutic Emphasis Area
Early	10–14	Developing communication skills for academic and personal-social purposes
Middle	14–16	Facilitation of communication skills for academic, personal-social, and vocational goals
Late	16–20	Developing communication skills for personal-social and vocational purposes

Source: Adapted from *Treatment Resource Manual for Speech-Language Pathology* (2nd ed.) by F. P. Roth and C. K. Worthington. Copyright 2001 by Delmar. Adapted with permission.

Within the confines of the different disorders, one can generally say that therapy for adolescents should focus on critical thinking strategies, listening skills (particularly important since most high school teaching models revolve around lectures), and written and oral language comprehension and production. In other words, it is particularly important that children in this age group be taught *how* to learn as opposed to *what* to learn. McKinley and Larson (1985) reported that when therapy focuses on teaching learning strategies, the child is more likely to "generalize basic skills across situations, settings, and curricula" (p. 4).

As presented in Chapter 10, it is critical to involve the adolescent in the stages of therapy by explaining the diagnostic and therapeutic processes and addressing the adolescent regarding the results of the assessment and development of therapy goals. The goals must be ones that are meaningful to the adolescent if he or she is expected to willingly participate in the therapeutic process. In addition, it is critical for the speech-language pathologist to stress the impact of achieving the set goals on future schooling and employment.

■ ADDRESSING WRITTEN LANGUAGE PROBLEMS IN CHILDREN WITH LANGUAGE-BASED LEARNING DISABILITIES

Written language poses a different set of problems than does oral language. Wong and colleagues (1991) identified problems these children have with written language as including "lower-order cognitive problems in spelling, punctuation, and grammar, and higher-order cognitive and metacognitive problems in planning, writing fluency, revising, and awareness of audience" (p. 117). They proposed an interactive teaching model to assist children with written language assignments. In an interactive model, the clinician engages the older elementary children or adolescents in oral discourse to help them clarify the theme of their writing, and to help them identify any ambiguous statements in their written narratives. Therapy for written language is best implemented in a collaborative approach involving the academic teachers and the speech-language pathologist.

■ MULTICULTURAL ISSUES IN LANGUAGE THERAPY

One of the first questions the clinician should ask when faced with serving a student whose first language is not English is, "Am I prepared to assess and work with students of other cultures who have various language-learning difficulties?" Providing treatment for multicultural students goes beyond knowing the child's native language. Clinicians must understand the child's native culture as well. Thus, it is important for clinicians to update their knowledge and skills with regard to cultural diversity. Another major question is, "How do I encourage positive interaction between myself and the client?" The answer to this question takes on extra meaning when we review the culturally accepted practices that affect pragmatics and interactions in non-English-speaking students. For example, in some cultures, it is considered a major transgression to touch someone's head. This could certainly have an impact on a clinician who is putting ear phones on a student or performing an oral-facial examination. Clinicians must be aware of verbal and nonverbal rules used by the student who speaks a minority language to avoid inadvertent insults, thus damaging the client-clinician relationship.

The ultimate goal in providing therapy to students from non-English-speaking backgrounds is equity. That is, it is important to give all students what they need to perform equally well in their academic and social pursuits. Addressing both verbal and nonverbal pragmatics is necessary when teaching multicultural students.

Impact of Theories of Language Development

Skinner espoused the behavioristic theory of language development. This viewpoint emphasizes the form of language, not necessarily the cognitive processes that underlie language and abstract thinking. Using behavioristic theory, language is taught in a stimulus-response paradigm. Although this type of theoretical approach to language therapy has a role in some therapies, it can be disastrous for students who have limited English proficiency (LEP) because it ignores many of the pragmatic issues that form a foundation for communication.

The nativist viewpoint of language development states that children have innate structures that enable language to develop when stimulated by the environment. Chomsky was the major proponent of the nativist theory, but as with the behavioristic approach, the emphasis is on form, and, in this case, syntax in particular.

Proponents of the interactionist theory of language development believe that language development interacts with cognition. In this theory, having a great variety of experiences means that there are greater opportunities to learn language. The interactionist approach is the most effective one to use with individuals who are learning English as a second language. The ability to address form, content, and use through a pragmatic approach to learning a second language should not be underestimated. However, the clinician should keep in mind that narrative performances "among various cultural, ethnic, and linguistic groups may differ greatly" (Owens, 1995, p. 62). Standard English relies primarily on word order to convey meaning, whereas many other languages tend to use more inflectional morphemes to convey meaning

(Nelson, 1993). Also, speakers in other cultures tend to use more paralinguistic devices than does most of the American culture (Owens, 1995).

A Continuum of Proficiency in English

The American Speech-Language-Hearing Association (ASHA) (1985) has outlined a continuum of proficiency in English:

1. Bilingual English proficient

2. Limited English proficient

3. Limited in English and the minority language

The association has also developed clinical competencies needed to serve each of these three groups. Clients who are bilingual English proficient are equally or more fluent in English than in their native language. If the communication disorder is in English, the speech-language pathologist does not have to be proficient in the minority language. However, the clinician must have enough base knowledge to distinguish between dialectical differences influenced by the minority language and the communication disorder. This would include knowing the rules that govern the use of the minority language and knowledge of contrastive phonological, grammatical, semantic, and pragmatic features of the minority language. The clinician must also be knowledgeable about nondiscriminatory testing procedures (ASHA, 1985).

The second group on the continuum includes persons who are considered to be limited English proficient. These are the students who are proficient in their native language but have limited mastery of the English language. In these cases, assessment and treatment must be conducted in the native language. Thus, the clinician must have native or near-native fluency in the minority language and English. He or she must also know normative processes for speech and language acquisition in the minority language, both oral and written. The clinician must be able to administer and interpret formal and informal assessment procedures to distinguish between a language difference and a language disorder. Again, the clinician should be sensitive to cultural factors affecting communication and its remediation (ASHA, 1985).

Students who are limited in both English and their minority language constitute the third group on the continuum. In these cases, the clinician must be fluent in English and the child's native language. It is important to assess the child in both languages to determine if one is dominant over the other. The same competencies required for working with students who have limited English proficiency apply to this segment of the continuum. Which language is used for intervention will depend on the assessment results (ASHA, 1985).

Language Education

School-based clinicians may provide services in the instruction of English as a second language or in teaching a nonstandard dialect. For most of these students, therapy will be considered an elective service, stemming from a desire to acquire more standard English production. Therefore, unless a disorder is present in the native language, the child will not qualify for services in the schools under Section 504 of the Rehabilitation Act, or under IDEA. However, funding from other sources within the district may be used to cover the costs of providing therapy.

To provide these therapeutic services, the clinician must be competent and knowledgeable in at least three areas. First, the clinician must be familiar with linguistic features of the child's dialect. Second, he or she must understand linguistic contrastive analysis. Third, the clinician must have an appreciation of the effects of attitudes toward dialects.

Therapy must emphasize language structure, language use, and language as a facilitator of cognition. The practical use of the language in a variety of settings also must be emphasized (Taylor, 1992). As with almost all language instruction, a multimodality, multifunctional approach would be most beneficial. It is also important to remember that proficiency in English at the elementary ages does not guarantee successful use of English in middle school and high school because of the differences in the language demands and use at the different age levels (Nelson, 1993).

There are three philosophies regarding whether or not to provide dialect intervention to children in the schools. The "no intervention view" states that community dialects are culturally adequate. Therefore, the stance should be to forgo intervention and permit the children to use the language of their home speech community. Proponents of the "bidialectal view" believe that it is important to respect and preserve the students' native dialects, but that it is also important to teach them to master the prevalent dialect so they can use it when expected or required to do so. The third philosophy is the "eradication view." In this viewpoint, community dialects have no value and should not be preserved. The children should be taught the prevalent dialect and instructed to use it in all settings at all times. The school-based clinician must be aware of these philosophies and know if one philosophy takes precedence over another within his or her own school setting.

Knapp, Turnbull, and Shields (1990) addressed the issue of how children from poverty homes succeed in school. They found that these children can rise to the challenges presented by individuals in the academic setting when the following occur.

1. Teachers respect the students' cultural/linguistic backgrounds and communicate this appreciation to them in a personal way.

2. The academic program encourages students to draw and build on the experiences they have, at the same time that it exposes then to unfamiliar experiences and ways of thinking.

3. The assumptions, expectations, and ways of doing things in school—in short, its culture—are made explicit to these students by teachers who explain and model these dimensions of academic learning (p. 5).

When these conditions are met, not only will children from poverty benefit, but so will those from any minority culture.

NELB and LEP

NELB and LEP are acronyms used to identify children as being of "non-English language background" or "limited English proficient." Typically, these terms are used to refer to speakers of English as a second language. However, it is important to remember that a child could be of a non-English language background but still be proficient in English. Likewise, it is possible to be limited English proficient without being of a non-English language background. Although these thoughts may seem trivial, they point out that clinicians and educators should not make hasty assumptions about a child based on his or her dialect or knowledge of the English language when English is a second language.

The Pygmalion effect states that individuals will live up to expectations placed on them. Thus, if our expectations are lowered for children with dialects or language differences, it is probable that these children will show, in accordance with the expectations, limited progress in their academic and social skills. In a lecture to students at the University of Florida, Bernardo Garcia, Director of the Office of Multicultural Student Language Education in the Florida Department of Education, proposed that we rename the acronym LEP to represent a more positive perspective. For example, he proposed that LEP could stand for "language-enhanced pupils" because many educators equate LEP with "lower expectation pupil" (Garcia, 1994). It is certainly something to consider. The real issue is "How meaningfully does this individual communicate?" not how well his or her language represents the standard dialect.

■ SUMMARY

Individuals with language-based learning disabilities, especially those that affect reading, spelling, and writing, often face an uphill battle to overcome these deficits. When structuring the treatment for these students, clinicians must avoid fostering a sense of failure and helplessness. Learned helplessness can be decreased by rewarding completed work with positive reinforcement and meaningful feedback. Promoting active involvement in the learning process and scheduling breaks to avoid mental fatigue also help to improve the student's abilities to sustain his or her attention on the task at hand. Teaching children to self-check their own work is likewise critical in decreasing learned helplessness because the children learn to rely on themselves for positive feedback instead of relying on others. Similarly, of critical importance, is teaching about the learning disability (Goldsworthy, 1996). Teach the student and his or her classmates what it means to have a learning disability and how it affects reading, spelling, writing, and communication. The more a student understands his or her disability, the more he or she can learn about strategies to overcome it.

Knowledge and personal understanding of the nature of the learning disability can help to prevent the depression and feelings of frustration that often become overriding factors. This is critical to understand because there are times when the depression and frustration can overwhelm the child and interfere with remediation of the problems. An effective, comprehensive program will focus on the strategies needed for effective reading, spelling, and writing but will not be limited to the mechanics of these skills. It is just as important to teach the children to concentrate, listen, and control their attention so that they can persist with a task until it is completed successfully.

In conclusion, there are a variety of techniques that can be used for intervention, but they all have a common set of goals. Specifically, the "critical steps of all of these curriculum-based language intervention strategies are to (1) identify zones of significance (contextually based needs); (2) analyze the communicative demands of the event or situation; (3) observe the individual's current attempts to meet those demands; (4) provide intervention to assist the individual to acquire new knowledge, skills, and strategies: (5) mediate the contextual demands to make them more accessible; and (6) keep in mind the desired outcome of independent functioning in the real world" (Nelson, 1998, p. 433).

CASE STUDY

History

D is a 9-year-old male who was diagnosed at the University of Florida Speech and Hearing Clinic as having developmental dyslexia. His diagnosis was based on a discrepancy between test scores of oral language and test scores of reading, spelling, and phonological awareness. He has been in dyslexia therapy for one semester. He was scheduled for 22 sessions between January and April and attended all sessions. Therapy was based on the Lindamood Phoneme Sequencing Programs (LiPS).

D is in the fourth grade at a Pine Hills Elementary School. He is an average student, getting mostly Bs and Cs on his report card. He is quite social and has several friends. He plays baseball in the local youth league, and also plays soccer.

Behavioral Observations During Therapy

D cooperated and worked diligently in all therapy sessions. He was very motivated to succeed. He responded well to verbal reinforcement. His mother observed each session and practiced his therapy goals at home between therapy sessions. She requested a set of LiPS cards to use at home to practice the LiPS labels, mouth movements, and corresponding sounds and symbols.

Long-Term Goals

1. D will complete all levels of the LiPS program. This includes (1) all voiced/unvoiced consonants, (2) all vowels, (3) tracking, spelling, and reading one-syllable words, and (4) tracking, reading, and spelling multisyllabic words.

2. D will improve his scores on the Lindamood Auditory Conceptualization test (LACT).

3. D will improve his scores on the Test of Phonological Awareness (TOPA).

Short-Term Goals

The LiPS program is a multisensory, multifaceted program of phonemic awareness training, based on a phonological foundation and rooted in the motor-articulatory feedback theory. This program facilitates perception of contrasts between speech sounds and the order of sounds in syllables in words, a critical skill needed for reading and spelling. A distinctive feature of the program is that the student is taught to self-correct, rather than be given the right answers.

1. Lip Poppers: D will say the sound, label, and write the symbols for the sounds /p/ and /b/ with 85% accuracy.

2. Tongue Tappers: D will say the sound, label, and write the symbols for the sounds /t/ and /d/ with 85% accuracy.

3. Tongue Scrapers: D will say the sound, label, and write the symbols for the sounds /k/ and /g/ with 85% accuracy.

4. Lip Coolers: D will say the sound, label, and write the symbols for the sounds /f/ and /v/ with 85% accuracy.

5. Skinny Air Sounds: D will say the sound, label, and write the symbols for the sounds /s/ and /z/ with 85% accuracy.

6. Tongue Coolers: D will say the sound, label, and write the symbols for the sounds /th/ (voicless) and /th/ (voiced) with 85% accuracy.

7. Fat Air Sounds: D will say the sound, label, and write the symbols for the sounds /sh/ and /zh/ with 85% accuracy.

8. Fat Pushed Air Sounds: D will say the sound, label, and write the symbols for the sounds /ch/ and /j/ with 85% accuracy.

9. Nose Sounds: D will say the sound, label, and write the symbols for the sounds /m/, /n/, and /ng/ with 85% accuracy.

10. Wind Sounds: D will say the sound, label, and write the symbols for the sounds /w/, /h/, and /wh/ with 85% accuracy.

11. Lifters: D will say the sound, label, and write the symbols for the sounds /l/ and /r/ with 85% accuracy.

12. Round Vowel Sounds: D will say the sound, label, and write the symbols for the sounds /oo/ (as in the words "book" and "look") and /oe/ with 85% accuracy.

13. Open Vowel Sounds: D will say the sound, label, and write the symbols for the sounds /o/ and /au-aw/ with 85% accuracy.

14. Smile Vowel Sounds: D will say the sound, label, and write the symbols for the sounds ee, I, e, ae, a, and u with 85% accuracy.

15. Slider Vowel Sounds: D will say the sound, label, and write the symbols for the sounds ie, ue, ou-ow, and oi-oy with 85% accuracy.

Results

Goals	Accuracy	Goal met (+)/not met(−)
Lip Poppers:		
Say	100%	+
Label	100%	+
Write	100%	+
Tongue Tappers:		
Say	100%	+
Label	100%	+
Write	100%	+

Tongue Scrapers

Say	100%	+
Label	100%	+
Write	100%	+

Lip Coolers:

Say	100%	+
Label	100%	+
Write	100%	+

Skinny Air Sounds:

Say	100%	+
Label	100%	+
Write	100%	+

Tongue Coolers:

Say	100%	+
Label	100%	+
Write	100%	+

Fat Air Sounds:

Say	92%	+
Label	100%	+
Write	100%	+

Fat Pushed Air Sounds:

Say	100%	+
Label	100%	+
Write	100%	+

Nose Sounds:

Say	100%	+
Label	100%	+
Write	100%	+

Wind Sounds:

Say	100%	+
Label	100%	+
Write	100%	+

Lifters:

Say	100%	+
Label	100%	+
Write	100%	+

Round Vowel Sounds:

Say	95%	+
Label	100%	+
Write	100%	+

Open Vowel Sounds:

Say	100%	+
Label	100%	+
Write	100%	+

Smile Vowel Sounds:

Say	100%	+
Label	100%	+
Write	100%	+

Slider Vowel Sounds

Say	92%	+
Label	100%	+
Write	100%	+

Procedures

In the LiPS program, D labeled, described, and categorized sounds and the symbols associated with the sounds. He also tracked one-syllable words with colored blocks. D played games during the second half of each therapy session to enforce the sounds, symbols, and labels that he was learning. The following is a list of the games D played in therapy:

1. D played "Memory" using the sounds he was currently learning in therapy. The symbols that he was learning in therapy were written on individual pieces of colored construction paper. Then, these pieces of paper were turned face down on the table. D took turns with the clinician turning over two pieces of paper at a time to try and find a match. Every time D turned a card over he was asked to produce the sound that the symbol represents and to label what group it was in.

2. D played "Go Fish" using the sounds he was currently learning in therapy. The symbols that D was learning in therapy were written on individual pieces of colored construction paper. These pieces of paper were then distributed to D and the clinician. The object was to get matches by asking the other player for certain sounds. For example, D might ask the clinician if she has an /l/. For every match made by either player, D was asked to produce the sound that corresponded to the symbol and to label what group it was in.

3. Pictures of different objects were presented to D who was then asked to name the object or picture, produce the initial sound in the word in isolation, and label the sound. He was given three different symbols to choose from.

4. D played a game in which he jumped to letter symbols on the floor after the clinician produced a sound. All the sounds were previously learned in therapy, so this was a review game.

5. D played "Guess Who" in which he answered a question about something he was working on in therapy in order to get a turn.

6. D played "Bingo" using the sounds he learned in therapy.

Summary of Results of Short-Term Goals

D met all of his short-term goals for this semester. He has now mastered all the consonant sounds and vowel sounds. D loved playing games, so incorporating games into his therapy sessions proved to be a valuable method to reinforce what he had learned. It was quite apparent that he practiced at home with his mother, and this was a major factor in his rapid progress.

Recommendations

It was recommended that D attend intensive individual summer therapy to complete the LiPS program for reading and spelling. It is also recommended that D's mother continue to practice at home with him to reinforce what is learned in therapy.

Therapy goals for next semester should include the following:

1. Review the vowels: round sounds, open sounds, smile sounds, and sliders.

2. Introduce the Crazy Rs.

3. Practice auditory recognition and discrimination for the initial sounds in words. One way to do this is to present D with an object or picture, then ask him to name it, produce the initial sound of the word in isolation, and label the sound. For example, when shown a picture of a cat, D will respond, "That's a cat, it starts with /k/ which is a tongue scraper."

4. Practice counting the number of syllables in words by clapping or pounding each syllable beat on the table as he says the word aloud.

▓ REVIEW QUESTIONS

1. Which of the following are form(s) of direct therapy?
   a. Consultation
   b. Pull-out model
   c. Collaborative model
   d. a and c
   e. b and c
   f. a and b

2. When does the emphasis in traditional reading instruction shift from basic skills to content acquisition?
   a. Grade 3
   b. Grade 4
   c. Grade 5
   d. Grade 6

3. Which of the following represent the domains which must be addressed on a child's education plan at school?
   a. Curriculum
   b. Independent functioning
   c. Social and personal
   d. Communication
   e. All of the above
   f. a, b, and d
   g. a, c, and d

4. An _____ must be written annually for school-age children receiving speech-language services in the schools.
   a. Individualized Family Service Plan (IFSP)
   b. Individualized Education Plan (IEP)
   c. Interventional Plan of Education (IPE)
   d. Progress Report, such as a SOAP note

5. Generalization is the gradual withdrawal of prompts and guidance to allow the stimulus to elicit the response.
   a. True
   b. False

6. Forward chaining is often used to teach academics.
   a. True
   b. False

7. The measured level of ability prior to intervention is
   a. Documentation of soft signs
   b. Baseline
   c. Task analysis
   d. Sensory integration

8. Exclusional criteria for determining placement in therapy is based on

   a. The gap between the child's expected level of achievement and his or her intellectual and social achievement levels compared to his or her language abilities

   b. The presence of a documented language and/or learning problem in the absence of cognitive, sensory, or physical handicaps

9. Which of the following theories on dialect intervention in the schools is most ethical?

   a. The no intervention view

   b. The bidialectal view

   c. The eradication view

10. Of the three models of language intervention described by Olswang and Bain, the _____ model is the most structured.

    a. Milieu teaching

    b. Joint action routines

    c. Inductive teaching

■ REFERENCES

American Speech-Language-Hearing Association (ASHA). (1985). Clinical management of communicatively handicapped minority language populations. *ASHA Desk Reference, 4,* IV-2–IV-6.

American Speech-Language-Hearing Association (ASHA). (1989, March). Issues in determining eligibility for language intervention. *ASHA, 31,* 113–118.

American Speech-Language-Hearing Association (ASHA). (1991). A model for collaborative service delivery for students with language-learning disorders in public schools. *ASHA,* 33(Suppl. 5), 44–50.

Bashir, A., Kuban, K., Kleinman, S., & Scavuzzo, S. (1983). Issues in language disorders: Considerations of cause, maintenance, and change. In J. Miller, D. Yoder, & R. Schiefelbush (Eds.), *ASHA Reports,* 92–106.

DiMeo, J., Merritt, D. D., & Culatta, B. (1998). Collaborative partnerships and decision-making. In D. D. Merritt & B. Culatta (Eds.), *Language intervention in the classroom* (pp. 37–96). San Diego: Singular Publishing Group.

Garcia, B. (1994). Personal communication.

Goldsworthy, C. L. (1996). *Developmental reading disabilities: A language-based treatment approach.* San Diego: Singular Publishing Group.

Hegde, M. N. (1996). *A coursebook on language disorders in children.* San Diego: Singular Publishing Group.

Knapp, M. S., Turnbull, B. J., & Shields, P. M. (1990). New directions for educating the children of poverty. *Educational Leadership, 48*(1), 4–8.

Larson, V. L., & McKinley, N. (1995). *Language disorders in older students: Preadolescents and adolescents.* Eau Claire, WI: Thinking Publications.

Lewis, P. (1987, December). A case for teaching functional skills. *TASH Newsletter* (The Association for Persons with Severe Handicaps).

McKinley, N. L., & Larson, V. (1985). Neglected language-disorder adolescents: A delivery model. *Language, Speech and Hearing Services in Schools, 16,* 2–15.

Merritt, D. D., & Culatta, B. (1998). *Language intervention in the classroom.* San Diego: Singular Publishing Group.

Naremore, R. C., Densmore, A. E., & Harman, D. R. (1995). *Language intervention with school-age children: Conversation, narrative, and text.* San Diego: Singular Publishing Group.

Nelson, N. W. (1993). *Childhood language disorders in context: Infancy through adolescence.* New York: Macmillan Publishing Company.

Nelson, N. W. (1998). *Childhood language disorders in context: Infancy through adolescence* (2nd ed.). New York: Macmillan Publishing Group.

Olswang, L., & Bain, B. (1991). Intervention issues for toddlers with specific language impairments. *Topics in Language Disorders, 11*, 69–86.

Owens, Robert E. (1995). *Language disorders: A functional approach to assessment and intervention.* Boston: Allyn and Bacon.

Owens, Robert E. (1999). *Language disorders: A functional approach to assessment and intervention* (3rd ed.). Boston: Allyn and Bacon.

Reed, V. A. (2005). *An introduction to children with language disorders* (3rd ed.). Boston: Allyn and Bacon.

Roth, F. P., & Worthington, C. K. (2001). *Treatment resource manual for speech-language pathology* (2nd ed.). Albany, NY: Delmar.

Sanger, D. D., Hux, K., & Griess, K. (1995). Educators' opinions about speech-language pathology services in the schools. *Language-Speech-Hearing Services in the Schools, 26*(1), 75–86.

Snyder, L. (1984). Developmental language disorders: Elementary school age. In A. Holland (Ed.), *Language disorders in children: Recent advances* (pp. 129–158). San Diego: College-Hill Press.

Taylor, J. S. (1992). *Speech-language pathology services in the schools* (2nd ed.). Boston: Allyn and Bacon.

Van Hattum, R. (1985). *Organization of speech-language services in schools: A manual.* San Diego: College-Hill Press.

van Kleeck, A. (1994). Metalinguistic development, In G. P. Wallach & K. G. Butler (Eds.), *Language learning disabilities in school-age children and adolescents: Some principles and applications* (2nd ed., pp. 53–98). Boston: Allyn and Bacon.

Wallach, G. P., & Liebergott, J. W. (1984). Who shall be called "learning disabled?" Some new directions. In G. P. Wallach & K. C. Butler (Eds.), *Language learning disabilities in school-age children.* Baltimore: Williams & Wilkins.

Warren, S. F., & Yoder, P. J. (1994). Communication and language intervention: Why a constructivist approach is insufficient. *Journal of Special Education, 28*, 248–258.

Wong, B. Y., Wong, R., Darlington, D., & Jones, W. (1991). Interactive teaching: An effective way to teach revision skills to adolescents with learning disabilities. *Learning Disabilities Research & Practice, 6*, 117–127.

LANGUAGE DISORDERS IN ADULTS

Many language disorders seen in school-age children may persist into adulthood. This certainly includes reading and spelling disorders, traumatic brain injury, and ADD or ADHD. Some people live with these disorders without having them identified at an earlier age. When they arrive in college, these students may seek assistance in identifying possible learning disabilities for the first time. Thus, understanding the effects of these disorders on higher learning, and vocations, cannot be underestimated. Even when disorders are identified, many adolescents do not follow through with treatment suggestions. However, when they reach adulthood and find that the possibilities of employment may be affected by the disorders, they have a motivation to follow through with remediation efforts.

In addition to the disorders that persist into adulthood, the two most common language disorders in the adult population are aphasia and dementia. Chapter 12 focuses on language disorders associated with dementia, and in Chapter 13, various aphasia syndromes are discussed.

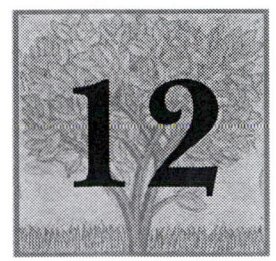

Alzheimer's Disease and Other Types of Dementia

■ LEARNING OBJECTIVES

After completion of this chapter, the reader will be able to

1. Define dementia and list its defining characteristics.

2. Differentiate between and give examples of cortical and subcortical dementias.

3. Describe language of patients at the three primary stages of Alzheimer's disease.

4. Describe neuropathological changes in the brain of patients with dementia, particularly Alzheimer's.

5. Describe dementia associated with the following: Pick's disease, Huntington's disease, multi-infarction disease, and Parkinson's disease.

6. Describe the role of the speech-language pathologist in the assessment and management of dementia.

■ INTRODUCTION

Approximately 10% of individuals aged 65 to 80 years have Alzheimer's, and 47% of the population over 85 years of age have the diagnosis of Alzheimer's disease. According to the National Alzheimer's Association, as of 2001 there were 4 million cases of Alzheimer's disease. The elderly population is the fastest growing age group in America, and it is estimated that by 2050 there will be 14 million individuals with Alzheimer's disease (Hopper & Bayles, 2001; Alzheimer's Association, 2004). Katzman (1998) writes that Alzheimer's disease accounts for 70% of the cases of dementia. According to the DSM-IV (American Psychiatric Association, 1994), Alzheimer's disease is present in the absence of other central nervous system disorders, psychiatric disorders such as schizophrenia or depression, systemic conditions, or substance-induced disorders. Gradual decline of cognitive functions and impairments of short- and long-term memory with progressive deterioration are characteristic of Alzheimer's dementia.

Research in geriatric medicine, neurology, speech-language pathology, and psychiatry is analyzing the differences among the various types of dementia and symptoms of normal aging. Using batteries of psychological assessments, structured interviews, functional assessments, and case history information, researchers are determining the early signs of dementia and becoming better able to predict who will or will not have Alzheimer's disease or other types of dementia.

■ WHAT IS DEMENTIA?

Dementia is defined as a "heterogeneous constellation of signs and symptoms of central nervous system degeneration that is often difficult to discern from other neurogenic language impairments such as aphasia" (Bayles et al., 1989, p. 100). According to Bayles and Kaszniak (1987), the diagnosis of dementia is complicated because the patients have "varied dementia symptomalogy because of patient age, disease onset, site of pathology, rate of disease, or because of family history" (Bayles & Kaszniak, 1987, p. 100). It is a syndrome marked by significant deterioration of memory and a minimum of one cognitive function to the degree that activities of daily living cannot be carried out independently (Hopper & Bayles, 2001). Regardless of its cause, dementia causes progressive deterioration in communicative functioning, personality traits, and intellectual functioning (Payne, 1997).

The assessment of language and communication in dementia should include comprehensive language evaluation, assessment of semantics, assessment of pragmatics, and evaluation of morphology, syntax, and memory (Ripich, 1991).

With regard to its impact on language features, dementia has its most damaging effects on semantics. Specifically, four areas of deterioration appear to occur in semantics: (1) breakdowns in **generative** and **confrontational naming**, (2) a progressively diminishing lexicon, (3) a decrease in the ability to either demonstrate an object's use or name an item that the clinician pantomimes, and (4) disintegration of word association skills. Phonology, morphology, and syntax are rarely affected, perhaps because these are more automatic language structures than semantics (Lass et al., 1988).

■ TYPES OF DEMENTIA

Dementias can be categorized as reversible or irreversible. Table 12–1 lists etiological factors in reversible dementias, and Table 12–2 lists factors associated with irreversible dementias.

According to Bayles (1986),

> A simple way to predict whether a particular communicative function will be impaired early in the demential syndrome is to consider the degree to which the function is routine and dependent on environmental sensitivity and memory. Communicative functions such as object naming, reciting the alphabet, and sentence completion are not likely to be affected, whereas functions involving semantic analysis, the ability to relate meaning to situation, and generation of names of items within a category are affected. (Bayles, 1986, p. 537)

Dementia. A conglomeration of signs and symptoms of central nervous system degeneration that result in progressive and persistent deterioration of intellectual functioning.

generative naming. The client names as many items as he/she can think of in a specified category and in a specified time period.

Confrontational naming. The naming of items as the child is confronted with the item by the clinician.

TABLE 12–1. Etiological factors in reversible dementias.

Depression

Drug toxicity

Infection

Normal pressure hydrocephalus

Nutritional deficiencies

Cardiopulmonary disorders

Resectable brain lesions

Source: Adapted from *Sourcebook of Medical Speech Pathology* (2nd ed.), by L. C. Golper, 1998, p. 153. San Diego: Singular Publishing Group. Copyright 1998 Singular Publishing Group.

TABLE 12–2. Etiological factors in irreversible dementias.

AIDS

Alzheimer's disease

Pick's disease

Alcoholic dementia syndromes

Cerebrocerebellar degenerations

Creutzfeldt-Jakob disease

Huntington's chorea

Multi-infarction diseases

Source: Adapted from *Sourcebook of Medical Speech Pathology* (2nd ed.), by L. C. Golper, 1998, p. 153. San Diego: Singular Publishing Group. Copyright 1998 Singular Publishing Group.

Bayles further summarizes the effects of dementing illness on communication in Table 12–3.

The Reversible Dementias

Reversible dementias may be caused by the ingestion of toxins, by drug interactions, and by some metabolic disorders (Johnson, 1997). Reversible dementias may not be reported initially because of the "common belief that old age is associated with illness, loss of independence, and feeling sick" (Payne, 1997, p. 135). A complicating issue is the fact that depression and subsequent loss of vitality and vigor may mask the symptoms of a reversible dementia. In addition, many persons are afraid to find out that something is wrong and would prefer not to have that knowledge. Thus, they do not report the symptoms to their physicians (Payne, 1997).

TABLE 12–3. Effects of dementing illnesses on communication.

Early Stages

Sounds:	Used correctly
Words:	May omit a meaningful word, usually a noun, when talking in sentences. May report trouble thinking of the right word. Vocabulary is shrinking.
Grammar:	Generally correct
Content:	May drift from the topic. Reduced ability to generate series of meaningful sentences. Difficulty comprehending new information. Vague
Use:	Knows when to talk, although may talk too long on a subject. May be apathetic, failing to initiate a conversation when it would be appropriate to do so. May have difficulty understanding humor, verbal analogies, sarcasm, and indirect and nonliteral statements.

Middle Stages

Sounds:	Used correctly
Words:	Difficulty thinking of words in a category. Anomia in conversation. Difficulty naming objects. Reliance on automatisms. Vocabulary noticeably diminished.
Grammar:	Sentence fragments and deviations common. May have difficulty understanding grammatically complex sentences.
Content:	Frequently repeats ideas. Forgets topic. Talk is about events of past or trivia. Fewer ideas.
Use:	Knows when to talk. Recognizes questions. May fail to greet. Loss of sensitivity to conversational partners. Rarely corrects mistakes.

Late Stages

Sounds:	Generally used correctly, but errors are not uncommon.
Words:	Marked anomia. Poor vocabulary. Lack of word comprehension. May make up words and produce jargon.
Grammar:	Some grammar is preserved but sentence fragments and deviations are common. Lack of comprehension of many grammatical forms.
Content:	Generally unable to produce a sequence of related ideas. Content may be meaningless and bizarre. Subject of most meaningful utterances is the retelling of a past event. Marked repetition of words and phrases.
Use:	Generally unaware of surroundings and context; insensitive to others. Little meaningful use of language. Some patients are mute. Some are echolalic.

Source: From "Management of Neurogenic Communication Disorders Associated with Dementia," by K. A. Bayles, in *Language Intervention Strategies in Adult Aphasia* (3rd ed., p. 542), by R. Chapey (Ed.), 1986, Baltimore: Williams & Wilkins. Copyright 1986 by Williams & Wilkins. Reprinted with permission.

The Irreversible Dementias

Multi-infarction diseases. Diseases that result in many focal necrotic lesions, causing widespread damage in cortical functioning.

Of the irreversible dementias, Alzheimer's disease is the most common. **Multi-infarction diseases** are the second most common cause of dementia. Other etiologies associated with irreversible dementias include Parkinson disease and vascular dementia that is frequently associated with hypertension and strokes. Berg and colleagues (1982) delineated the key features needed for a diagnosis of dementia:

1. A sustained deterioration of *memory*, plus a disturbance in at least three of the following areas: (a) orientation in time and place; (b) judgment and problem solving (dealing with everyday situations); (c) community affairs (shopping, handling finances); (d) home and avocations; and (e) personal care

2. A gradual onset and progression

3. A duration of at least six months or longer (Haynes & Pindzola, 1998, pp. 270–271).

Dementia should not be confused with aphasia. Although these disorders can occur simultaneously, they are separate entities. In the early stages, some dementias resemble fluent aphasias. However, as the dementia progresses, there is a simultaneous decline in language and cognitive functions. In aphasia, once the patient is stable, there is no further decline in the language functions, and the cognitive functions are usually intact in persons with aphasia. Table 12–4 delineates the communicative and cognitive differences between dementia and aphasia.

TABLE 12–4. Cognitive and communicative differences between aphasia and dementia.

Variable	Aphasia	Dementia
Progression	There is rapid onset; improvement is typical.	There is slow onset and progressive deterioration.
Cognition	Cognition is generally intact.	Cognition is mildly to profoundly impaired; it worsens with the condition; problem solving is poor.
Memory	Memory is generally intact.	Memory ranges from mildly forgetful to profoundly impaired or amnesic; it worsens with the condition.
Emotionality	Mood is typically appropriate with occasional periods of depression or frustration.	Person is typically labile; is apathetic and withdrawn; intermittently shows agitation; and can exhibit depression or mania.

Variable	Aphasia	Dementia
Pragmatics	Socially appropriate skills are evident despite some comprehension failures; communication efforts typically show relevance.	Social skills are mildly to severely affected; inappropriate behaviors and irrelevant comments are typical; thought processes are disorganized.
Repetition	This ability is slightly to severely impaired.	This ability is generally intact unless the condition is severe.
Semantics	Word retrieval difficulties can be mild to severe; semantic and literal paraphasias may be used.	Impairment ranges from mild word-retrieval difficulties to severe vocabulary reductions.
Syntax	Syntax is affected to varying degrees; it can be classified as fluent or nonfluent based on length of utterance.	Syntax is intact when disorder is mild; there is reduction of syntactic complexity as the disorder progresses.
Phonology	Phonology is impaired in nonfluent aphasia; it may be present as literal paraphasia in fluent aphasia.	Phonology is intact unless the condition is severe; dysarthria is possible.

Source: From Haynes, W. O., and Pindzola, R. H., *Diagnosis and Evaluation in Speech Pathology*, 5th ed. Published by Allyn and Bacon, Boston. Copyright © 1998 by Pearson Education. Reprinted by permission of the publisher.

Cortical and Subcortical Dementias

Another diagnostic dichotomy is the classification of dementia as cortical or subcortical, based on the site of the lesion or the site of neurological degeneration. Lesions associated with cortical dementias typically are located in the hippocampus and the neocortical association areas (Johnson, 1997). Alzheimer's and Pick's diseases are examples of cortical dementias. Subcortical dementias are associated with lesions in the basal ganglia, rostral brain stem, and thalamus. Patients with cortical dementias rarely demonstrate impaired motor function (until the late stages). On the other hand, those with subcortical dementias associated with Parkinson's disease and Huntington's disease show early motor involvement, including **dysarthria** and **bradykinesia** (Johnson, 1997). Impairment of cognitive function in cortical and subcortical dementias is contrasted in Table 12–5. A patient can also have a mixed dementia that involves cortical and subcortical lesions as in multi-infarct dementia.

Patients' awareness of their deficits is another diagnostic differentiator between cortical and subcortical dementias. Persons with cortical dementias tend to be indifferent about their deficits. However, those with subcortical dementias are more apt to be concerned about their difficulties and may demonstrate depression as a result of their awareness (Johnson, 1997).

Dysarthria. Speech disorder resulting from generalized weakness of the oral musculature due to pathology in the central and/or peripheral nervous system.

Bradykinesia. Slow motor movements.

TABLE 12–5. Comparison of impaired cognitive functions in cortical and subcortical dementias.

Cortical Dementia	Subcortical Dementia
Aphasia	Psychomotor retardation
Poor abstraction abilities	Forgetfulness
Agnosia	Cognitive dilapidation
Amnesia	Impaired insight
Acalculia	Poor strategy formulation
Visuospatial disturbances	

Source: Adapted from "Mental Status and Aging: Cognition and Effect," by D. J. Johnson, in *Aging and Communication*, by B. B. Shadden and M. A. Toner (Eds.), 1997. Austin, TX: Pro-Ed. Copyright 1997 by Pro-Ed.

ACQUIRED IMMUNODEFICIENCY SYNDROME (AIDS)

Over 50% of patients with human immunodeficiency virus (HIV) develop central or peripheral neurological complications. AIDS-related dementia typically develops in the later stages of the disease process (Payne, 1997). Marked language impairment is not noted until the terminal stage of AIDS. However, patients often demonstrate reduced concentration, increased forgetfulness, and possible apathy. As the body loses strength, speech becomes more effortful (Navia, Jordan, & Price, 1986).

ALZHEIMER'S DISEASE

Alzheimer's disease is the most prevalent cause of dementia and is the result of biochemical and structural changes in the brain. The fourth leading cause of death in the United States, Alzheimer's disease is estimated to afflict 4,000,000 people in this country (Johnson, 1997). It is characterized by short-term and long-term memory impairment, breakdowns in higher cortical functions, impaired abstract thinking and judgment, and personality changes. These changes interfere with normal activities and relationships (Payne, 1997). Risk factors for the disease are listed in Table 12–6.

According to the American Psychiatric Association (1994), dementia of the Alzheimer's type is characterized by an insidious onset with a generally progressive deteriorating course that affects cognition, memory, and language.

TABLE 12–6. Risk factors for Alzheimer's disease.

Family history of dementia

Family history of Down syndrome

Family history of Parkinson's disease

Late onset of depression

Head injury

Hypothyroidism

Maternal age greater than 40 years at birth

Source: Adapted from "Mental Status and Aging: Cognition and Effect," by D. J. Johnson, in *Aging and Communication,* 1997, p. 80, by B. B. Shadden and M. A. Toner (Eds.), Austin, TX: Pro-Ed. Copyright 1997 by Pro-Ed.

In addition, the syndrome excludes all other specific causes of dementia by history, physical examination, and laboratory studies (American Psychiatric Association, 1994). The diagnostic criteria for dementia of the Alzheimer's type are listed in Table 12–7.

Stages of Alzheimer's Disease

Alzheimer's disease typically is characterized by seven overlapping stages which are delineated in Table 12–8. The early onset is characterized "by memory problems that are more severe than those seen in normal aging adults" (Payne, 1997, p. 109). For example, a normally aging adult may forget where he or she has placed the keys, but a person with Alzheimer's disease will forget what the keys are for (Overman & Geoffrey, 1987a). The person with Alzheimer's disease also will become disoriented in unfamiliar locations and have difficulty remembering recent events or names. This stage typically lasts from one to three years (Overman & Geoffrey, 1987a). The patients may use pauses, circumlocution, nonspecific pronouns, and word substitutions to compensate for naming problems. They also may self-correct their naming errors (Payne, 1997).

During the early stages of Alzheimer's disease, the patient's long-term and short-term memories are already affected. Early memory systems that are deficient are working memory and episodic memory (Hopper & Bayles, 2001). The patient may be disoriented with regard to time, but not to person or place. During casual conversations, the patient appears to do fairly well but may digress or ramble during interactions with others. They may have word retrieval deficits, and difficulty interpreting sarcasm and humor (Murray & Chapey, 2001). While they may have enjoyed the company of

TABLE 12–7. Diagnostic criteria for dementia of the Alzheimer's type.

A. The development of multiple cognitive deficits manifested by both

  (1) memory impairment (impaired ability to learn new information or to recall previously learned information)

  (2) one (or more) of the following cognitive disturbances:

    (a) aphasia (language disturbance)

    (b) apraxia (impaired ability to carry out motor activities despite intact motor function)

    (c) agnosia (failure to recognize or identify objects despite intact sensory function)

    (d) disturbance in executive functioning (i.e., planning, organizing, sequencing, abstracting)

B. The cognitive deficits in Criteria A1 and A2 each cause significant impairment in social or occupational functioning and represent a significant decline from a previous level of functioning.

C. The course is characterized by gradual onset and continuing cognitive decline.

D. The cognitive deficits in Criteria A1 and A2 are not due to any of the following:

  (1) other central nervous system conditions that cause progressive deficits in memory and cognition (e.g., cerebrovascular disease, Parkinson's disease, Huntington's disease, subdural hematoma, normal-pressure hydrocephalus, brain tumor)

  (2) systemic conditions that are known to cause dementia (e.g., hypothyroidism, vitamin B12 or folic acid deficiency, niacin deficiency, hypercalcemia, neurosyphilis, HIV infection)

  (3) substance-induced conditions

E. The deficits do not occur exclusively during the course of a delirium.

F. The disturbance is not better accounted for by another Axis I disorder (e.g., Major Depressive Disorder, Schizophrenia).

Source: Reprinted with permission from the *Diagnostic and Statistic Manual of Mental Disorders.* Copyright 2000. American Psychiatric Association.

others throughout their life, many people with Alzheimer's may withdraw from others and eventually have a lonely lifestyle, as seen in Figure 12–1.

Several studies have looked at discourse parameters in individuals with early Alzheimer's disease when compared to normal elderly individuals. Mentis, Briggs-Whittaker, and Gramigna (1995) compared 12 patients with senile dementia of the Alzheimer's type (SDAT) with 12 control subjects (NE) who were matched by level of education, age, and sex. A speech-language pathologist conducted a 20-minute casual conversation with each subject and then analyzed the videotape of the conversation to evaluate topic management. Their results indicated that there are significant differences in the abilities of individuals with SDAT with regard to topic introduction and topic

TABLE 12–8. Behavioral characteristics of the seven primary stages in progression of Alzheimer's disease.

fact sheet

alzheimer's ᗯ association

About the stages of Alzheimer's disease

Experts have documented common patterns of symptom progression that occur in many individuals with Alzheimer's disease and developed several methods of "staging" based on these patterns. Progression of symptoms corresponds in a general way to the underlying nerve cell degeneration that takes place in Alzheimer's disease. Nerve cell damage typically begins with cells involved in learning and memory and gradually spreads to cells that control other aspects of thinking, judgment and behavior. The damage eventually affects cells that control and coordinate movement.

Staging systems provide useful frames of reference for understanding how the disease may unfold and for making future plans. But it is important to note that all stages are artificial benchmarks in a continuous process that can vary greatly from one person to another. Not everyone will experience every symptom and symptoms may occur at different times in different individuals. People with Alzheimer's live an average of 8 years after diagnosis, but may survive anywhere from 3 to 20 years.

The framework for this fact sheet is a system that outlines key symptoms characterizing seven stages ranging from unimpaired function to very severe cognitive decline. This framework is based on a system developed by Barry Reisberg, M.D., Clinical Director of the New York University School of Medicine's Silberstein Aging and Dementia Research Center.

Within this framework, we have noted which stages correspond to the widely used concepts of mild, moderate, moderately severe and severe Alzheimer's disease. We have also noted which stages fall within the more general divisions of early-stage, mid-stage, and late-stage categories.

Stage 1: No cognitive impairment
Unimpaired individuals experience no memory problems and none are evident to a health care professional during a medical interview.

Stage 2: Very mild decline
Individuals at this stage feel as if they have memory lapses, especially in forgetting familiar words or names or the location of keys, eyeglasses, or other everyday objects. But these problems are not evident during a medical examination or apparent to friends, family, or co-workers.

Stage 3: Mild cognitive decline
Early-stage Alzheimer's can be diagnosed in some, but not all, individuals with these symptoms

Friends, family or co-workers begin to notice deficiencies. Problems with memory or concentration may be measurable in clinical testing or discernible during a detailed medical interview. Common difficulties include:
- Word- or name-finding problems noticeable to family or close associates
- Decreased ability to remember names when introduced to new people
- Performance issues in social or work settings noticeable to family, friends or co-workers
- Reading a passage and retaining little material
- Losing or misplacing a valuable object
- Decline in ability to plan or organize

Stage 4: Moderate cognitive decline (Mild or early-stage Alzheimer's disease)
At this stage, a careful medical interview detects clear-cut deficiencies in the following areas:
- Decreased knowledge of recent events
- Impaired ability to perform challenging mental arithmetic—for example, to count backward from 100 by 7s
- Decreased capacity to perform complex tasks, such as marketing, planning dinner for guests, or paying bills and managing finances
- Reduced memory of personal history
- The affected individual may seem subdued and withdrawn, especially in socially or mentally challenging situations

TABLE 12–8. (*continued*)

Stage 5: Moderately severe cognitive decline (Moderate or mid-stage Alzheimer's disease)

Major gaps in memory and deficits in cognitive function emerge. Some assistance with day-to-day activities becomes essential. At this stage, individuals may:

- Be unable during a medical interview to recall such important details as their current address, their telephone number, or the name of the college or high school from which they graduated
- Become confused about where they are or about the date, day of the week or season
- Have trouble with less challenging mental arithmetic; for example, counting backward from 40 by 4s or from 20 by 2s
- Need help choosing proper clothing for the season or the occasion
- Usually retain substantial knowledge about themselves and know their own name and the names of their spouse or children
- Usually require no assistance with eating or using the toilet

Stage 6: Severe cognitive decline (Moderately severe or mid-stage Alzheimer's disease)

Memory difficulties continue to worsen, significant personality changes may emerge, and affected individuals need extensive help with daily activities. At this stage, individuals may:

- Lose most awareness of recent experiences and events as well as of their surroundings
- Recollect their personal history imperfectly, although they generally recall their own name
- Occasionally forget the name of their spouse or primary caregiver but generally can distinguish familiar from unfamiliar faces
- Need help getting dressed properly; without supervision, may make such errors as putting pajamas over daytime clothes or shoes on wrong feet
- Experience disruption of their normal sleep/waking cycle
- Need help with handling details of toileting (flushing toilet, wiping and disposing of tissue properly)
- Have increasing episodes of urinary or fecal incontinence

- Experience significant personality changes and behavioral symptoms, including suspiciousness and delusions (for example, believing that their caregiver is an impostor); hallucinations (seeing or hearing things that are not really there); or compulsive, repetitive behaviors such as hand-wringing or tissue shredding
- Tend to wander and become lost

Stage 7: Very severe cognitive decline (Severe or late-stage Alzheimer's disease)

This is the final stage of the disease when individuals lose the ability to respond to their environment, the ability to speak, and, ultimately, the ability to control movement.

- Frequently individuals lose their capacity for recognizable speech, although words or phrases may occasionally be uttered
- Individuals need help with eating and toileting and there is general incontinence of urine
- Individuals lose the ability to walk without assistance, then the ability to sit without support, the ability to smile, and the ability to hold their head up. Reflexes become abnormal and muscles grow rigid. Swallowing is impaired.

There is currently no cure or prevention for Alzheimer's disease, but the Alzheimer's Association is fighting on your behalf to give everyone a reason to hope. For more information about Alzheimer research, treatment and care, please contact the Alzheimer's Association.

Contact Center **1.800.272.3900**
TDD Access **1.312.335.8882**
Web site **www.alz.org**
e-mail **info@alz.org**
Fact sheet prepared **October 13, 2003**

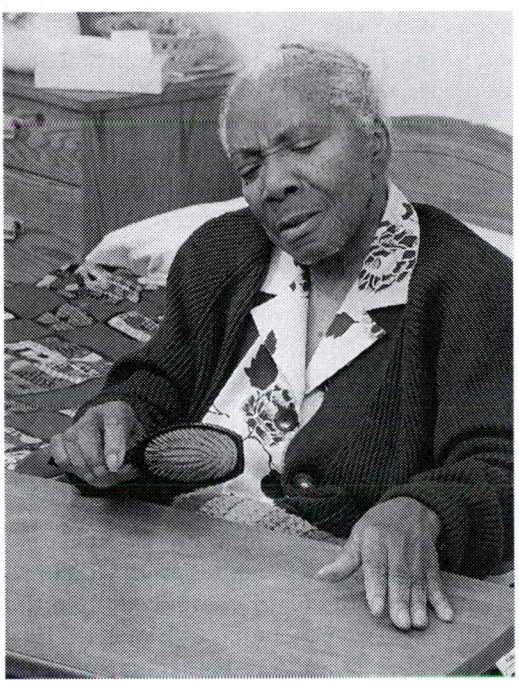

FIGURE 12–1. Dementia can lead to withdrawal from social settings and other persons.

maintenance. Specifically, they found that "the topic management profiles of the SDAT subjects were characterized by a reduced ability to change topics while preserving the discourse flow, difficulty in actively contributing to the prepositional development of the topic, and a failure to consistently maintain topic in a clear and coherent manner" (p. 1054). The problems exhibited by the SDAT subjects were evident across multiple aspects of language such as cognitive, linguistic, and discourse-pragmatic domains. At the cognitive level, patients with SDAT experience difficulties with problem solving, reasoning, memory, attention, and world knowledge (Mentis et al., 1995) Discourse-pragmatic problems may be due in part to deficits in the rules and principles that govern topic management. Pragmatic deficits in individuals with SDAT have been documented (Blanken et al., 1987; Heller, Dobbs, & Rule, 1992), and the findings of Mentis and colleagues support that finding. There also may be linguistic breakdowns centered around knowledge of semantic relations and syntactic and morphological rules and structures.

There is conflicting evidence as to whether or not syntax and morphology are spared or impaired in SDAT. Blanken and colleagues (1987) and Glosser and Deser (1990) reported that in patients with mild to moderate SDAT, syntax and morphology are relatively spared. However, Emery (1988) and Kirshner and Freemon (1982) found that syntax in patients with SDAT is not spared and syntactic deficits negatively impact the ability of these patients to use complex linguistic forms. Lexical semantics are problematic for individuals with SDAT and also have a negative impact on topic management (Bayles & Tomoeda, 1983; Martin & Fedio, 1983; Mortensen, 1992; Mentis et al., 1995). In summary, Mentis and colleagues (1995) found that topic management skills are problematic for patients with SDAT. Specifically, "the profiles of the SDAT subjects were characterized by a reduced ability to change topics while preserving the discourse flow, difficulty in actively contributing to the prepositional development of the topic, and a failure to consistently maintain topics in a clear and coherent manner" (p. 1061). However, there was substantial variability within the SDAT subject group; possibly this was due to varying levels of impairment amongst the subjects with SDAT.

The middle moderate stages of Alzheimer's disease typically last from 2 to 10 years. During this time, affected persons have difficulty with accurate and efficient completion of complex tasks. They may experience social withdrawal and exhibit a flat affect. They show increased errors on naming, with no efforts to self-correct. Semantic paraphasias, as seen in patients with aphasia, also are common during the middle stages, along with misuse of syntactic forms (Payne, 1997). Bollinger, Berg, and LeWitt (1994) reported on a study by Hungerford in which he found that meaning disintegrates more than language structure in patients with Alzheimer's disease. This may be due to the fact that syntax and phonology are more automatic and less vulnerable to the cortical damage associated with Alzheimer's disease. Bayles (1984) also pointed out that individuals experience a loss of judgment, initiative, and tact. Thus, the patient may become less able to stay alone owing to safety concerns that arise as a result of the loss of judgment.

Patients in the middle stages frequently have difficulty orienting to time and place. They have increasing difficulty abiding by pragmatic rules that govern conversation, exhibiting problems with turn-taking, topic shifts, and topic maintenance. During the middle stages, the patient will begin to have problems with reading and auditory comprehension. They continue to lose semantic abilities with their language becoming "vague, empty, perseverative, and often irrelevant" (Murray & Chapey, 2001, pp. 70–71).

Orange, Lubinski, and Higginbotham (1996) cite Bayles and Kaszniak's (1987) description of conversations by individuals in the middle stages of Alzheimer's in their article on conversational repair by patients with Alzheimer's. Orange and colleagues wrote that

> individuals in the middle clinical stage of dementia of the Alzheimer's type ask few questions of their partner, infrequently comment on their own utterances, digress, produce overly long vague answers to questions, offer few clarification requests, infrequently repair their own utterances, and experience difficulty producing and responding to requests for clarification. (p. 881)

In addition, since individuals with Alzheimer's frequently use nonspecific references, unexpectedly shift topics and digress, conversational partners report having difficulty following a conversation with an individual who has Alzheimer's. Repair strategies normally used by the nonimpaired population typically are employed to clarify, correct, and resolve any miscommunications in the conversational process. However, individuals with middle- to late-stage Alzheimer's generally do not employ repair strategies. Orange and colleagues studied conversational repair tactics in a control group of nonimpaired adults, a group of adults in the early stages of Alzheimer's disease (EDAT), and a group in the middle stages of Alzheimer's (MDAT). They found that "less than a fifth of the control groups' utterances were problematic, nearly one quarter of the EDATs' utterances and one third of the MDATs' utterances involved repair" (Orange et al., 1996, p. 891). This indicates that as the dementia increases over time, the ability of the patient to repair discourse becomes more impaired. However, in contrast to previous beliefs, Orange and colleagues also found that "the EDAT and MDAT dyads generated problem-free conversation over 75% and 64% of the time, respectively, demonstrating a notable measure of linguistic, pragmatic, and discourse competency through these two clinical stages of DAT" (p. 891).

Kempler, Almor, and MacDonald (1998) studied the role of semantic impairments and memory in the comprehension of sentences. Their subjects were 11 patients with mild to moderate dementia, and 9 age-matched controls who were healthy. The researchers presented 20 sentence pairs, with the difference between the two being how well the final word was semantically and grammatically appropriate. For example, an introductory sentence ("Kevin learned something new today.") was followed by "Many people wash their————" (coherent condition) and "Many insects wash their————" (anomalous condition). The reading target was "KNIVES." The sentences were presented via an on line task(visual), and through a high-quality loudspeaker with the volume adapted for each subject. The subjects in the Alzheimer's group and in the control group had similar performances on the task with regard to appropriateness of the target word, and the continuation word in the context of the sentence. This suggests that it is memory, not semantic impairments, that contribute to poor sentence comprehension by patients with Alzheimer's disease.

In the later stages of Alzheimer's disease, naming becomes severely impaired. Expressive language often is limited to jargon and repetition, and the individual has difficulty attending to structured tasks (Payne, 1997). Patients often use circumlocution to mask the word-finding problem and may use an increased number of indefinite pronouns in place of the substantive words. Paraphasias and **neologisms** may be used (Murdoch, 1990), similar to patients with fluent aphasias. Difficulties with reading and writing also emerge in the later stages of the disease (Overman & Geoffrey, 1987b). In

Neologisms. Unintended substitution of an invented or nonsense word that contains no similarities to the target (intended) word.

addition to deficits in episodic and working memory, patients with late stage Alzheimer's disease have problems with semantic memory and procedural memory (Hopper & Bayles, 2001). They are disoriented with regard to person, place, and time, and are dependent for most self-help and daily activities (Murray & Chapey, 2001).

As the disease moves into the final stages, patients become totally dependent, even needing assistance with routine daily living skills. Cognitively, the patients become unable to recall names, events, and places. Typically, they do not initiate conversations, and language skills are severely impaired (Gelfer, 1996). The individual becomes progressively weaker, bedridden, and incontinent, and primitive reflexes will reemerge (Lauter, 1985). In many ways, the person seems to revert to infancy. Patients often die from heart failure or pneumonia. A summary of the progression of Alzheimer's disease is given in Table 12–8.

Hearing Loss in Patients with Alzheimer's Disease

Many studies have been done which have found a relationship between cognitive decline and hearing loss, with a correlation between the severity of the cognitive decline and the degree of hearing sensitivity (Hodkinson, 1973; Kay, Beamish, & Roth, 1964; Peters, Potter, & Scholer, 1988; Uhlmann et al., 1989). Either disorder alone can have a significant impact on an individual's social and vocational life; together the effects are compounded. Palmer and colleagues (1999) report on studies showing that individuals with a hearing loss have feelings of depression, helplessness, passivity, and negativism (Herbst & Humphrey, 1980; Weinstein & Ventry, 1982).

Hearing-impaired individuals may have difficulty adjusting to life events and may have changes in their social life (Birren, 1964; Palmer et al., 1999). This difficulty is more notable in those individuals who also suffer from Alzheimer's disease. Patients with Alzheimer's disease frequently have signs of forgetfulness as evidenced by asking a conversational partner to repeat what he or she has said, or by searching for an answer. These same signs also may be attributed to a possible hearing loss. In a study by Palmer and colleagues (1999), the authors studied the management of hearing loss in patients with Alzheimer's disease, collecting data on treatment compliance (as measured by the number of hours the patient used his or her hearing aid) and reduction in problem behaviors that were reported by the patients' caregivers.

In a previous study cited by Palmer and colleagues (1999), Bourgeois, Burgio, and Schulz (1992) asked caregivers to count problem behaviors in their spouses who had Alzheimer's disease. They found that half of the 10 most frequently reported problem behaviors could potentially be due to hearing loss as opposed to dementia. Yet, patients with Alzheimer's remain underreferred for audiological testing and management for a variety of reasons including lack of understanding of the nature of hearing loss, the belief that patients with Alzheimer's cannot be reliably tested, lack of referral from physicians, and poor use of technology and access to audiologists for management (Palmer et al., 1999).

Numerous studies have shown that patients with Alzheimer's disease can be reliably tested (Uhlmann et al., 1989; Durrant et al., 1991). In addition, Palmer's study demonstrated that caregivers are reliable in their identification of problem behaviors when their observations were compared to those of the clinical observers. As a result of hearing management, the caregivers reported fewer problem behaviors in the spouses with Alzheimer's. Thus, it appears that management of hearing impairment in patients with Alzheimer's disease is worthy of consideration and may improve the life functioning of these individuals.

Neuropathology of Alzheimer's Disease and Other Dementias

Although the neuropathology of the dementias varies, nearly all dementias include brain atrophy and neurochemical deficiencies (Hegde, 1996). Until recently, Alzheimer's disease was thought to be the result of diffuse damage in the brain. However, current research indicates that a multifocal pathologic pattern instead of a diffuse pattern is the basis for the disease (Davis, 1993). Patients with Alzheimer's disease demonstrate multifocal infarcts causing a multitude of symptoms. Davis (1993) discusses the presence of neurofibrillary tangles in the inferior temporal lobe and the posterior association regions of the brain. **Neurofibrillary tangles** are defined by Davis (1993, p. 142) as "unusual triangular and looped fibers in the cytoplasm of nerve cells." He also cites research that has demonstrated the existence of **neuritic plaques**, which are "granular deposits and remains of degenerated nerve fibers" (Davis, 1993, p. 142).

Definitive diagnosis of Alzheimer's disease can only be made post mortem. Thus, patients typically are diagnosed as having "probable dementia of the Alzheimer's type" in accordance with criteria developed at the National Institutes of Health. Neuropsychological testing can be done to identify symptom patterns; however, definitive diagnosis can be made only through autopsy findings. Autopsy findings include the presence of the neurofibrillary tangles and numbers of plaques that exceed what would be expected on the basis of the person's age (Davis, 1993). Other findings include multifocal lesions throughout the white matter of the brain. In fact, autopsy studies reveal reduced amounts of white and gray matter in the brains of patients with dementia, with a loss of approximately 10% of the brain's weight in comparison to the brains of people without dementia. Most of this loss is in the frontal and temporal regions of the brain (Hegde, 1996).

Neurofibrillary tangles. Twisted and tangled neurofibrils in the body of the nerve cells.

Neuritic plaques. Minute areas of degeneration of cortical and subcortical tissues in the brain, also known as senile plaques.

Differentiating Alzheimer's Disease from Aphasia

In aphasia, the language problem is "disproportionately severe when compared to overall intellectual and memory abilities" (Bollinger, Berg, LeWitt, 1994, p. 12). In Alzheimer's disease, language deteriorates along with cognitive and memory skills. Language deficits that occur after a stroke typically improve with treatment. However, in patients with Alzheimer's disease, improvement is not likely. In treating patients with aphasia, clinicians can use intact cognitive processes to reorganize the language system. Because cognitive functions and processes deteriorate in patients with Alzheimer's disease, this type of cognitive reorganization is not possible, particularly in the middle and late stages of the disease process (Bollinger et al., 1994). In short, even though some of the language symptoms in Alzheimer's disease resemble those in aphasia, a progressive and severe decline is typical of the patient with Alzheimer's disease, which is not seen in patients with aphasia (Gelfer, 1996).

A telling example offered by Davis (1993) is that the patient with aphasia will recognize a family member even if he or she cannot recall the name of the family member. In contrast, the patient with Alzheimer's disease not only will fail to remember the person's name but also will fail to recognize the person.

■ PICK'S DISEASE

Pick's disease resembles Alzheimer's disease in its symptoms but has a different etiology. Pick's disease is a "progressive neurologic disease associated with a gradual decrease in brain mass, especially in the temporal and frontal lobes" (Hegde, 1996, p. 333). Early symptoms include changes and deterioration in social behaviors. Patients may display uninhibited mannerisms, such as making offensive comments and telling inappropriate jokes. They often repeatedly engage in meaningless and ritualistic behaviors. Patients with Pick's disease also display intellectual disturbances similar to those seen in patients with Alzheimer's disease. They, too, develop impaired judgment. Another common symptom in the early stages is excessive eating and an accompanying weight gain (Hegde, 1996).

In the later stages of Pick's disease, the patients continue to demonstrate a progressive deterioration of intellectual functioning. Echolalia and meaningless repetition of phrases is common. Naming problems accompanied by circumlocution also are common (Hegde, 1996). In contrast to the person with Alzheimer's disease, the patient with Pick's disease is more likely to show a deterioration in the form of language (morphology, syntax, and phonology) than in the content of language. **Auditory agnosia** is common.

Auditory agnosia.
Inability to make sense of incoming auditory stimuli.

As the disease progresses, anomia and impaired speech fluency become evident, and the patient demonstrates symptoms consistent with a primary progressive aphasia. However, language comprehension and nonverbal cognition frequently are preserved (Payne, 1997). Typically, the patient's condition progresses to a point of mutism, total disorientation, and confusion (Hegde, 1996).

■ MULTI-INFARCTION DISEASES

Approximately 20% of patients diagnosed as having some form of senile dementia will have multi-infarction disease. This disorder is typically the result of several small strokes involving areas throughout the cortex, resulting in the loss of blood flow to the damaged areas (Boone & Plante, 1993). Based on this disease process, multi-infarction diseases (MID) often are referred to as vascular dementia, and the patient typically has a history of hypertension. The patient with MID is frequently emotionally fragile and depressed (Payne, 1997). MIDs are characterized by the "loss of intellectual functioning due to significant cerebrovascular disease and repeated infarctions" (Payne, 1997, p. 128). The etiology is frequently **hypertension** with **arteriosclerosis**. The patient may have a history of stroke with a sudden onset of mental decline and an uneven decline of other functions (Payne, 1997). Impulse control and personality also are affected in most cases (Tonkovich, 1988). Payne (1997) notes that "neurological characteristics are multiple areas of softening of brain tissue and may involve possible pathological alterations in cerebral blood vessels" (p. 128). The presence of multiple infarcts resulting in damaged subcortical structures is sometimes seen in Binswanger's disease (Hegde, 1996).

Hypertension. High blood pressure.

Arteriosclerosis. Hardening of the arteries.

Cognition in MID is characterized by inconsistent memory lapses and gradual intellectual loss (Payne, 1997). Memory, abstract thinking, and judgment frequently are affected (Tonkovich, 1988).

Language disorders in MID are dependent on the site of the lesion or lesions. For example, if the lesion is in the left middle cerebral artery, the clinician can expect to see aphasia, **apraxia**, and dementia. If the lesion is in the right middle cerebral artery, visuospatial disorders are common. When the lesion occurs in the posterior middle artery, the patient typically displays fluent aphasia, and **alexia** with **agraphia** (Payne, 1997).

Apraxia. Inability to coordinate the limb or oral musculature to perform voluntary movements.

Alexia. Inability to read, possibly due to neurological impairment.

■ SUBCORTICAL DEMENTIAS

Parkinson's Disease

There are approximately one million cases of Parkinson's disease in the United States. Symptoms are associated with a deterioration of the substantia nigra that leads to a disruption of subcortical and cortical processes (Murray, 2000). The dementia associated with Parkinson's disease is a subcortical dementia. Basically, these dementias are distinguished from those of cortical origin by the presence of motor disturbances accompanying the dementia

Agraphia. Inability to write.

(Davis, 1993). In fact, the motor disturbances precede the associated dementias. Patients with subcortical dementia typically will demonstrate resting tremor, hypokinetic dysarthria, gait disturbances, weak vocal intensity, a stooped posture, and difficulties with the rate of speech. They also may have difficulties with pitch and articulation. With regard to cognition, in the early stages patients with Parkinson's disease frequently display problems with executive functioning, attention, and memory, regardless of whether dementia is present. Murray (2000) goes on to say that patients with Parkinson's disease exhibit language impairments including "high level comprehension impairments such as difficulties processing sentences with metaphoric, ambiguous, or implied information or with complex grammar" (p. 1351). These findings are also true of individuals with Huntington's disease which is discussed later in this chapter (Murray, 2000). With regard to quantity of language output, patients with Parkinson's disease have been shown to say as much as adults without brain damage, although they may produce a smaller proportion of sentences that are grammatical when compared to control groups (Murray, 2000; Illes, 1989; Illes et al., 1988). Furthermore, over time, the patients produced fewer utterances as the disease progresses.

Up to 40% to 50% of patients with Parkinson's disease suffer from problems with word-finding, cognition, and memory. However, only 10% to 20% of people with Parkinson's disease will have full-blown dementia (Tison et al., 1995). If the dementia occurs early in the disease process, involvement of the brain may be more extensive with degenerating neurons, creating an "extended" form of Parkinson's disease. (Duvoisin et al., 1996). Due to neuropathology in the basal ganglia, patients with Parkinson's disease (with or without the presence of dementia) typically have difficulty with tasks that require new procedural learning (Saint-Cyr, Taylor, & Lang, 1988). These problems typically occur later in the disease process and in older patients with Parkinson's disease. Nonetheless, the symptoms are still milder than those associated with Alzheimer's disease.

Similarly, confusion may be a problem, although it is sometimes difficult to determine if the confusion is related to the disease process or is a side-effect of the anti-Parkinsonian medications that are taken by many of the patients (Duvoisin et al., 1996). Finally, as indicated earlier, depression is more common in patients with subcortical dementias. Typically, the mood remains relatively normal in cortical dementias (Lass et al., 1988). Even so, the support of family as depicted in Figure 12–2 is critical.

Huntington's Disease

Huntington's disease (also called Huntington's chorea) is another neurological disease that is frequently associated with subcortical dementia. Chorea, a dominant sign of Huntington's disease, is defined by Hegde as

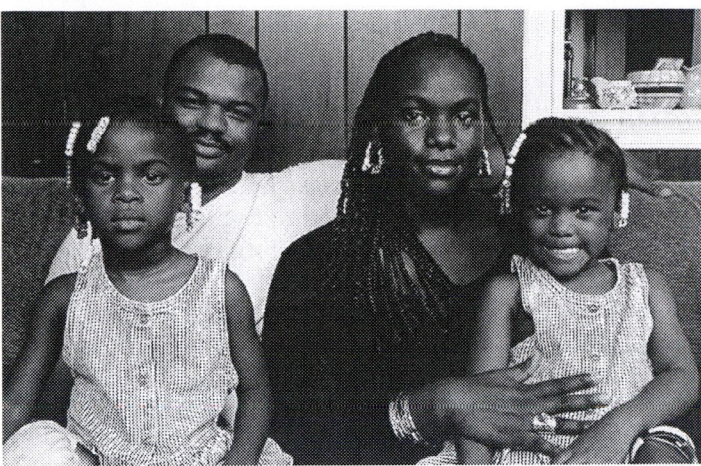

FIGURE 12–2. The support of family members is critical in caring for a family member with dementia.

"irregular, spasmodic, jerky, complex, rapid, and involuntary movements of the limb and facial muscles" (Hegde, 1996, p. 242). Genetic in origin, Huntington's disease affects men and women equally and has been identified in children as young as 4 years of age. There are approximately 30,000 cases of Huntington's disease in the United States. Symptoms are associated with a deterioration of the caudate nucleus that leads to a disruption of subcortical and cortical processes (Murray, 2000).

In the early stages, the patient undergoes gradual changes in behavior and personality. The changes can include depression, anxiety, and irritability. Emotional outbursts are common. The patient may have a false sense of superiority, be suspicious, and show complaining behaviors and nagging. The patient may have problems with abnormal motor movements that resemble fidgeting. Speech becomes disorganized, and problems with memory, **executive functions**, and judgment may be seen (Hegde, 1996).

Executive functions. Activities such as setting goals, initiating tasks, self-monitoring, self-evaluating, keeping schedules, and managing time well.

Advanced symptoms include a worsening of the deficits that appeared early in the disease process. Chorea becomes generalized, and intellect deteriorates. The patient will have attention deficits, confusion, and disorientation. Language impairments frequently associated with dementia also appear and progress to the profoundly impaired level. Typically, patients with Huntington's disease have less verbal output when compared to control subjects. It has also been found that patients with Huntington's disease "produce shorter utterances, a smaller proportion of grammatical utterances, a larger proportion of simple sentences, and fewer embeddings per utterance" (Murray, 2000, p. 1360) when compared to control subjects and to patients with Parkinson's disease. (Murray, 2000; Illes, 1989; Gordon & Illes, 1987). Murray (1999) writes that it is important to note that language deficits in both Huntington's disease and Parkinson's disease can occur prior to signs of dementia.

Murray (2000) also found that patients with Huntington's disease (as well as with Parkinson's disease) often had the same spoken quantity as control subjects, but the content of their speech was less informative than that of the controls. Another study by Murray and Stout found that patients with Huntington's disease and Parkinson's disease had more problems with discourse comprehension than did control subjects (1999). This would lend further support to the hypothesis that these patients' apparent language problems are due to not only motor speech deficits as many previous researchers believed, but also to specific language deficits. In addition, **hyperkinetic dysarthria** is exhibited by patients with Huntington's disease. Death typically occurs within 10 to 20 years after onset.

Hyperkinetic dysarthria. Dysarthria characterized by involuntary movements, disorders of loudness and rate, interruptions in phonation, and abnormal muscle tone.

■ THE ROLE OF THE SPEECH-LANGUAGE PATHOLOGIST

The primary role of the speech-language pathologist in cases of dementia is to aid in the assessment of the disorder. The first task is to obtain a reliable history that includes identifying information, medical history, cognitive and communication status, and psychosocial parameters. It may be necessary to rely on family members to obtain the history.

The second task is to differentiate between language disorders associated with dementia and other types of language disorders frequently seen in the elderly population. The clinician also must distinguish language and cognitive deficits associated with dementia from those seen in cases of depression, confusion, and other reversible dementias (Payne, 1997).

Dementias can arise from cortical, subcortical, and mixed etiological factors. Thus, the assessment process should focus on identifying the language disorders associated with the different etiological considerations. This will include determining the level of the language deficits and the progression of the dementia (Payne, 1997). In the early and middle stages of Alzheimer's dementia, the speech-language pathologist can provide communication strategies that the family members can use to facilitate communication with their affected family member. In the subcortical dementias, patients may experience dysarthria. In these cases, the speech-language pathologist should be actively involved in helping the patient with techniques designed for remediation of the symptoms of dysarthria. However, in most other factors related to dementia, the speech-language pathologist's role is limited to assessment and counseling of the patient and his or her family (Boone & Plante, 1993).

As stated many times in previous chapters, one purpose of assessment is to determine a baseline that can be used to measure progress in therapy. In cases of reversible dementias, this same purpose can be subsumed. However, in cases of irreversible dementia, the baseline may be a guideline against which to measure progressive deterioration with repeated testing (Payne, 1997).

It is also critical to evaluate the patient's communication needs in his or her daily environment. As part of this evaluation, the amount of environmental support that is available to the patient needs to be assessed. This information, combined with the patient's age, gender, severity at time of diagnosis, and existing deficits all become determining factors in the patient's prognosis. Once all of this information is gathered by the clinician, he or she should ascertain the presence of any barriers that would lead to noncompliance, then select the therapy goals (Payne, 1997).

Published tests for the assessment of dementia include the Arizona Battery for Communication Disorders of Dementia (ABCD) (Bayles & Tomoeda, 1993), which results in a profile of a patient's abilities based on performance on 14 subtests used to assess five primary areas: (1) mental status; (2) visuospatial construction; (3) linguistic expression; (4) linguistic comprehension; and (5) episodic memory (Bayles & Tomoeda, 1993). The ABCD was developed to assess the communication functioning of individuals with mild to moderate dementia. The Functional Linguistic Communication Inventory (FLCI; Bayles & Tomoeda, 1994) can be used to assess communication in those individuals with more severe dementia. Another test is the Global Deterioration Scale for Age-Related Cognitive Decline and Alzheimer's Disease Primary Degenerative Dementia (GDS) (Reisberg et al., 1982). The GDS is based on a seven-stage scale with defining levels of clinical characteristics delineated for each stage. The stages range from "No Cognitive Decline" (marked by no complaints or evidence of memory loss) to "Very Severe Cognitive Decline" (characterized by the loss of all verbal abilities, including speech, and the loss of all basic psychomotor and self-care skills). Intellectual functioning can also be tested using the Wechsler Adult Intelligence Scale-Revised (Ripich, 1991). The Mini-Mental State Examination (MMS; Folstein, Folstein, & McHugh, 1975) can also be used to screen for dementia and to stage it based on severity of symptoms.

■ TREATMENT SUGGESTIONS

For many adult patients suffering from dementia, therapy should probably focus more on teaching compensation strategies than on restoring function. As with all other disorders, the identification of cognitive and language skills that are relatively spared can be used as the foundation for treatment of patients with dementia, regardless of the etiology of the dementia.

Depending on the setting and the personal philosophy of the clinician, direct therapy may or may not be provided to a patient with declining function due to Alzheimer's disease and other types of dementia. Most therapy suggestions are designed to facilitate interaction, so the clinician may choose to use a collaborative model of intervention (similar to the collaborative model in the public schools). In nearly every instance, however, time will need to be spent with the patient's family, providing them with information on how to facilitate maximum communication performance in the family member with dementia. Caregivers become more objective and less angry at the patient when they have explanations related to the confusion, memory lapses, depression, apathy, and forgetfulness demonstrated by the affected family member (Bayles, 1986).

One suggestion is to be sure to establish contact with the patient prior to initiating conversation. This can be done by touching the patient to direct his or her attention to the communication partner. The communication partner should use short sentences and speak slowly to facilitate the exchange of information. It is also helpful to use frequent repetitions of phrases and sentences. Closed-ended questions that contain clues are similarly helpful. For example, instead of asking, "What did you have for breakfast?" the communication partner should ask, "What kind of eggs did you have for breakfast?"

Bayles and Tomoeda (1997) have made several suggestions with regard to the treatment of patients with Alzheimer's disease. Since episodic and working memory systems are the most affected, tasks that rely on these systems should be reduced. The patient should be taught to rely more on nondeclarative memory because it is less affected. They also suggest that activities designed to enhance lexical and conceptual associations should be incorporated into therapy, as well as the use of sensory cues "that evoke positive fact memory, action, and emotion" (Hopper & Bayles, 2001).

If the patient still has the capacity to read and understand substantive words, it may help to use cue cards to remind him or her of daily activities. Frequently, patients with dementia need assistance in activities of daily living. This may even progress to the point of having to remind the patient to chew and swallow after having placed food in his or her mouth. Other interventions to help facilitate daily activities, such as dressing, include buying shoes that close with Velcro instead of shoelaces and using pants that have elastic at the waistline instead of zippers and buttons.

Spaced-Retrieval Training (SRT) has been shown to have success in teaching new and forgotten behaviors and information to patients with dementia. Hopper and Bayles (2001) describe SRT as follows:

> In SRT, a patient is told a piece of information and then is asked to recall that information repeatedly and systematically over time. Intervals are manipulated to facilitate production of a high number of correct responses to the stimulus question and retention of information over increasingly longer periods of time. (p. 837)

According to Schacter, Rich, and Stampp (1985), SRT has a low cognitive demand, making it a successful technique to employ in the treatment of patients with dementia.

Some success has been seen in providing toy therapy and pet therapy for patients with dementia. This may be accompanied by art therapy and music therapy. One suggestion is to play music from the patient's "youth era" and dance with the patient. Another is to spend time looking at old photos and reminding the patient of the names of the persons in the pictures.

Periodic retesting of the patient's cognitive and communicative abilities is also paramount. This should include a hearing evaluation approximately every six months. Hearing loss is a side effect of aging, and symptoms due to hearing loss can be remediated if they are not mistaken as symptoms of a progressing dementia. The use of assistive listening devices or hearing aids may be beneficial, particularly in the early stages of dementia.

Day-care facilities for patients with dementia are becoming more common and provide a valuable resource for caregivers. Originally, day-care facilities were limited to caring for those individuals who were in the early stages of dementia. However, centers are now opening their doors to patients in the middle and late stages of dementia. Day-care facilities provide a valuable respite for families. In some cases, this often allows the family members to maintain work and other daily functions that were no longer possible without the respite care. However, the benefits are not limited to the caregivers. Workers in day-care centers report that the patients seem to derive some enjoyment from talking with each other even though seemingly little content is being shared. Families also report that the patients sleep better at night because of the high activity level in the day-care facilities. The staff members at the facilities work hard at keeping the patients awake and active during their time at the day-care sites. This precludes catnapping and leads to better sleep at night. This, in turn, facilitates the family's ability to care for the patient. In many cases, the day-care facilities have members of a multidisciplinary team on staff, so the patients can receive physical therapy, occupational therapy, speech therapy, and other interventions as needed. Thus, the cognitive, emotional, and physical needs of the patients can be met in the day-care facilities.

■ SUMMARY

Adult patients with dementia present a special challenge to the speech-language pathologist, who has two major roles with this population. The first role is to assist the multidisciplinary team with an assessment of the patient's language and cognitive status. The second role is to be available to the patient's family to help structure the environment to facilitate the best communication possible. This requires a great deal of patient and family education about the disorder of dementia and a willingness to listen to the family members as they adapt to their roles in the rehabilitation process. Because of the devastating implications of the diagnosis of dementia, it is important for speech-language pathologists to work closely with other professionals and family members to ease the transitions that accompany the progressive dementia.

CASE STUDY

R is a 79-year-old woman who has been in good physical health for most of her life. In 2001 she suffered a mild heart attack, with only mild residual deficits. She is being treated with pharmaceuticals for hypertension, and the question of a possible vascular dementia has been raised. Approximately two years ago, R began to suffer mental lapses such as forgetting that she had put soup on to cook after a Christmas meal with her family. Her memory slowly declined until she was having difficulty remembering names of acquaintances and recent events. In the last year, she has suffered episodes of becoming disoriented in space and time, often forgetting where she is when she awakens when staying over with friends or family. When driving, she forgets her destination and/or how to get to it. She is able to recognize that she is forgetful, often saying, "My memory is shot" and "Getting old is for the birds." She has pragmatic deficits, often rambling tangentially to a conversation, and repeating the same stories three to four times in a single conversation. Approximately one year ago, her physician prescribed Aricept that she takes on a daily basis.

R is now in the early days of the middle/moderate stage of Alzheimer's. She has experienced increased irritability, and is showing some signs of paranoia. For example, when she sees two to three family members in a discussion, she will say, "Are you plotting against me?" She is no longer permitted to drive and has difficulty remembering to take her medications. In addition, she questions the need to take her medications, saying that she doesn't need them. She is no longer able to live alone due to lapses in judgment and safety concerns. She is unable to manage her finances.

R has a strong support system in her family, so this has helped to provide the needed supervision of her finances and daily living. Due to the personality changes and the steady deterioration of her cognitive and language skills, it is suspected that R has senile dementia of the Alzheimer's type. Speech-language testing revealed a moderate impairment of both short-term and long-term memory, decreased attention span, and moderate difficulty with abstract reasoning. Intervention focused on short-term memory and working with the family to develop strategies for communication.

■ REVIEW QUESTIONS

1. Which of the following statements is most true?
   a. All dementias eventually reveal themselves as a form of Alzheimer's disease.
   b. Just as in stroke victims, the language problems associated with dementia do improve with appropriate treatment.
   c. An individual with dementia associated with Alzheimer's disease will have language deficits that are disproportionately severe compared to his or her overall intellectual capabilities.
   d. There is some evidence that language content disintegrates more than does language structure in patients with Alzheimer's disease.

2. Progressive and irreversible dementias result from
   a. Metabolic conditions and Alzheimer's disease
   b. Hydrocephalus and metabolic conditions
   c. Multi-infarct dementia and metabolic conditions
   d. Alzheimer's disease and multi-infarct dementia

3. Which of the following sets of memory are most affected in the early/middle stages of Alzheimer's?
   a. Episodic and working
   b. Semantic and procedural
   c. Episodic and semantic
   d. Semantic and working

4. Which of the following is most characteristic of dementias associated with Parkinson's disease?
   a. Word finding is less impaired than in Alzheimer's disease.
   b. Depression rarely occurs.
   c. Cognition is more impaired than in dementia associated with Alzheimer's.
   d. Speech is characterized by apraxia with rate and pitch difficulties.

5. Which of the following about Pick's disease is most true?
   a. There is no decrease in brain mass.
   b. Deterioration of language form is more likely than deterioration of content.
   c. In the late stages, all aspects of language and cognition deteriorate.
   d. Judgment remains intact.

6. Declarative memory consists of which of the following sets of skills?
   a. Semantic, episodic, lexical
   b. Semantic, motor, episodic
   c. Motor, procedural, lexical
   d. Semantic, cognitive procedural, lexical

7. Huntington's chorea is associated with

   a. Dysarthria with weak vocal intensity
   b. Cortical deficits
   c. Jerky, involuntary movements of the limbs and facial muscles
   d. Intact judgment

8. Dementias associated with Parkinson's and Huntington's diseases are typically cortical dementias.

   a. True
   b. False

9. Abnormal protein deposition in the neurons of brain cells has been identified as a causative factor in the disease mechanism of Alzheimer's disease.

   a. True
   b. False

10. The Mini-Mental State Examination can be used to screen for dementia and to stage it based on the severity of the symptoms.

    a. True
    b. False

■ REFERENCES

Alzheimer's Association (2004). Alzheimers is the death of the mind before the death of the body. http://www.efmoody.com/longterm/alzheimers.html.

American Psychiatric Association. (1994). *Diagnostic and statistic manual of mental disorders* (4th ed). Washington, DC: Author.

Bayles, K. A. (1984). Language and dementia. In A. L. Holland (Ed.), *Language disorders in adults: Recent advances* (pp. 209–243). San Diego: College-Hill Press.

Bayles, K. A. (1986). Management of neurogenic communication disorders associated with dementia. In R. Chapey (Ed.), *Language intervention strategies in adult aphasia* (3rd ed.) Baltimore, MD: Williams & Wilkins.

Bayles, K. A., Boone, D. R., Tomoeda, C. K., Slauson, T. J., & Kaszniak, A. W. (1989). Differentiating Alzheimer's patients from the normal elderly and stroke patients with aphasia. *Journal of Speech and Hearing Disorders, 54,* 74–87.

Bayles, K. A., & Kaszniak, A. W. (Eds.) (1987). *Communication and cognition in normal aging and dementia.* Boston: College-Hill Press.

Bayles, K. A., & Tomoeda, C. K. (1983). Confrontation naming impairments in dementia. *Brain and Language, 19,* 98–114.

Bayles, K. A., & Tomoeda, C. (1993). *Arizona battery for communication disorders of dementia* (Research ed.). Tucson, AZ: Canyonlands Publishing.

Bayles, K. A., & Tomoeda, C. K. (1994). *The functional linguistic communication inventory.* Tucson, AZ: Canyonlands Publishing.

Bayles, K. A., & Tomoeda, C. K. (1997). *Improving function in dementia and other cognitive-linguistic disorders.* Tucson, AZ: Canyonlands Publishing.

Berg, L., Hughes, C. P., Cohen, L. A., Danzinger, W. L., & Martin, R. L. (1982). Mild senile dementia of Alzheimer type: Research diagnostic criteria, recruitment, and description of a population study. *Journal of Neurology, Neurosurgery, and Psychiatry, 45,* 962–968.

Birren, J. (1964). *The psychology of aging.* Englewood Cliffs, NJ: Prentice Hall.

Blanken, G., Dittmann, J., Haas, J. C., & Wallesch, C. W. (1987). Spontaneous speech in senile dementia and aphasia: Implications for a neurolinguistics model of language production. *Cognition, 27,* 247–274.

Bollinger, R., Berg, L., & LeWitt, P. (1994). Communication issues in Alzheimer's and dementia. *Advance, 4*(19), 12–13.

Boone, D. R., & Plante, E. (1993). *Human communication and its disorders* (2nd ed.). Englewood Cliffs, NJ: Prentice Hall.

Bourgeois, M., Burgio, L., & Schulz, R. (1992, November). *Teaching caregivers of spouses with Alzheimer's disease to modify problem behaviors in the home.* Presentation at the GSA Convention, Washington, DC.

Chapey, R. (2001) *Language intervention strategies in aphasia and related neurogenic communication disorders* (4th ed.). Philadelphia: Lippincott Williams & Wilkins.

Davis, G. A. (1993). *A survey of adult aphasia and related language disorders* (2nd ed.). Englewood Cliffs, NJ: Prentice Hall.

Durrant, J., Gilmartin, K., Holland, A., Kamerer, D., & Newall, P. (1991). Hearing disorders management in Alzheimer's disease patients. *Hearing Instruments, 42,* 32–35.

Duvoisin, R. C., Golbe, L. I., Mark, M. H., Sage, J. I., & Walters, A. S. (1996). *Parkinson's disease handbook: A guide for patients and their families.* Staten Island, NY: The American Parkinson Disease Association, Inc.

Emery, O. B. (1988). Language and memory processing in senile dementia Alzheimer's type. In L. H. Light & D. M. Burke (Eds.), *Language, memory and aging* (pp. 221–243). New York: Cambridge University Press.

Folstein, M. F., Folstein, S. E., & McHugh, P. R. (1975). "Mini-Mental State": A practical method for grading the cognitive state of patients for the clinician. *Journal of Psychiatric Research, 36,* 216–220.

Gelfer, M. P. (1996). *Survey of communication disorders: A social and behavioral perspective.* New York: McGraw-Hill.

Glosser, G., & Deser, T. (1990). Patterns of discourse production among neurological patients with fluent language disorders. *Brain and Language, 40,* 67–88.

Golper, L. C. (1998). *Sourcebook of medical speech pathology* (2nd ed.). San Diego: Singular Publishing Group.

Gordon, W. P., & Illes, J. (1987). Neurolinguistic characteristics of language production in Huntington's disease: A preliminary report. *Brain and Language, 31,* 1–10.

Haynes, W. O., & Pindzola, R. H. (1998). *Diagnosis and evaluation in speech pathology* (5th ed.). Boston: Allyn and Bacon.

Hegde, M. N. (1996). *PocketGuide to assessment in speech-language pathology.* San Diego: Singular Publishing Group.

Heller, R. B., Dobbs, A. R., & Rule, B. G. (1992). Communicative function in patients with questionable Alzheimer's disease. *Psychology and Aging, 7,* 395–400.

Herbst, K., & Humphrey, C. (1980). Hearing impairment and mental state in the elderly living at home. *British Medicine Journal of Clinical Research, 281,* 903–905.

Hodkinson, H. (1973). Mental impairment in the elderly. *JR College of Physicians London, 7,* 305.

Hopper, T., & Bayles, K. A. (2001). Management of neurogenic communication disorders associated with dementia. In R. Chapey (Ed.), *Language intervention strategies in aphasia and related neurogenic communication disorders* (4th ed.). Philadelphia: Lippincott Williams & Wilkins.

Illes, J. (1989). Neurolinguistic features of spontaneous language production dissociate three forms of neurodegenerative disease: Alzheimer's, Huntington's, and Parkinson's. *Brain and Language, 37*, 628–642.

Illes, J., Metter, E. J., Hanson, W. R., & Iritani, S. (1988). Language production in Parkinsons's disease: Acoustic and linguistic considerations. *Brain and Language, 33*, 146–160.

Johnson, D. J. (1997). Mental status and aging: Cognition and affect. In B. B. Shadden & M. A. Toner (Eds.), *Aging and communication.* Austin, TX: Pro-Ed.

Katzman, R. (1998, May). Diagnosis and etiology of related disorders. Paper presented at the meeting of the University of California, San Diego School of Medicine, Alzheimer's Disease Research Center, San Diego, CA.

Kay, D., Beamish, P., & Roth, M. (1964). Old age mental disorders in Newcastle upon Tyne: II. A study of possible social and medical causes. *British Journal of Psychiatry, 110*, 668.

Kempler, D., Almor, A., & MacDonald, M. C. (1998, February). Teasing apart the contribution of memory and language impairments in Alzheimer's disease: An online study of sentence comprehension. *American Journal of Speech-Language Pathology, 7*(1), 61–67.

Kirshner, H., & Freemon, F. (1982). *The neurology of aphasia.* Lisse, Holland: Swets and Zeitlinger.

Lass, N. J., McReynolds, L. V., Northern, J. L., & Yoder, D. E. (1988). *Handbook of speech-language pathology and audiology.* Philadelphia: B. C. Decker.

Lauter, H. (1985). What do we know about Alzheimer's disease today? *Danish Medical Bulletin, 3*, 1–21.

Martin, A., & Fedio, P. (1983). Word production and comprehension in Alzheimer's disease: The breakdown of semantic knowledge. *Brain and Language, 19*, 124–141.

Mentis, M., Briggs-Whitaker, J., & Gramigna, G. D. (October, 1995). Discourse topic management in senile dementia of the Alzheimer's type. *Journal of Speech and Hearing Research, 38*(5), 1054–1066.

Mortensen, L. (1992). A transivity analysis of discourse in dementia of the Alzheimer's type. *Journal of Neurolinguistics, 7*, 309–321.

Murdoch, B. (1990). *Acquired speech and language disorders: A neuroanatomical and functional neurological approach.* London: Chapman & Hall.

Murray, L. L. (2000, December). Spoken language production in Huntington's and Parkinson's diseases. *Journal of Speech, Language, and Hearing Research, 43*(6), 1350–1366.

Murray, L. L., & Chapey, R. (2001). Assessment of language disorders in adults. In R. Chapey, (Ed.). *Language intervention strategies in aphasia and related neurogenic communication disorders,* 4th ed. (pp. 55–128). Philadelphia: Lippincott Williams & Wilkins.

Murray, L. L., & Stout, J. C. (1999, May). Discourse comprehension in Huntington's and Parkinsons's diseases. *American Journal of Speech-Language Pathology, 8*(2), 137–148.

Navia, B. A., Jordan, B. D., & Price, R. W. (1986). The AIDS dementia complex: I. Clinical features. *Annals of Neurology, 19*, 517–524.

Orange, J. B., Lubinski, R. B., & Higginbotham, D. J. (1996, August). Conversational repair by individuals with dementia of the Alzheimer's type. *Journal of Speech and Hearing Research, 39*(4), 881–895.

Overman, C. A., & Geoffrey, V. C. (1987a). Alzheimer's disease and other dementias. In H. G. Mueller & V. C. Geoffrey (Eds.), *Communication disorder in the aging:*

Assessment and management (pp. 271–297). Washington, DC: Gallaudet University Press.

Overman, C. A., & Geoffrey, V. C. (1987b). Alzheimer's disease and other dementias. In H. G. Mueller & V. C. Geoffrey (Eds.), *Communication disorders in the aging: Assessment and management* (pp. 3–35). Washington, DC: Gallaudet University Press.

Palmer, C. V., Adams, S. W., Bourgeois, M., Durrant, J., & Rossi, M. (1999, April). Reduction in caregiver-identified problem behaviors in patients with Alzheimer disease post-hearing-aid fitting. *Journal of Speech, Language, and Hearing Research, 42*(2), 312–328.

Payne, J. C. (1997). *Adult neurogenic language disorders: Assessment and treatment.* San Diego: Singular Publishing Group.

Peters, C., Potter, J., & Scholer, S. (1988). Hearing impairment as a predictor of cognitive decline in dementia. *Journal of the American Geriatrics Society, 36,* 981–986.

Reisberg, B., Ferris, S. H., DeLeon, M. J., & Crook T. (1982). The global deterioration scale for assessment of primary degenerative dementia. *American Journal of Psychiatry, 139,* 1136–1139.

Ripich, D. N. (1991). Differential diagnosis and assessment. In R. Lubinski (Ed.), *Dementia and communication.* Philadelphia: B. C. Decker.

Saint-Cyr, J. A., Taylor, A. E., & Lang, A. E. (1988). Procedural learning and neostriatal dysfunction in man. *Brain, 111,* 941–959.

Schacter, D. L., Rich, S. A., & Stampp, M. S. (1985). Remediation of memory disorders: Experimental evaluation of the spaced-retrieval technique. *Journal of Clinical and Experimental Neuropsychology, 7,* 79–96.

Shadden, B. B., & Toner, M. A. (Eds.). (1997). *Aging and communication.* Austin, TX: Pro-Ed.

Tison, F., Dartigues, J. F., Auriacombe, S., Letenneur, I., Boller, F., & Alperovitch, A. (1995). Dementia in Parkinsons' disease: A population based study in ambulatory and institutionalized individuals. *Neurology, 45,* 705–708.

Tonkovich, J. L. (1988). Communication disorders in the elderly. In B. B. Shadden (Ed.), *Communication behavior and aging: A sourcebook for clinicians* (pp. 197–218). Baltimore, MD: Williams and Wilkins.

Uhlmann, R., Larson, E., Rees, T., Koepsell, T., & Duckert, L. (1989). Relationship of hearing impairment to dementia and cognitive dysfunction in older adults. *Journal of the American Medical Association, 261,* 1916–1919.

Uhlmann, R., Rees, T., Psaty, B., & Duckert, L. (1989). Validity and reliability of auditory screening tests in demented and non-demented older adults. *Journal of General Internal Medicine, 4,* 90–96.

Weinstein, B., & Ventry, I. (1982). Hearing impairment and social isolation in the elderly. *Journal of Speech and Hearing Research, 25,* 593–599.

Wechsler, D. (1981). *Wechsler adult intelligence scale-revised.* New York: The Psychological Corporation.

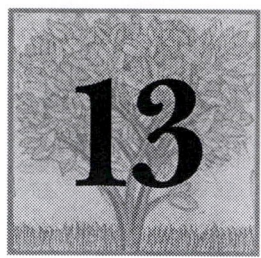

13

Aphasia in Adults

LEARNING OBJECTIVES

After completion of this chapter, the reader will be able to

1. Differentiate between and discuss causes and etiologies of stroke.

2. Explain the time course (clinical presentation) of strokes.

3. Identify questions that should be addressed by a diagnostic team when assessing a patient for neurological deficits.

4. Show mastery of terminology associated with adult onset aphasia.

5. Explain five different imaging techniques used to identify neurological structures and deficits in adult-onset aphasia.

6. Discuss the four primary features used for differential diagnosis of aphasia.

7. Differentiate between the different types of aphasia.

8. Describe the decision-making process to determine if a patient with aphasia is suitable for therapy.

INTRODUCTION

Most language disorders in the adult population are related to cerebrovascular disorders, accidents resulting in traumatic brain injury, disease processes, and aging. In the United States, approximately 700,000 individuals per year will have a stroke which translates into approximately 80,000 new cases of aphasia every year. Of the 700,000 strokes per year, approximately 500,000 are first strokes, and 200,000 are recurrent attacks. In 2002, 162,672 people died as a result of a stroke (National Institute of Neurological Disorders and Stroke, 2005).

In the United States, stroke is the third leading cause of death. Only heart disease and cancer are more fatal than a stroke. The pie chart in Figure 13–1 shows a percentage breakdown of deaths from cardiovascular disease in the United States. The risk of a first occurrence stroke in African-American males is almost twice that of Caucasians, and the African-American males have the highest death rate of all populations of stroke patients (U.S. News and World Report, 2006). Long-term disability is often associated with stroke. Prevalence figures from the American Heart Association (2005) indicate that there are approximately 5,400,000 people in the United States who survived a stroke and are living with the subsequent disabilities associated with stroke. These incidence and prevalence figures do not include the countless family members and friends who are affected when a spouse, parent, or friend has **aphasia**.

Aphasia. Impairment of the abilities to comprehend and express language resulting from acquired neurological damage.

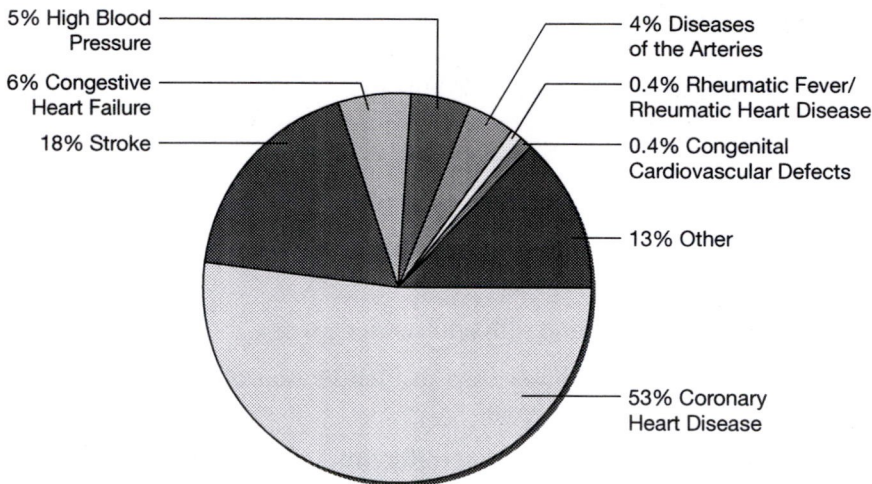

Source: CDC/NCHS.

FIGURE 13–1. Percentage breakdown of deaths from cardiovascular diseases. (Reproduced with permission. *Heart Disease and Stroke Statistics—2005 Update.* © 2005, American Heart Association.)

Diagnosis of language disorders in the adult population typically involves a team approach, with at least the speech-language pathologist, the neurologist, and the family as core members of the team. If the patient has physical anomalies in association with the language disorder, the team will also include the physical therapist and the occupational therapist. Other members of the team typically include nurses, rehabilitation medicine physicians (physiatrists), psychologists, and social workers. To understand and treat aphasia, all of the professionals on the team must have a working knowledge of the neuroanatomy and physiology of aphasia. An in-depth discussion of these topics is beyond the scope of this book. However, readers are strongly encouraged to carefully review the basics of neuroanatomy and physiology in order to fully comprehend the nature of this disorder (Kent, 1997; Seikel, King, & Drumright, 1997; Webster, 1997).

Some general guidelines as to aphasia treatment are offered later in this chapter. However, specific information will also be offered in the sections dedicated to each type of aphasia syndrome.

■ WHAT IS APHASIA?

Aphasia is an impaired ability to comprehend or express linguistic symbols, or both. It can lead to deficits in auditory comprehension and retention of information. It can also result in deficits in visual comprehension and written expression. Verbal expression is frequently problematic and is usually described as being either **nonfluent aphasia** or **fluent aphasia**. Aphasia is an acquired disorder, with many of the same etiological factors as those discussed in Chapter 7. Usually, in adults, the primary etiological factor is **stroke**. Murray and Chapey (2001) define aphasia as "an acquired impairment in language production and comprehension and in other cognitive processes that underlie language" (p. 55). They go on to point out that it is a multimodality disorder that affects speaking, reading, listening, and gesturing abilities.

Strokes occur from numerous causes. In some cases the onset is sudden, whereas in others it is more progressive. The most common form is a cerebral vascular accident (CVA). CVAs are usually of sudden onset and involve a blockage of blood flow to the brain. Frequently, they result from the presence of cerebrovascular occlusive disease due to high blood pressure, arteriosclerosis (hardening of the arteries), or space occupying lesions (tumors). Three major types of cerebrovascular accidents are recognized: (1) thrombotic, (2) embolic, and (3) hemorrhagic. In each case, a lesion in the cerebral cortex causes the aphasia (Davis, 1993). **Thrombotic strokes** occur as a result of the build-up of fatty plaque and atherosclerotic platelets on the inner walls of a vessel (Davis, 1993). This build-up, which blocks the flow of blood, is sometimes called a clot. It may take minutes or weeks for a thrombosis to completely block the flow of blood through an artery. The associated dysfunction has a sudden onset but can worsen progressively over time. This progressive worsening is a "stroke in evolution" (Davis, 1993).

An **embolic stroke** results from the traveling of the clot from the location at which it forms (such as the heart, carotid artery, or aorta) to an artery in the brain (typically the middle cerebral artery). Frequently, these clots consist of platelets and plaque that break off from the wall of a vessel where a thrombus is developing. Occlusion occurs much more quickly after an embolism because the clot becomes lodged in a smaller cerebral artery than the one where it originated. Thus, when the occlusion occurs, it is fairly rapid, creating a complete disruption in the blood flow in seconds or minutes (Davis, 1993). Sometimes, it is difficult to determine if the blockage is due to embolism or thrombosis; thus, strokes are sometimes referred to as thromboembolic in the patient's medical charts.

Hemorrhagic stroke occurs when a bursting of the arterial walls occurs due to stretching and weakening in the wall of the blood vessel. The stretching and weakening of the wall is called an aneurysm. The aneurysm and rupture in the brain frequently are the result of aging (loss of elasticity of the vessel walls) or high blood pressure. The rupture results in intense inflammation and swelling of surrounding brain tissue. The accumulation of blood in the brain is called a **hematoma**. The hematoma expands rapidly and will compress or displace the adjacent brain tissues, or both. The patient who has a hemorrhagic stroke

---

Nonfluent aphasia. Aphasia characterized by slow, labored speech, word retrieval deficits, and motor planning deficits.

Fluent aphasia. Aphasia in which the initiation and production of speech are intact, but deficits occur in semantics and comprehension.

Stroke. A condition caused by blockage or bursting of an artery, leading to disruption of blood flow to the brain and resulting in neurologic damage to the area of the brain that is supplied by that artery.

Thrombotic stroke. A stroke occurring after the build-up of plaque on the inner walls of a vessel, which blocks the flow of blood.

Embolic stroke. A stroke that results from the traveling of a clot from the location at which it forms.

Hemorrhagic stroke. A stroke occurring after the bursting of the arterial walls in the brain due to aging or high blood pressure.

Hematoma. The accumulation of blood below the skin or within the brain.

often will complain of a headache and nausea prior to losing consciousness and/or suffering from cognitive impairment (Davis, 1993).

Lesions may be **parenchymal** or **ischemic**. Parenchymal refers to matter within the brain tissue. Since thromboses and embolisms are within the vessels, they are not parenchymal. However, since a hemorrhagic stroke results in blood escaping into the brain tissue, it is known as a parenchymal event. Ischemia refers to a deficiency of blood, caused by blockage or constriction, usually from within an artery. Thus, since thromboses and emboli involve the formation of clots, or blockages, they are known as ischemic attacks. Metabolism is defined by Davis (1993) as "the exchange of nutrients and 'digestive' waste products between the circulatory system and neural tissue." When this metabolism is disrupted for more than two minutes, necrosis (or death) of the neural tissue occurs. The necrotic tissue is referred to as an **infarct** (Davis, 1993). In most cases of thrombotic or embolic strokes, the infarct is focal.

Other etiological factors that can result in aphasia are closed head injury, tumors, anoxia (lack of oxygen in the brain), hypertension (high blood pressure), and aging. Strokes also can occur as a result of progressive neurological diseases, such as Parkinson disease, Pick disease, or infectious diseases.

When classifying a CVA, the clinician must take into account the time course and the site of the primary disease. With regard to the time course, which is sometimes called the clinical presentation, strokes fall within one of four categories: (1) a transient ischemic attack (TIA), (2) a reversible ischemic neurological deficit (RIND), (3) a stroke in evolution, or (4) a completed stroke. A TIA is a rapidly resolving event. The patient may report a momentary loss of consciousness, dizziness, blurring of the vision, weakness on one side of the body, or speech difficulty. TIAs usually last only a few minutes. However, they may last up to an hour and are defined as completed within 24 hours (Davis, 1993). Frequently, by the time the patient seeks medical attention, the incident has resolved. TIAs do not leave behind any residual effects, although they may reoccur. Recurring TIAs may be an early warning sign of a more serious stroke.

RINDs typically last longer than TIAs and may leave some mild residual deficits. These deficits can last for days or weeks; over the course of time, minimal, partial, or no residual neurological deficits may be the result of a RIND (Aronson, 1991).

A stroke in evolution is a classic, full stroke from which the person can expect residual problems, including physical weakness and language deficits such as aphasia. In a full stroke, the symptoms persist longer than 24 hours and an associated progressive deterioration occurs in the patient's neurological status (Aronson, 1991). The amount of residual damage will depend on

Parenchymal lesions. Those which extend to matter within the brain tissue such as those that occur as a result of a hemorrhagic stroke.

Ischemic. A deficiency of blood caused by blockage or constriction, and usually from within an artery.

Infarct. Necrotic, or dead, tissue that occurs as a sequela to an ischemic attack.

whether the lesion is focal or diffuse and on the severity of the attack. With focal lesions, the residual deficits are limited to a small area of brain tissue. Diffuse lesions, such as those that result from a hemorrhagic stroke, leave more widespread damage because of more extensive involvement of the brain tissue as the blood spreads into the tissues.

The completed stroke refers to one in which the deterioration stops and the patient's condition stabilizes. Neurological deficits remain, but typically they do not worsen once the patient's condition is medically stable. The symptoms may evolve from one type of aphasia into another, but they do not worsen in terms of the time course or the area of damage.

■ DIAGNOSTIC EXAMINATION

Aronson (1991) developed a series of questions that should be addressed by the neurological team when evaluating patients with neurological deficits. This team includes the speech-language pathologist, the neurologist, and, possibly, a neurosurgeon. The questions are listed in Table 13–1.

Questions 3 through 6 primarily address the issue of the lesion, so these questions are the purview of the neurologist or neurosurgeon, or both. The other three questions focus mainly on the malfunction, and the speech-language pathologist can be a contributor to the answering of these questions. The answer to question 1 relates to the patient's complaints. The answer to question 2 is based on the clinician's observations. The entire intervention team should address question 7, with the answer based on the patient's weaknesses and strengths (the four-box system helps here), test results, and medical stability.

TABLE 13–1. Prerequisite questions to guide the evaluation of patients with neurological deficits.

1. What is malfunctioning?
2. How is it malfunctioning?
3. Is a lesion causing the malfunction?
4. Where is the lesion?
5. What is the lesion?
6. What can be done to reduce or eliminate the lesion?
7. What can be done to reduce or eliminate the malfunction?

Source: From "Neurology for the Medical Speech-Language Pathologist," by A. E. Aronson, 1991. Workshop presented in Tampa, Florida.

Preassessment Interview

The preassessment interview should serve as a time for the clinician to provide release and support for the client's frustrations. A major goal of the initial interview should be to remove discomfort by promoting a sense of well-being and acceptance. Most likely, the patient is going through a time of stress and confusion. The job of the clinician at this stage is to convey interest and support of the client as a person and to show empathy. This enables the clinician to form a bond of identification with the patient, which becomes the basis for the relationship in which the clinician can assist the patient in resolving his or her difficulties. This requires the setting of the proper tone for the interview. The atmosphere must foster communication. The clinician should immediately empower the family to be part of the evaluation and treatment processes by defining the roles that each individual will have in working through the communication disorder.

Next, it is important to explain the purpose of the interview so that everyone is clear as to why the information is being gathered and how it will be used in the evaluation and treatment process. It is critical that the clinician maintain a relaxed, natural posture and affect, with good eye contact and listening skills. Empathy is based on understanding, not identification, so the clinician should not make the mistake of saying that he or she knows how the patient or family member feels. Even if the clinician has had a family member who has similar problems, the effects are different on each individual. The clinician can share the experience he or she has had, but it is still a mistake to say that he or she knows how the patient feels.

Questions should be structured to promote the exchange of information. Sudden shifts in the content and purpose of the questions should be avoided. Yes-no and either-or questions fail to yield much information, so they should not be used in the interview process. In addition, the clinician should not use questions with inhibitive phrasing such as, "You don't have periods when you can't recall names, do you?" The clinician needs to remember that the interview is to be an exchange of information, not a one-sided dialogue. The clinician should employ open-ended questions and active listening skills to encourage the client to provide as much useful information as possible.

The importance of using of active listening skills cannot be overemphasized in any discussion about diagnostic interviewing. When using active listening, the clinician often paraphrases the words of the patient or family member to help form a psychological link to show that he or she is listening. Active listening does not involve asking a lot of questions. Rather, it is structuring the environment so that the patient and family members feel secure in sharing information with the clinician.

With the elderly, the clinician should be alert to failing eyesight or hearing and to fatigue. Many victims of stroke or a traumatic brain injury have low stamina, which could interfere with the diagnostic and therapeutic sessions. Also, the patient and the family members may spend time reviewing the past. It is very important to listen to the stories because they familiarize the clinician with the patient as a person, not as a stroke victim. This familiarization may play a role in enhancing the patient's self-esteem. The sharing of their memories is also an opportunity to let the family begin their involvement in the diagnostic process.

The Neurological Examination

General Observations and Mental Status

Much of the neurological examination can be obtained while the clinician and physician are taking the patient's history, because a good neurological examination relies heavily on clinical observation skills. Initially, the patient's behavior should be analyzed. Does the patient interact appropriately? What kind of mood and affect does the patient generate? Is the patient clean and neat? What thought processes does the patient exhibit? Does the patient appear to be anxious or confused? (Helm-Estabrooks & Albert, 1991).

In addition to behavior, the patient's gait and posture should be observed, looking for signs of asymmetry, unsteadiness, or weakness. The patient's mental status likewise should be evaluated during the history-gathering process. For example, is the patient alert and attentive to the examiner's questions and comments? What is the memory status of the patient? Memory can be assessed informally by teaching the patient a list of four unrelated items, then asking him or her to recall the list after a five-minute interlude of other questions and conversation. Recall of immediate events ("Tell me what happened to you") and recall of major events from the past ("Are you married? How many children do you have?") similarly are important aspects of memory to assess (Helm-Estabrooks & Albert, 1991). Knowledge of recent nonpersonal events should be explored, depending on the patient's areas of interest. For example, if the patient likes baseball, questions such as, "Who won the World Series this year?" would be a way to explore memory.

Cranial Nerve Examination

The cranial nerve examination is done by the neurologist, although the speech-language pathologist can contribute to this portion of the evaluation. Humans have 12 pairs of cranial nerves that are divided into sensory nerves, motor nerves, and mixed nerves (Table 13–2). Simple tests to use when assessing the patency of the cranial nerves involved in speech are outlined in

TABLE 13–2. The cranial nerves.

I	Olfactory	Sensory
II	Optic	Sensory
III	Oculomotor	Motor
IV	Trochlear	Motor
V	**Trigeminal**	**Sensory and motor**
VI	Abducens	Motor
VII	**Facial**	**Sensory and motor**
VIII	Acoustic	Sensory
IX	**Glossopharyngeal**	**Sensory and motor**
X	**Vagus**	**Sensory and motor**
XI	**Spinal Accessory**	**Motor**
XII	**Hypoglossal**	**Motor**

Nerves in boldface type are most frequently involved in speech.

Afferent fibers.
Sensory nerve fibers that carry the impulses that arise from sensory stimulation of the sensory end organs to the central nervous system.

Hemianesthesia. The lack of sensation on either the right or the left side of the body.

Agnosia. The inability to perceive, integrate, and attach meaning to incoming sensory stimuli.

Efferent fibers. Motor nerve fibers that carry impulses from the central nervous system to the muscles and other organs.

Table 13–3. While assessing the cranial nerves, the astute physician and clinician will also evaluate the patient's motor skills, the status of his or her sensory system, and the presence and absence of reflexes.

Sensory Nerves. Cranial nerves consist of afferent and efferent fibers. The **afferent fibers** are the sensory fibers. They carry the impulses that arise from sensory stimulation of the sensory end organs to the central nervous system (Goss, 1973). It is not unusual for individuals with aphasia to have visual deficits because the visual tracks cross through Wernicke's and Broca's areas. The patient also may complain of **hemianesthesia**, which is the lack of sensation on either the right or the left side of the body. In addition, the patient may have **agnosia**, which is the inability to perceive, integrate, and attach meaning to incoming stimuli.

Motor Nerves. **Efferent fibers**, or motor fibers, carry impulses from the central nervous system to the muscles and other organs (Goss, 1973). The motor nerves are a two-neuron system. The upper motor neurons, also known as the central neurons, constitute the cortical bulbar tract. Damage to the upper motor neurons results in hypertonia and pervasive spasticity. Hypertonia and spasticity are characterized by too much tone in the muscles, which creates a tightness throughout the muscle. If early and adequate physical and occupational therapy are not provided, the patient may have contractures and be unable to move the extremity in which the hypertonia occurs. When damage occurs to the central neurons, the patient will also

TABLE 13–3. General tests for the assessment of cranial nerves involved in speech (nerves V, VII, IX, X, XI, XII).

Nerve	Tests
Trigeminal (V)	Check sensation with cotton wisps, pinpricks, warm and cold objects
	Ask if patient can sneeze
	Check ability to chew
	Palpate masseters and temporal muscles with jaw clamped tightly
	Look for wasting of masseter on affected side and deviation of the mandible to one side when lowering jaw against resistance
Facial (VII)	Check ability to smile
	Check ability to whistle
	Check results of EMG studies[*]
	Offer taste tests (sweet with sugar; sour with citric acid; bitter with quinine; salty with salt)
	Look for facial symmetry at rest
	Look for facial symmetry during voluntary facial movement
Glossopharyngeal (IX)	Elicit pharyngeal gag (stroking of affected side does not produce gagging if the nerve is injured)
	Ask patient to say "ah" (look for presence of constriction of pharyngeal wall)
	Administer taste tests on the posterior one third of the tongue
Vagus (X)	Perform a laryngoscopic examination to check motor status of the larynx and pharynx
	Check sensory status of the larynx and pharynx (gag reflex)
Accessory (XI)	Check ability of patient to shrug shoulders and rotate head against resistance
	Complete objective examination for muscle atrophy and shoulder drop
	Evaluate EMG results
Hypoglossal (XII)	Test tongue strength by having patient push tongue tip against the cheek against clinician's finger resistance
	Check for deviation of the tongue upon protrusion
	Notice atrophy or tremors of the tongue
	Evaluate EMG stimulation of tongue muscles

[*]EMG, electromyography

have hyperactive reflexes. This includes the oral reflexes, so the patient may have related difficulties with eating and swallowing.

Peripheral nerve involvement involves the lower motor neurons. The effect of this involvement is the opposite of that seen with upper motor neuron deficits. The patient in this case has hypoactive reflexes, hypotonia, and flaccidity in specific motor groups. This means the reflexes do not provide the protection they should with regard to eating and swallowing, and there is a "floppiness" in the muscles. The patient with hypotonia will have difficulty maintaining an upright position, so he or she will need assistance in standing and sitting.

Brain Imaging Techniques

Several different types of brain imaging techniques can be used to determine the location and extent of damage after a stroke or head injury. The speech-language pathologist should be familiar with these techniques for a variety of reasons. One major reason is that the patient and family members may ask questions about it, and the speech-language pathologist should understand the general procedures and purposes of the tests. It is also important to understand the advantages and disadvantages of the different procedures.

Angiography

Angiography. An x-ray study to evaluate the flow of blood in the arteries.

Angiography, one type of arteriography, is an x-ray technique used to study the flow of blood, as, for example, in the neck and head arteries. Dye (an iodinated opaque fluid) is inserted into the head and neck arteries and the movement of the dye through the arteries is tracked on the x-ray. This helps to determine the site of the occlusion, or blockage, of the blood flow because the dye will not be evident beyond the site of the blockage. The blockage can come from within the blood vessel, as in a thrombosis or embolism, or from pressure on the blood vessel from a space-occupying lesion. Whether from within or without, the angiogram will show any disruption of the arterial blood flow.

Radioisotope Scanning

Radioisotope scanning of the brain is synonymous with a brain scan, isotope scanning, radionuclide scanning, and cerebral scintigraphy. Although it is invasive, this technique is relatively safe. In radioisotope scanning, the progress of the isotopes through the brain is tracked. Radioisotope scanning is not precise in locating lesions.

Computerized Tomography

Otherwise known as the **CT scan**, computerized tomography (also known as computerized axial tomography), is a safe, easy, and noninvasive technique. CT scans provide an accurate computerized reconstruction of the cerebral structures (Murdoch, 1988; Patronas, Deveikis, & Schellinger, 1987). Narrow x-ray beams focus on a single plane as the scanner rotates around the patient's head. Computer displays reveal the intensity of the beam, then calculate the absorption coefficients, which indicate tissue densities. Areas of altered density indicate pathology. An infarct will show up as decreased density, and a hemorrhage will be revealed as an area of increased density where the blood has invaded the brain tissues, owing to differences in tissue composition. The procedure typically takes about 30 minutes to complete. Clinically, the CT scan shows good resolution of the lesion. Also, it can be used to detect past CVA damage. If further information is needed, dye can be injected and tracked as it progresses through the vascular system (Davis, 1993).

CT scans. A computerized reconstruction of structures, as in the head, created when narrow x-ray beams focus on a single plane as the scanner rotates around the patient's head.

Magnetic Resonance Imaging

MR imaging, or magnetic resonance imaging, is also noninvasive. MR imaging has also been called nuclear magnetic resonance (NMR). MR images can differentiate between white matter, which is primarily neurons and related processes and gray matter (bundles of nerve fibers). Large electromagnets manipulate the spin of the hydrogen molecules. MR images are superior to CT scans in studying brain symmetries and asymmetries. They are more sensitive to subtle kinds of neuropathology, and they are better at early detection of neurophysiological changes (Davis, 1993).

Functional Magnetic Resonance Imaging

Functional magnetic resonance imaging (fMRI) can be used to "map" brain anatomy and physiology, including brain activity, using MRI. It takes the images from MRI one-step further enabling physicians to identify small rapid metabolic changes in the brain. Using fMRI, the radiologist can monitor the autoregulation of blood flow in the cerebrum and changes that occur in the magnetic properties of blood due to increased blood flow. fMRI can be used to "visualize the inner workings of the human brain in a completely noninvasive way; there is no radiation or injections. (Shaywitz, 2003, p. 69). fMRI can be used to identify, investigate, and monitor changes in the brain due to stroke, tumors, and CNS disorders such as Parkinsons's disease. It is possible to detect these changes at an earlier stage than with more conventional imaging techniques. In fMRI, the patient is asked to perform specific tasks while an MRI is being done. Radiologists are able to pinpoint more precisely where special functions, including speech and language, are handled in the brain by identifying where chemical changes, expansion of blood vessels, and delivery of extra oxygen to the brain take place. These markers are indicative of brain activity to process information and issue commands to the rest of the body. This information can be used to make a more precise diagnosis that can be helpful in determining treatment methods including surgery and radiation treatments.

Positron Emission Tomography (PET)

PET scan. The observation of patterns of radioactivity in the brain through position emission tomography.

PET scans enable the clinician to visualize metabolic activity in the cerebral cortex. Small amounts of radioactive chemicals are injected into the patient, and the "patterns of subsequent radioactivity are recorded over the brain" (Helm-Estabrooks & Albert, 1991, p. 64). The patient is asked to do a series of cortical tasks, and the activity of the radioactive nutrients is visualized and compared with metabolic activity at rest (Davis, 1993).

Hemispheric Differentiation Testing

The Wada test, electroencephalograms (EEGs), dichotic listening tasks, and cortical mapping are examples of hemispheric differentiation testing. In the **Wada test**, named after Jean Wada, sodium amytal is injected into the left or right carotid artery to temporarily paralyze one hemisphere. The patient then does automatic speech tasks (Davis, 1993).

Wada test. The administration of automatic speech tasks after the injection of sodium amytal into the left or right carotid artery to temporarily paralyze one hemisphere.

EEGs measure electrical activity of brain through electrodes placed on the patient's scalp. EEGs are useful in the diagnosis of convulsive disorders and can also be used to detect focal lesions, which are manifested as abnormal neurologic signs (Davis, 1993).

EEG. The measurement of electrical activity of the brain taken from electrodes placed on the scalp to detect abnormal neurological signs.

In dichotic listening tasks, the patient is stimulated with auditory signals in both ears, but he or she has to respond to information presented in either the left or right ear, or has to inform the clinician through which ear the stimulus is better received. In cortical mapping tasks, the patient receives electrode stimulation during surgery to determine areas of cortical activity when a variety of stimuli are given.

Language Testing

Generally speaking, the purpose of assessment of adult language deficits is the same as for children, that is, to determine the patient's strengths and weaknesses, to describe the existing problems, to define "factors that facilitate the comprehension, production, and use of language (Murray & Chapey, 2001, p. 57), and to delineate treatment goals (Murray & Chapey, 2001). In addition, the reader is referred to Chapter 3 for a review of the diagnostic process based on the scientific model to help guide the process of

TABLE 13–4. Specific goals of assessment.

Etiologic Goals

---

1. Determination of the presence or absence of aphasia

2. Identification and definition of complicating conditions that have precipitated or are maintaining the communication impairment to determine if they can be eliminated, reduced, or changed

Cognitive, Linguistic, and Pragmatic Goals

(For each of the following goals, behaviors are analyzed
to specify the nature and extent of the strengths
and weaknesses in that particular behavior)

3. Analysis of cognitive abilities

4. Analysis of the ability to comprehend language content

5. Analysis of the ability to comprehend language form

6. Analysis of the ability to produce language content

7. Analysis of the ability to produce language form

8. Analysis of pragmatic abilities

Treatment Goals

---

9. Determination of candidacy for and prognosis in treatment

10. Specification and prioritization of treatment goals

Source: From "Assessment of Language Disorders in Adults" by L. L. Murray and R. Chapey, pp. 55–126 in *Language Intervention Strategies in Adult Aphasia and Related Communication Disorders* (4th ed.) by R. Chapey (Ed.). © Lippincott, Williams & Wilkins, 2001.

assessing the adult patient with aphasia. Murray and Chapey (2001) outlined ten goals of assessment. These goals are summarized in Table 13–4.

As with all other testing, a critical component is observation of the patient by health-care professionals as well as by the family. In 1989, Lomas and colleagues developed the Communicative Effectiveness Index (CETI). The CETI contains 16 items on which the family member(s) rate the family member who has had a stroke. They judge these items on a scale ranging from "not at all able" to "as able as before the stroke." A listing of these 16 items can be found in Table 13–5.

It is also important to observe the patient interacting with family members in natural settings such as mealtime at home. This enables the clinician to document possible strategies the family members may be able to use to facilitate interaction and communication. Murray and Chapey (2001) also advocate the use of moderately structured observations that incorporate the use of

TABLE 13–5. The sixteen items of the Communication Effectiveness Index (CETI).

Please rate _____'s performance for that particular communication situation.

1. Getting somebody's attention.
2. Getting involved in group conversations that are about him or her.
3. Giving yes and no answers appropriately.
4. Communicating his or her emotions.
5. Indicating that he or she understands what is being said to him or her.
6. Having coffee-time visits and conversations with friends and neighbors (around the bedside or at home).
7. Having a one-to-one conversation with you.
8. Saying the name of someone whose face is in front of him or her.
9. Communicating physical problems such as aches and pains.
10. Having a spontaneous conversation (i.e., starting the conversation and/or changing the subject).
11. Responding to or communicating anything (including yes or no) without words.
12. Starting a conversation with people who are not close family.
13. Understanding writing.
14. Being part of a conversation when it is fast and there are a number of people involved.
15. Participating in a conversation with strangers.
16. Describing or discussing something in depth.

Source: From Lomas, J., Pickard, L., Bester, S., Elbard, H., Finlayson, A., and Zoghaib, C. (1989). "The Communicative Effectiveness Index: Development and Psychometric Evaluation of a Functional Communication Measure for Adult Aphasia." *Journal of Speech and Hearing Disorders, 54,* pp. 113–124. Reprinted by permission. Copyright 1989, the American Speech-Langauge-Hearing Association.

predetermined questions and scenarios such as "ordering in a restaurant and paying the bill" and asking the patient "How do you make a cake?". Furthermore, highly structured observations such as bedside screening tests can be used to form an initial impression of the patient's abilities. Typically, screening tests are relatively short because the patient's stamina may be compromised. Examples of aphasia screening tests that are standardized include the Aphasia Language Performance Scales (ALPS) by Keenan and Brassell (1975). There is a screening version of the Porch Index of Communicative Ability (SPICA) developed by Holtzapple and colleagues in 1989, and the Minnesota Test for Differential Diagnosis of Aphasia (Powell et al., 1980). More recent screening tests include the Quick Assessment for Aphasia (Tanner & Culbertson, 1999), and the Frenchay Aphasia Screening Test (Enderby et al., 1987; Enderby & Crow, 1996).

TABLE 13–6. Criteria for test selection.

Does the test provide information that cannot be obtained by interviewing or by less structured observation?

Is it possible to convey the instructions without lengthy and complicated explanations?

Is the test relatively easy to administer and score?

Is the test economical in terms of the client's time and energy?

Are the theoretical constructs upon which the test is constructed congruent with the examiner's beliefs?

Does the test permit objective scoring?

Will the test actually make a difference in setting the goals and objectives for therapy?

Does the test violate the client's integrity?

Does the diagnostic tool permit the development of clearly defined and reportable concepts regarding the client and his or her communication disability?

Does the test yield clinically relevant descriptive information about the person's problem?

Is the test reliable?

Is the test valid?

In what manner was the test standardized?

Source: Adapted from *Diagnosis and Evaluation in Speech Pathology* by L. L. Emerick and W. O. Haynes, 1986, Englewood Cliffs, NJ: Prentice Hall. Copyright 1986 by Prentice Hall.

Criteria for test selection are outlined in Table 13–6. It is critical to address these questions in addition to such obvious criteria as the purposes of the evaluation and the amount of time available. The nature of the client's presenting problem, the client's age and level of intelligence, the constraints of the setting, and the diagnostician's training, also are important issues to address when selecting the tests to be used in assessing adult language disorders.

Four primary features are used for differential diagnosis of aphasia: (1) naming, (2) conversational speech, (3) auditory comprehension, and (4) word or sentence repetition. The first step in differential diagnosis is to establish the presence of **anomia**, which is the absence of the ability to name familiar objects and people. If anomia is not present, the patient does not have aphasia. Thus, anomia is a hallmark symptom of aphasia.

Anomia. Lack of the ability to recall names of people, common objects, and places.

Naming

When checking the patient's naming abilities, the clinician must consider word frequency, the semantic category, and the nature of the task. The patient may do more poorly on less commonly used words than on more familiar words, although he or she will probably struggle to some degree with both familiar and unfamiliar words. With regard to semantic category, the categories of words that present difficulty for the patient should be documented. For example, the clinician should note whether the patient has more difficulty with verbs than with nouns.

The nature of the task also is important. Naming can be assessed using confrontational naming and free recall. In confrontational naming, the patient is shown a series of objects or pictures and asked to provide the name of the object or picture. In free recall, the patient is asked to list members of a specific category, usually under a time limit, as for example the names of all the animals the patient can think of in 60 seconds.

Word Fluency

Paraphasia. The unintentional substitution of an incorrect word for an intended word.

Word fluency in conversational speech can be assessed during informal interactions with the patient. The clinician should note whether or not the patient has difficulty initiating speech. This difficulty is typical of a nonfluent aphasia. Another aspect of word fluency is the analysis of the patient's use of paraphasias. A **paraphasia** is the unintended substitution of one word for another. Paraphasia can be phonemic, semantic, or neologistic. In phonemic paraphasias, the patient substitutes a sound for another sound in a word ("stoon" for "spoon"). In semantic paraphasias, the patient substitutes one categorically related word for another. Using the same example as before, instead of saying "spoon," the patient may give a semantically related word, such as "fork" or "knife." Neologisms are invented words that the patient creates and uses in place of the target word. Again, using the spoon as an example, a patient may call it a "stumple"—an invented word to represent "spoon."

Spontaneous speech should be analyzed further to determine if it is more or less fluent across topics, tasks, contexts, and conversational partners. Simmons-Mackie (1997) writes that

> information on language competence can be derived from partially structured tasks, such as picture descriptions, question-answer formats, barrier activities (i.e., describing a picture or object not visible to the listener), narratives (i.e., describing an event), or role-playing, while samples of genuine social communication provide data on the types and success of communication strategies used, methods of repair, effects of context, ability to initiate and terminate conversations, and strategies for maintaining the flow of interaction. (p. 74)

Auditory Comprehension

Auditory comprehension should be tested initially using single word identification. In this task, the clinician asks the patient to respond with single

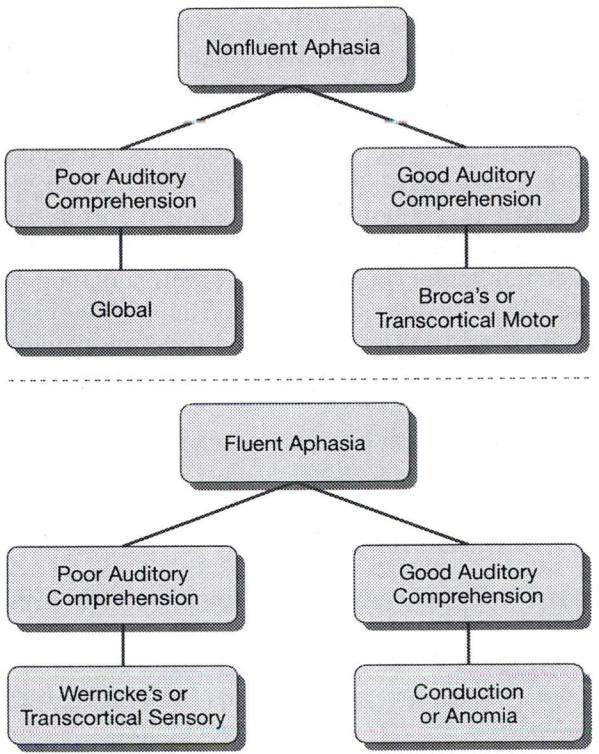

FIGURE 13–2. Diagnosis based on auditory comprehension.

words to identify or describe an object, a picture, or an action. A second task is to have the patient follow simple commands. Finally, the patient should be asked a series of questions. These questions should explore four different types of interactions. The first set of questions should relate to personal information. For example, the patient may be asked to tell the clinician his or her name and address. The next set of questions should relate to impersonal questions such as, "Is it raining outside today?" or "Who is President of the United States?" Third, the clinician should ask questions related to well-known stories such as "Little Red Riding Hood" or "The Three Little Pigs." Finally, the clinician should ask about more obscure facts, such as "Who was the first person to walk on the moon?"

The relationship between performance on auditory comprehension tasks and the diagnostic label is diagrammed in Figure 13–2.

Repetition Skills

Just as the difficulty of the questions is increased systematically, so should the content of the repetition tasks. The single words used in the initial testing of repetition skills should be selected from a wide variety of semantic categories. The words should progress from single to multi-syllabic words and from simple to complex words with regard to their phonetic content. Initially, the clinician should ask the patient to repeat words that are used frequently, then low frequency words. The clinician should then use emotional words (e.g., happy, home, sad, angry) and neutral words (e.g., car, weather). After assessing the patient's repetition skills at the single word level, the clinician should have the patient repeat phrases and sentences. These phrases should include short, common phrases, such as "Sit down," and longer everyday sentences, such as, "Go to the store and buy some milk." After using the familiar phrases and sentences, the clinician should have the patient repeat short unfamiliar phrases followed by long unfamiliar phrases.

The relationship between performance on repetition tasks and the diagnostic label is diagrammed in Figure 13–3.

Standardized Assessment Tools

Several diagnostic tools are available in this field. The Western Aphasia Battery (WAB) (Kertesz, 1982) provides a profile of the various aphasia syndromes based on specific test scores. It also provides summary scores the clinician can use to track the patient's progress. The WAB consists of two main sections, the oral section, and the visual language section, along with optional subtests assessing nonverbal skills. Naming, repetition, auditory comprehension, and spontaneous speech (both fluency and content) are assessed on the oral section. The visual language section consists of subtests assessing reading, writing, praxis, and calculation skills. The WAB yields three scores. The aphasia quotient (AQ), measures the degree of language impairment and is scored based on the oral section. The cortical quotient (CQ) is a "summary score of the cognitive functions measured by the entire WAB. The scores from all WAB subtests are factored into the calculation of the CQ" (Kearns, 1997, p. 21). The language quotient (LQ) is based on all of the language subtests in addition to the reading and writing subtests.

The Boston Diagnostic Aphasia Examination (BDAE) (Goodglass, Kaplan, & Barresi, 2001) also profiles aphasia syndromes. The test battery consists of 27 subtests used to assess auditory comprehension, conversational speech, expository speech, reading comprehension, oral expression, and writing. There are also some supplementary nonlanguage and language tasks that can be administered at the clinician's discretion. The BDAE has a Rating Scale of Speech Characteristics that is used to rate the patient's speech characteristics, auditory comprehension, and repetition abilities. It also has an Aphasia Severity Rating Scale that ranges from 0 ("no usable speech or auditory comprehension") to 5 "minimal discernible speech handicaps; patient may have subjective difficulties that are not apparent to listener" (Goodglass et al., 2001). The newest version also assesses the patient's narrative speech, reading

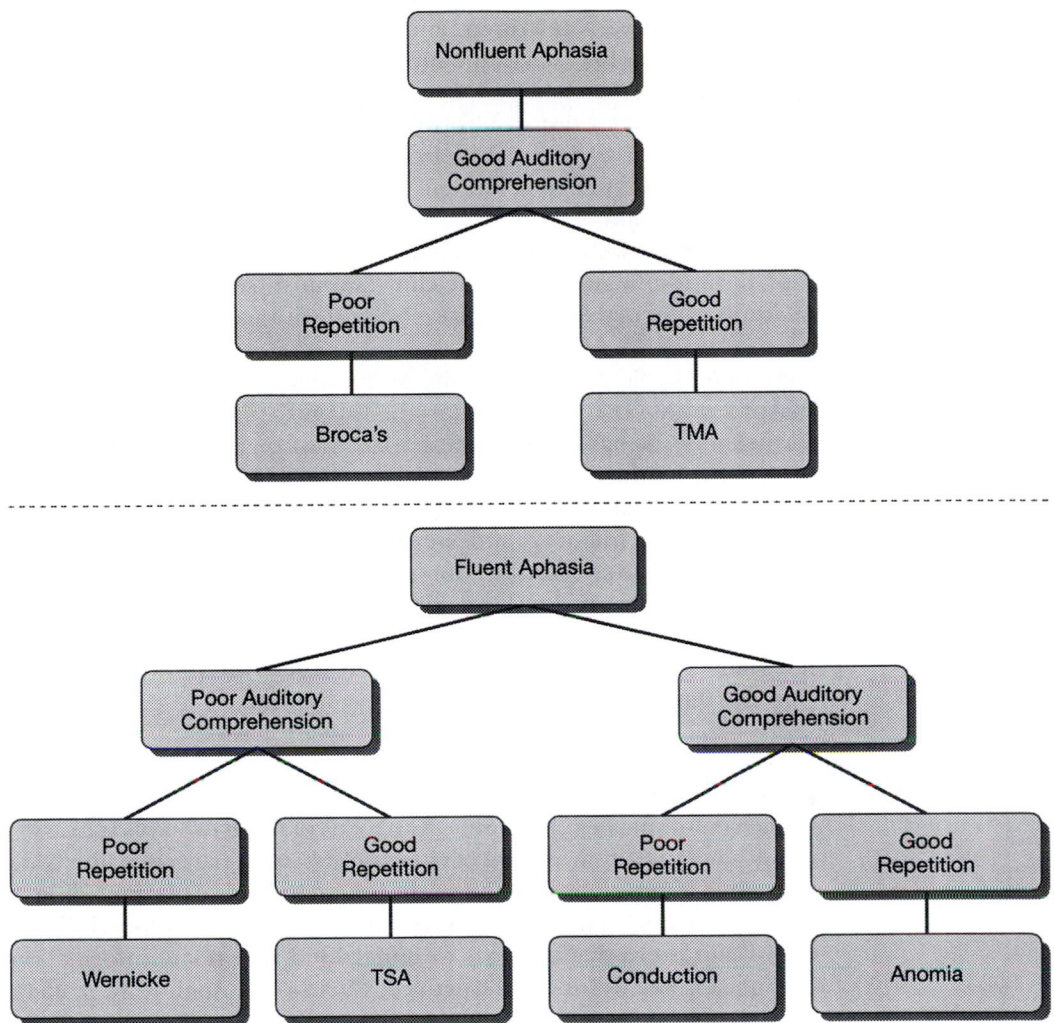

TMA = Transcortical Motor Aphasia
TSA = Transcortical Sensory Aphasia

FIGURE 13–3. Diagnosis based on repetition tests.

skills, category-specific word comprehension, and syntax comprehension. In addition, there is a short form of the BDAE in this latest version.

The Boston Naming Test (Kaplan, Goodglass, & Weintraub, 1983) has long been a staple for the assessment of naming abilities.

The Porch Index of Communicative Ability (PICA) (Porch, 1981) attempts to quantify a prediction for recovery. It consists of 18 subtests that permit a comparison of verbal, written, and gestural language. It uses the same 10 common objects for each of the subtests. These objects are a cigarette, comb, fork, key, knife, matches, pen, pencil, quarter, and toothbrush. "The PICA is best described as a test of information processing in which the systematic manipulation of tasks reveals deficits at various levels of processing and degrees of severity" (Tsing & McNeil, 1997, p. 184). As a side note, there is also a pediatric version of the PICA known as the Porch Index of Communicative Ability for Children (PICAC). While the PICA is a very useful assessment tool, it should be noted that the clinician must participate in approximately 40 hours of formal training before using it with patients.

Developed by Schuell (1965), the Minnesota Test of Differential Diagnosis of Aphasia (MTDDA) also profiles the various aphasia syndromes including, for example, aphasia with visual impairment or aphasia with sensorimotor involvement (Murray & Chapey, 2001). The MTDDA consists of 46 subtests, most of which are based on plus/minus scoring. They cover written language, reading, listening, and speaking. There is also a severity rating scale (0–6) that provides quantification of the patient's performance on the four areas of language previously mentioned. Like the PICA, the MTDDA can also be used to predict the patient's recovery based on guidelines provided in the test manual by Schuell. The Revised Token Test by McNeil and Prescott (1978) provides information on auditory comprehension.

Two tests, the Communicative Ability in Daily Living (CADL) (Holland, 1980) and the Functional Communication Profile (Sarno, 1969) assess how an individual communicates in daily life. The focus of these two tests is to assess communication in daily living, not language accuracy. In particular, the CADL tests a variety of linguistic and nonlinguistic pragmatic behaviors, including "speech acts, humor and metaphor, numeric estimates and calculations, integration of verbal and nonverbal contexts to understand and relate information, role-playing, and the use of social language" (Newhoff & Apel, 1997, p. 258).

The Functional Assessment of Communicative Skills for Adults (ASHA FACS) is a tool for measuring aphasia that has been validated on patients with aphasia as well as patients with head trauma (Frattali et al., 1995). Covering a wide variety of domains, the ASHA-FACS can be used to track the progress a patient is making over time.

The Communication Profile: A Functional Skills Survey (Payne, 1994) is an interview-based protocol in which the patient is asked to rate 26 communication behaviors as to their importance in his or her daily life. The behaviors cover social and health-related behaviors. The subjects in the normative sample represent a wide variety of occupations, ethnic groups, income levels, and living situations.

Another test that is on the market is the Reading Comprehension Battery for Aphasia-2. Developed by LaPointe and Horner, this test provides a "systematic evaluation of the nature and degree of reading impairment in adolescents and adults with aphasia" (LaPointe & Horner, 1998, p. 1). The test utilizes silent reading on all of its subsets to measure comprehension.

It should be noted that the clinician is not limited to the use of tests dedicated to aphasia. These tests can be augmented with information from assessments designed to assess other language functions. A table showing these tests can be found in Table 13–7.

TABLE 13–7. Tests of specific language functions that may be used to augment or replace comprehensive aphasia batteries.

Language Function	Instrument	Source
Auditory Comprehension	Auditory Comprehension Test for Sentences	Shewan (1979)
	Functional Auditory Comprehension Task	LaPointe & Horner (1978)
	Discourse Comprehension Test	Brookshire & Nicholas (1997)
	Peabody Picture Vocabulary Test-3	Dunn & Dunn (1997)
	Psycholinguistic Assessments of Language Processing in Aphasia	Kay et al. (1997)
	Pyramids and Palm Trees	Howard & Patterson (1992)
	Revised Token Test	McNeil & Prescott (1978)
	Test for Reception of Grammar	Bishop (1983)
Verbal Expression	Action Naming Test	Obler & Albert (1979)
Naming	Boston Naming Test	Kaplan et al. (1983)
	Comprehensive Receptive and Expressive Vocabulary Test-Adult	Wallace & Hammill (1997)
	Controlled Oral Word Association Test	Benton et al. (1994)
	Object Naming Test	Newcombe et al. (1971)
	Psycholinguistic Assessments of Language Processing in Aphasia	Kay et al. (1997)
	Test of Adolescent and Adult Word-Finding	German (1990)
	The Naming Test	Williams (1996)
	The Word Test-Adolescent	Zachman et al. (1989)

(continued)

TABLE 13–7. (*continued*)

Language Function	Instrument	Source
Syntax	Northwestern Syntax Screening Test	Lee (1971)
	Shewan Spontaneous Language Analysis	Shewan (1988a, 1988b)
	The Reporter's Test	DeRenzi & Ferrari (1978)
Reading Comprehension	Gray Oral Reading Tests-3	Wiederholt & Bryant (1992)
	Johns Hopkins University Dyslexia Battery	Goodman & Caramazza (1986b)
	Peabody Individual Achievement Test-Revised	Markwardt (1988)
	Psycholinguistic Assessments of Language Processing in Aphasia	Kay et al. (1997)
	Nelson Reading Skills Test	Hanna et al. (1977)
	New Adult Reading Test	Nelson (1984)
	Reading Comprehension Battery for Aphasia-2	LaPointe & Horner (1998)
	Test of Reading Comprehension-3	Brown et al. (1995)
	Wide Range Achievement Test-3	Wilkinson (1993)
Writing	Johns Hopkins University Dysgraphia Battery	Goodman & Caramazza (1986a)
	Psycholinguistic Assessments of Language Processing in Aphasia	Kay et al. (1997)
	Test of Written Language-3	Hammill & Larson (1996)
	Thurstone Word Fluency Test	Thurstone & Thurstone (1962)
	Wide Range Achievement Test-3	Wilkinson (1993)
	Writing Process Test	Warden & Hutchinson (1993)
	Written Language Assessment	Grill & Kirwin (1989)
Gesture	Assessment of Nonverbal Communication	Duffy & Duffy (1984)
	Pantomime Recognition Test	Benton et al. (1993)
	Test of Oral and Limb Apraxia	Helm-Estabrooks (1991)

Source: From "Assessment of Language Disorders in Adults" by L. L. Murray and R. Chapey, pp. 55–126, in *Language Intervention Strategies in Adult Aphasia and Related Communication Disorders* (4th ed.), by R. Chapey (Ed.). © Lippincott, Williams & Wilkins, 2001.

■ APHASIA SYNDROMES

Subcortical Aphasias

The "subcortical" syndromes include (1) anterior capsular or putaminal aphasia; (2) posterior capsular or putaminal aphasia; (3) global capsular or putaminal aphasia; and (4) thalamic aphasia. The subcortical syndromes of aphasia are evaluated using the same four primary diagnostic categories in delineating the "cortical" aphasias. However, additional categories include verbal agility, nonverbal agility, and the presence of **hemiplegia** or **hemiparesis**. Most subcortical aphasias are believed to be due to "lesions in or surrounding the left basal ganglia or the left thalamus" (Hegde, 1994, p. 148).

Hemiplegia. The paralysis of either the right or left side of the body.

Hemiparesis. Weakness or incomplete paralysis on the right or left side of the body.

Fluent Cortical Aphasias

The first step in the diagnostic process is to determine the presence of anomia. The second task is to determine if the patient has signs or symptoms of a fluent aphasia, or a nonfluent aphasia. A comparison chart is found in Table 13–8.

Fluent Cortical Aphasias

The three fluent aphasias that will be discussed in this chapter are Wernicke's aphasia, conduction aphasia, and transcortical sensory aphasia. A chart comparing the primary diagnostic categories of these three primary fluent aphasias is found in Table 13–9.

TABLE 13–8. A comparison of fluent and nonfluent aphasias.

Fluent Aphasias	Nonfluent Aphasias
Voice onset time not impaired	Voice onset time often impaired
Phonemic substitutions used that differ by more than one feature	Phonemic substitutions usually differ from the target by a single feature
Many substitutions and additions of sounds	Timing errors or transition errors in speech
Transposition and sequencing errors	Prevalence of substitutions
Errors tend to be more toward the end of the word	Use of intrusive vowels and prolongations
Errors on vowels and consonants	Errors tend to be at the beginning of the words
	Primarily errors on consonants

TABLE 13–9. A comparison of the three primary fluent aphasias.

Diagnostic Entity	Wernicke's Aphasia	Conduction Aphasia	Transcortical Sensory Aphasia
Spontaneous speech	Fluent, but pauses for word retrieval; press of speech; lacks content; jargon; monologue-like	Fluent, but frequent use of inappropriate words; good intonation	Fluent; discourse incoherent and circumlocutory; lacks content; uses stereotypical phrases
Articulation	Good	Good	Good
Auditory comprehension	Poor to severely impaired	Good	Poor
Reading comprehension	Poor	Good	Poor
Naming	Poor; neologisms	Very poor	Very poor; produces long, unrelated sentences
Writing	Mechanically good but lacks content	Poor to dictation but good volitionally	Poor
Grammaticism	Word strings empty of content but syntactically correct	No problem	Word strings empty of content but syntactically correct
Error awareness	Little to none	Yes	Little to none
Echolalia	Doubtful	No	Present
Paraphasias	Semantic	Phonemic	Semantic or neologistic
Repetitions	Poor due to decreased auditory comprehension	Very poor	Good
Visual disturbances	Possibly	Variable	Frequently
Reading aloud	Poor	Poor	Good
Paralysis or paresis	No	Rare	Rare; mild if occurs

Sources: From Aronson (1991), Benson (1979), Davis (1993), Gonzalez-Rothi (1990), Helm-Estabrooks and Albert (1991), and Rubens (1976).

Wernicke's Aphasia. The lesion in Wernicke's aphasia causes damage to Wernicke's area and neighboring temporal and parietal regions (Figure 13–4) This area centers on the posterior third of the superior temporal gyrus (Helm-Estabrooks & Albert, 1991). When the lesion is in Wernicke's area and the inferior parietal area, fluent speech and phonemic paraphasias predominate. Lesions that occur in the more posterior angular gyrus and

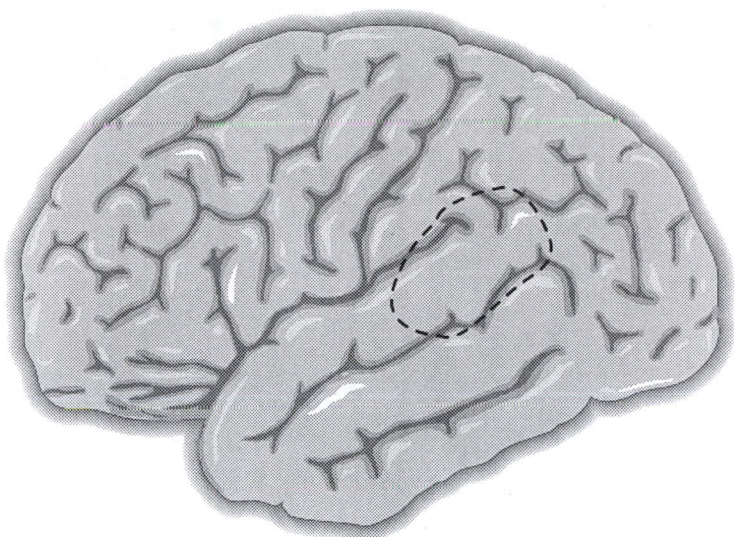

FIGURE 13–4. Location of lesions resulting in Wernicke's aphasia.

occipital area lead the patient to the use of verbal paraphasias, whereas lesions that are even more posterior lead to neologistic jargon.

Researchers and clinicians tend to disagree as to what truly constitutes Wernicke's aphasia and whether it really exists! Wertz (1986) wrote, "While we may not agree on what to call it, we seem to recognize it when we see it. This is fortunate, since we see a lot of it" (p. 767). With regard to diagnosis, there are a wide variety of aphasia tests which have been described previously in this chapter. Auditory comprehension is the most affected area in Wernicke's aphasia, so it should be assessed thoroughly (Graham-Keegan & Caspari, 1997). In addition to the previously described test, the Functional Auditory Comprehension Test (FACT; LaPointe & Horner, 1978) and the Revised Token Test (McNeil & Prescott, 1978) can be used to assess auditory comprehension. In measuring the relationship between these two tests and the CADL, LaPointe, Holtzapple, and Graham report that the FACT correlates highly with the CADL (Holland, 1980), but the Revised Token Test does not. In addition to standardized measures, auditory comprehension should be assessed using natural conversation based on real-life context. The redundancy and somewhat predictable nature of conversation will help the patient with Wernicke's aphasia to comprehend spoken language (Brookshire & Nicholas, 1980, 1982, 1985; Graham-Keegan & Caspari, 1997; Waller & Darley, 1978; Wilcox, Davis, & Leonard, 1978). Reading comprehension and written language should also be assessed although there are limited assessment devices in these areas that are standardized for use with aphasics. Reading,

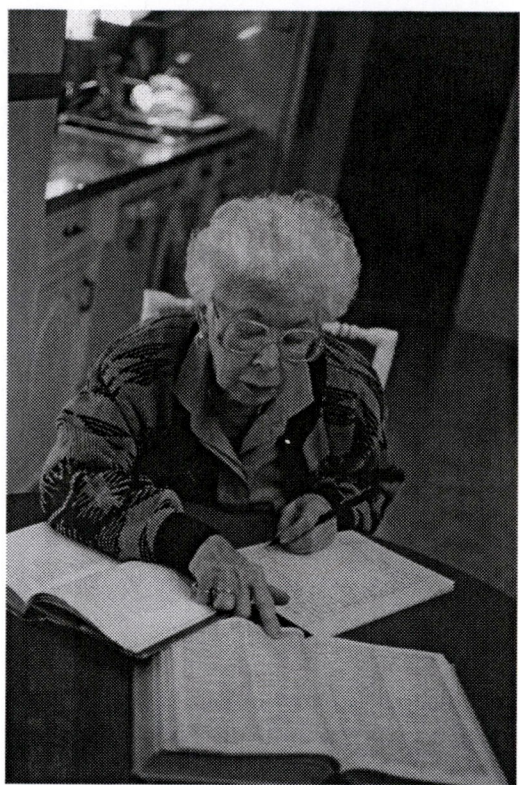

FIGURE 13–5. Because patients with Wernicke's aphasia typically have poor reading comprehension, what was once an enjoyable activity may no longer provide relaxation and pleasure.

while it may have been enjoyed prior to the stroke, may not provide pleasure to an individual with Wernicke's aphasia as depicted in Figure 13–5.

There is evidence that treatment is effective with patients with Wernicke's aphasia in spite of some controversy in the literature as to whether these patients will respond to treatment. A study was done by Weiller and colleagues (1995) who used PET to study activation of the right hemisphere in language tasks undertaken by patients with Wernicke's aphasia. The subjects were six individuals who were medically stable following an infarction that rendered the left posterior perisylvian language area essentially useless and had received speech-language therapy for the resultant aphasia. There were also six controls. All subjects were asked to repeat pseudowords and to generate verbs. Using PET, regional blood flow (rCBF) to the different hemispheres was analyzed. The results indicated that in the controls there was a strong activation of rCBF in both Broca's area and Wernicke's area in the left hemispheres, with very little activation in the right hemisphere. In contrast, the individuals with Wernicke's aphasia had preserved blood flow in the frontal areas of the brain and activation of the rCBF in the right hemisphere in the zones that were analogous to the language areas of the left hemisphere. This provides clear evidence of reorganization of hemispheric function and has implications for treatment of individuals who have left hemisphere damage (Code, 1994; Gainotti, 1995; Graham-Keegan & Caspari, 1997; Weiller et al., 1995)

Goodglass (1993) summarized the symptoms of Wernicke's aphasia as follows:

> Speech output is facile in articulation and sentence structure, tending to be filled with ill chosen words and poorly formed sentences (semantic paraphasia and paragrammatism). In severe cases, speech output consists only of neologistic jargon. Auditory comprehension is defective for the comprehension of common object names—it is even more defective for the comprehension of sentences. Word finding is severely restricted so that free conversation is often circumlocutory and empty. Patients' rate of speech is sometimes excessively rapid and they may be unaware of their many speech output errors. Early in the illness, patients who exhibit this pattern may incorporate words and phrases that are far afield from the presumed topic of conversation. Their output may consist largely of neologisms embedded in pseudogrammatical sentences with grammatical words, noun and verb inflections, providing a semblance of syntactic structure. (pp. 210–211)

With such a wide variety of deficit areas, the decision as to where to begin therapy could be difficult. However, improvement of auditory comprehension and self-monitoring would be the logical "first goals" due to their impact on the patient's ability to participate in other language-based activities. Patients with Wernicke's aphasia are typically not aware of their errors, so they may not understand the need for therapy. Thus, the first goal actually should be to gain the cooperation of the client and set up a reliable response mode. It is also necessary to work out a signal or gesture that the clinician can use to stop the normally verbose patient with Wernicke's aphasia. Since these clients typically demonstrate press of speech, the clinician may have a hard time getting in the instructions and stimuli for a listening task; hence there is a need for some type of signal to cue the patient to stop talking and listen (Graham-Keegan & Caspari, 1997). Marshall (1994) suggested using short and meaningful messages, increasing redundancy, and exaggerating gestures and facial expressions to facilitate auditory comprehension.

Conduction Aphasia. In conduction aphasia, the lesion is in the arcuate fasciculus (the white matter pathways), or the association tracts, that connect Wernicke's and Broca's areas (Helm-Estabrooks & Albert, 1991)

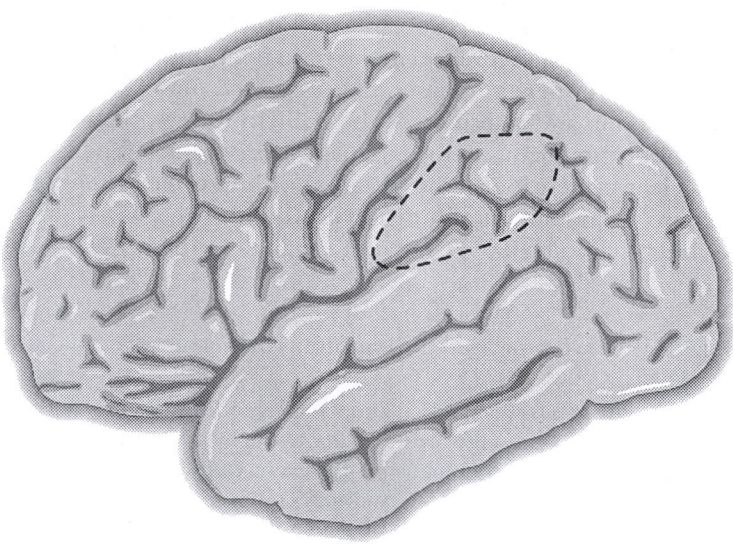

FIGURE 13–6. Location of lesions resulting in conduction aphasia.

(Figure 13–6). Typically damage occurs to the posterior superior temporal cortex and inferior parietal cortex (supramarginal gyrus) with infarction of deep white matter consistent with damage to the arcuate fasciculus. Conduction aphasia is so named because lesions in the arcuate fasciculus interfere with the conduction of the message from Wernicke's area to Broca's area (Geschwind, 1965). Although conduction aphasia is generally thought of as a fluent aphasia, the more anterior the lesion, the less fluent the speech.

The hallmark symptom of conduction aphasia is a significant deficit in verbal repetition, with the repetition being markedly poor when one considers the fluency of the patient's spontaneous speech and relatively intact auditory comprehension. In addition to the poor repetition, phonemic paraphasias are common. The spontaneous speech is not as fluent as that of patients with Wernicke's aphasia, with the speech of those who have conduction aphasia containing hesitations and attempts at self-correction (Goodglass & Kaplan, 1983a). They also have word retrieval deficits, particularly of substantive and content words. Compared to other types of aphasia, the incidence of conduction aphasia is rare, and the prognosis is usually good. "Because of the relatively good auditory comprehension, fairly copious verbal output, and an ability to supplement speech with gestural, melodic and facial information, these patients tend to function well in situations that do not require single-word accuracy or specific responses" (Simmons-Mackie, 1997, p. 71).

When assessing patients with aphasia, repetition is one of the major areas of the evaluation. The repetition items on the Boston Diagnostic Aphasia

Examination (BDAE) and the BDAE Supplementary Language Tests were selected based on conduction aphasia, making these subtests appropriate for the assessment of conduction aphasia. Areas of repetition that are particularly problematic for individuals with conduction aphasia are the repetition of multisyllabic words and lesser known phrases and words. When planning treatment, the clinician should study the impact of prompts and cues on repetition performance by the patient (Simmons-Mackie, 1997). The clinician is advised against using verbal repetition as a deblocking technique to improve word retrieval since "repetition is a primary deficit, it becomes a target of treatment rather than an approach to treatment" (Simmons-Mackie, 1997, p. 79). As with all types of treatment for all types of disorders, functional communication, including social conversation, should be the ultimate goal.

Transcortical Sensory Aphasia. Damage in the parietal-temporal junction area posterior to Wernicke's area is the main lesion in transcortical sensory aphasia (Benson, 1979) (Figure 13–7). Transcortical sensory aphasia strongly resembles Wernicke's aphasia with the exception that the ability to repeat remains intact. In fact, the repetition abilities are quite extraordinary. It is not unusual for global aphasia to resolve into transcortical sensory aphasia. In such cases, the patient initially may experience no comprehension and little or no verbal output. This is followed by a period of jargon replete with numerous neologisms. As the neologistic paraphasias decrease, words and meaningful phrases begin to appear, although they typically have little or no relationship to the clinician's questions or remarks. As the words and

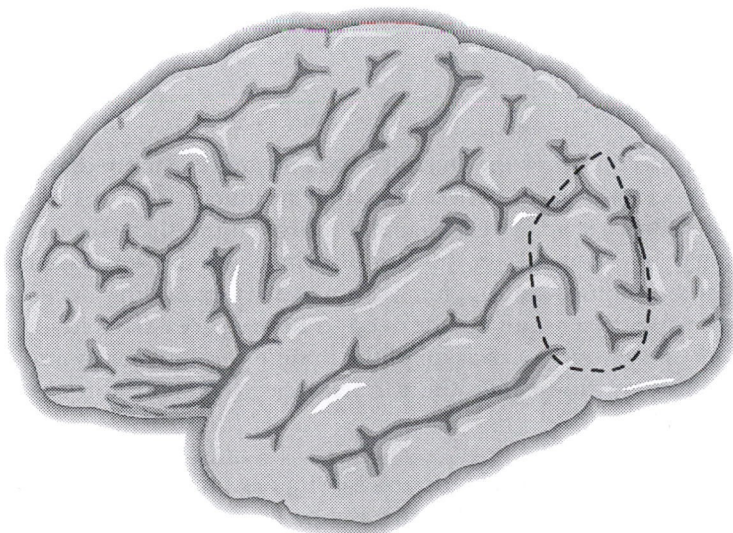

FIGURE 13–7. Location of lesions resulting in transcortical sensory aphasia.

phrases appear, the ability to repeat begins to emerge (Benson, 1979). This repetition ability becomes the hallmark symptom of transcortical sensory aphasia and can be used as a marker to differentiate Wernicke's aphasia from transcortical sensory aphasia.

As in Wernicke's aphasia, patients with transcortical sensory aphasia have limited auditory and visual comprehension of words, and have significant word-finding deficits. They patients can read aloud and repeat long, complex utterances, but they do not understand what is read or repeated (Gonzalez-Rothi, 1997).

The most common etiological factor in transcortical sensory aphasia is vascular disease, with occlusive problems being most causative. Typically, occlusion of the left internal carotid artery leading to infarction in the parietal-temporal junction area underlines transcortical sensory aphasia. Tumors in the same area also can produce transortical sensory aphasia (Benson, 1979).

The prognosis for patients with transcortical sensory aphasia is generally good (Gonzalez-Rothi, 1997).

Nonfluent Cortical Aphasias

Nonfluent aphasias are characterized primarily by the effort and difficulty the patient has in generating spoken language. A chart comparing the primary diagnostic categories of the three primary nonfluent aphasias is found in Table 13–10.

Broca's Aphasia

Broca's area comprises the third frontal convolution immediately anterior to the precentral gyrus. The lesion that produces what is commonly referred to Broca's aphasia is actually much larger than Broca's area. As illustrated in Figure 13–8, it typically "involves the left lateral frontal, prerolandic, suprasylvian region (Broca's area) extending necessarily into the periventricular white matter deep to Broca's area. This lesion is in the territory of the superior division of the middle cerebral artery and often extends posteriorly to include the parietal lobe" (Helm-Estabrooks & Albert, 1991, p. 21).

Broca's aphasia is a nonfluent aphasia that is characterized primarily by telegraphic speech. In other words, the patient omits most function words such as pronouns, auxiliary verbs, conjunctions, articles, and prepositions, making the speech sound like the wording in a telegram. Articulation is

TABLE 13–10. A comparison of the three primary nonfluent aphasias.

Diagnostic Entity	Broca's Aphasia	Global Aphasia	Transcortical Motor Aphasia
Spontaneous speech	Nonfluent; apraxic labored; telegraphic	Nonfluent and infrequent; stereotypic utterances	Nonfluent; decreased verbal output; paucity of speech; difficulty initiating speech
Articulation	Poor; many	Poor (scarce)	Poor
Auditory comprehension	Good	Very poor	Good
Reading comprehension	Usually good	Poor	Good
Naming	Poor	Poor	Poor
Writing	Mechanically poor; content like speech	Poor	Poor; letters are large and clumsily produced
Grammaticism	Agrammatism	Not applicable	Possibly agrammatic; reduced complexity
Error awareness	Yes	Probably not	Probably
Echolalia	Rare	Not likely	Maybe (not a true echolalia because will correct errors in the original statement)
Paraphasias	No	No	No
Repetitions	Mechanically poor	Poor	Excellent
Visual disturbances	No	Possibly	Rare
Reading aloud	Poor	Very poor	Poor
Paralysis or paresis	Yes	Possibly	Probably; often right hemiparesis

Source: From Aronson (1991), Benson (1979), Davis (1993), Gonzalez-Rothi (1990), Helm-Estabrooks and Albert (1991), and Rubens (1976).

inconsistent, even when the same phrase is repeated (Wertz, LaPointe, & Rosenbek, 1984). Since Wernicke's area is undisturbed, the patient with Broca's aphasia understands (for the most part) what is being said to him or her but has difficulty with the motor speech output. It takes effort to talk, and the speech is characterized by pauses that interfere with the fluency of the speech (hence the designation as a nonfluent aphasia). Reading comprehension is similar to auditory comprehension. Confrontation naming and the ability to repeat words and phrases is impaired. Writing is motorically compromised and errors are similar to those found in speech.

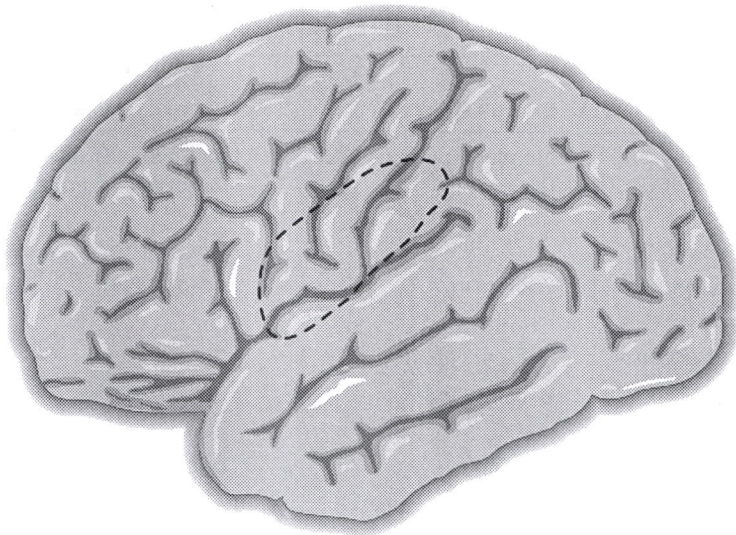

FIGURE 13–8. Location of lesions resulting in Broca's aphasia.

Global Aphasia

Global aphasia is the most devastating and pervasive of all the aphasia syndromes. Collins (1997) defines global aphasia as follows:

> a severe, acquired impairment of communicative ability, which crosses all language modalities, usually with no single communicative modality substantially better than any other. In addition, visual, nonverbal problem-solving abilities, as well as other cognitive skills, are often severely depressed, and are usually compatible with language performance. (pp. 133–134)

The damage in global aphasia is in the perisylvian region (along the sylvian fissure). Language functions around the sylvian fissure including the precentral and postcentral gyri area. CT scans of persons with global aphasia show lesions of the entire perisylvian fissure, including Broca's and Wernicke's areas (Davis, 1993).

Many of these lesions extend deep into the white matter below the cortex (Figure 13–9). The individual with global aphasia will have difficulty understanding speech as well as producing speech. Language functions will be devastated, including reading and auditory comprehension. According to Collins, there are three types of global aphasia. The first one is acute global aphasia in which the patient is still very ill, the aphasia is severe, and functional communication should not be presumed. Evolving aphasia is the term that is used during the patient's recovery as he regains some of his lost

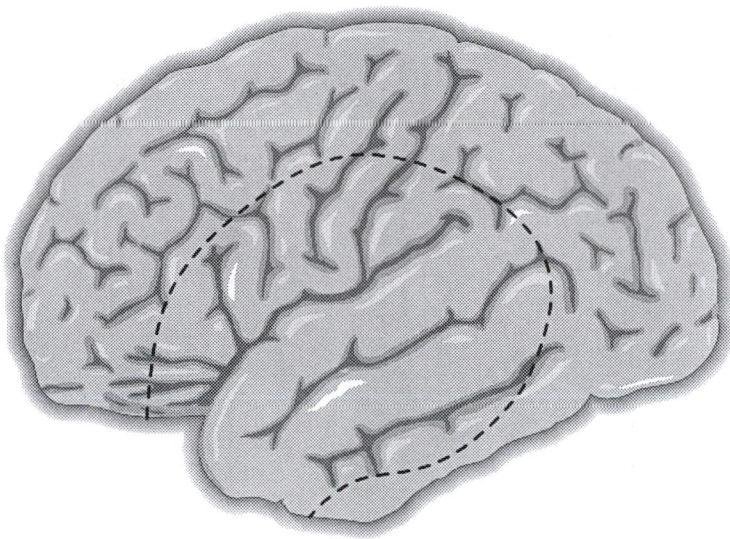

FIGURE 13–9. Location of lesions resulting in global aphasia.

language. In chronic global aphasia, the client is no longer medically or neurologically compromised, usually one week to one month post onset. There is little language, and the aphasia crosses all modalities.

Transcortical Motor Aphasia

Trauma and tumors are more common etiological factors in transcortical motor aphasia than are cerebrovascular disorders. When this type of aphasia is due to a cerebrovascular disorder, typically an intercerebral hematoma is the causative agent. Occlusion of the dominant anterior cerebral artery that results in medialfrontal damage also produces transcortical motor aphasia (DeMasio & Kassel, 1978; Rubens, 1976). The lesion in transcortical motor aphasia is located in the border zones of the perisylvian area, usually in the region of the brain that is anterior or superior to Broca'a area (Benson, 1979) (Figure 13–10). Both Broca's aphasia and transcortical motor aphasia are considered nonfluent aphasias, with some signs of dysarthria in both. However, in transcortical motor aphasia, the spontaneous speech resembles stuttering more than does the spontaneous speech in Broca's aphasia (Benson, 1979). Benson reports that many individuals with transcortical motor aphasia will have trouble initiating speech but will be able to complete a sentence or list once it has been started by someone else. For example, if asked to count, the patient may have difficulty saying "One." However, once the clinician gives the patient the first one or two numbers, the patient will be able to pick up on the series and complete it without further difficulty. Similarly, if the clinician starts a nursery rhyme or a common poem, the patient will be able to complete it almost

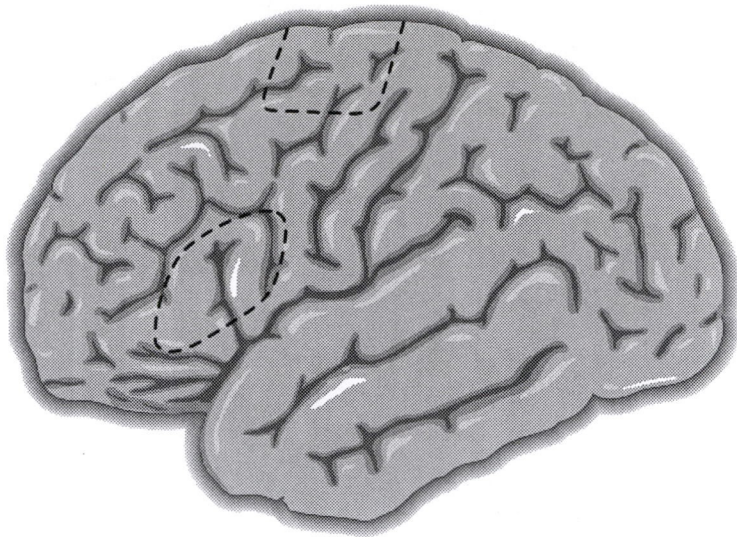

FIGURE 13–10. Location of lesions resulting in transcortical motor aphasia.

automatically. The patient with transcortical motor aphasia also will tend to have better reading comprehension than the patient with Broca's aphasia.

As in transcortical sensory aphasia, repetition is remarkably intact in patient with transcortical motor aphasia. A patient with transcortical motor aphasia will typically present with all or some of the characteristics of their nonfluency, including reduced quantity of speech, an absence of elaboration and variety of output, reduced complexity of sentences, and a lack of motoric precision when verbalizing (Gonzalez-Rothi, 1997).

Other nonlanguage symptoms frequently seen in patients with transcortical motor aphasia who have superior premotor involvement include rigidity of the upper extremity, transient urinary incontinence, and hemiparesis of the left leg (worse in leg than in arm) (Bogousslavsky & Regli, 1990). Those patients with lesions in the supplemental motor area may exhibit mutism that rapidly evolves into transcortical motor aphasia, akinesia, bradykinesia, and bilateral ideomotor apraxia (Watson et al., 1986).

Evaluation of patients with suspected transcortical motor aphasia should include a comparison of spontaneous speech with repetition tasks. In these patients, the speech associated with repetition tasks will be superior to that demonstrated in spontaneous speech. The repetition tasks should move from single words to sentences consisting of up to 10 words. The repetition will typically break down as complexity and length increases as well as with the use of less familiar words. After comparing speech in spontaneous and repetition tasks, the clinician should assess comprehension of auditory and orthographic information using any of the tests previously described. Finally, word fluency should be assessed by having the patient name all the words beginning with a letter specified by the clinician that he can think of in 60 seconds. This will typically be deficient when compared to naming words associated with a specific semantic category which remains relatively intact (Gonzalez-Rothi, 1997).

It has been suggested that treatment should focus on restoring motor function. With regard to language, there is little evidence that traditional language and speech therapy is effective with these patients, particularly the use of repetition and verbal cueing techniques (Alexander & Schmitt, 1980). Other researchers (Luria & Tsvetkova, 1968; Luria, 1977) have suggested substitutive strategies such as reorganization and relying on the right hemisphere to take over for the damaged left hemisphere.

Generally speaking, the prognosis for patients with transcortical motor aphasia is good (Gonzalez-Rothi, 1997).

Primary Progressive Aphasia (PPA)

PPA "is a clinical syndrome in which patients suffer progressive language deterioration despite unidentifiable stroke, tumor, infection, or metabolic disease and relative preservation of cognition and independence in activities of daily living" (Murray & Chapey, 2001, p. 71). Some argue that PPA cannot be differentiated from generalized dementias, while others maintain that it is a separate diagnosis based on the typical etiology and course of the disease. Patients with PPA usually have deficits in auditory comprehension, word-finding, and repetition. There are some studies (Westbury & Bub, 1997) showing that reading and writing skills stay intact for a substantial amount of time beyond the initial onset. McNeil and Duffy (2001) write that "aphasia can announce the presence of degenerative neurologic disease, and that is may be the only manifestation of the central nervous system for a substantial period of time or perpetually" (p. 472).

PPA is unlike other aphasias in that it is of slow onset, is gradually progressive, and does not initially affect nonlanguage computational abilities as may be seen in other aphasias. It may evolve into a dementia. In the initial stages, "PPA is a clinical syndrome and not a reflection of a particular underlying brain pathology" (McNeil & Duffy, 2001, p. 473). In fact, the neuropathology of PPA is unknown.

The following diagnostic criteria must be met for a diagnosis of PPA:

1. History of language decline for at least two years.
2. Preservation of most mental functions in the presence of marked language deficits.

3. Ability to independently perform activities of daily living.

4. No identified neurological insult such as a stroke, infection, or tumor.

5. Performance on neuropsychological and speech-language tests indicating language deficits (McNeil & Duffy, 2001).

Westbury and Bub (1997) found that the most frequently reported initial complaint is problems with word finding. The patients are aware of their deficits. Other than word finding, they do not complain of memory deficits. Unlike those with dementia, these patients do not typically undergo the personality changes, although they do express frustration due to their word-finding problems.

Patients with PPA may present with additional deficits, including nonverbal oral apraxia, weakness, and/or clumsiness in the extremities, verbal apraxia, dysarthria, dysphagia, and possibly limb apraxia. Neurologically, there is usually a progressive degeneration in the "language dominant perisylvian region of the brain" (McNeil & Duffy, 2001, p. 483). The neurological studies indicate left-hemisphere abnormalities. When abnormalities affect the right and left hemispheres, the deficits are greater in the left hemisphere. The initial presentation is different from Alzheimer's disease and other degenerative conditions in which the patient experiences cognitive decline in addition to the language deficits. It more closely resembles a stroke-induced language deficit but differs from stroke-induced aphasia with regard to time progression. Stroke produces immediate effects that often improve over time. PPA, as stated earlier, has an insidious onset over a two-year period (McNeil & Duffy, 2001).

Therapy should focus on the development of compensatory strategies, and include training on augmentative and alternative communication devices if apraxia of speech emerges (McNeill & Duffy, 2001).

■ RECOVERY AND GENERAL TREATMENT STRATEGIES

Many factors affect how well an individual will recover from a stroke or traumatic brain injury. General characteristics include the patient's age and general health and his or her physical condition prior to the onset. The younger a person is, the more likely he or she is to recover with few side effects and long-term sequelae. However, just as important as age, and perhaps more so, is the patient's general health and physical status. The healthier an individual is, regardless of his age, the better the likelihood of a good outcome after a catastrophic event. Other factors include the client's motivation, how the client dealt with challenges pre-onset, level of education, problem-solving skills, and prestroke intelligence (Holland et al., 1996). The extent and location of the brain damage certainly are major factors to consider, as are the quality and immediacy of the medical care received after onset.

Controversy exists regarding when to begin therapy. Some studies (Sarno, Silverman, & Sands, 1970; Sarno & Levita, 1971) determined that some patients benefited more from treatment provided several months after the event as opposed to immediate treatment. Wertz and colleagues (1986) delayed treatment for one of their therapy groups until three months postonset. Those patients did not demonstrate any negative effects from waiting to begin therapy. Several techniques for therapy have been developed to provide therapy for patients with chronic aphasia. These are outlined in Table 13–11.

TABLE 13–11. Representative treatment techniques.

General approaches to aphasia treatment

Traditional modality specific stimulus-response treatment: Wertz et al., 1981; Wertz et al., 1986

Language oriented therapy (LOT): Shewan & Kertesz, 1984; Shewan & Bandur, 1986

Group therapy: Springer, 1991

*Linguistic-specific treatment: Thompson, Shapiro, & Roberts, 1993

*Functional communication therapy: Aten, Caliguiri, & Holland, 1982.

*PACE: Davis & Wilcox, 1985; Springer, 1991

Augmentation approaches: Beukelman, Yorkston, & Dowden, 1985

*Cognitive neuropsychology approaches: Byng, 1988; Fink et al., 1993

*Programmer instructional approaches: Holland, 1970

Computerized approaches—Steele et al., 1989; Katz & Wertz, 1992.

Specific techniques of treatment

---

*Treating aphasic perseveration (TAP): Helm-Estabrooks, Emery, & Albert, 1987

*Melodic intonation therapy (MIT): Sparks, Helm, & Albert, 1974

*Visual action therapy (VAT): Helm-Estabrooks, Fitzpatrick, & Barressi, 1982

Response elaboration training: Kearns, 1985

Auditory comprehension training: Marshall & Neuburger, 1984

*Self-monitoring: Whitney & Goldstein, 1989

---

*Developed on patient's past spontaneous recovery period.

Source: "Treatment Efficacy in Aphasia," by A. Holland, D. Fromm, F. DeRuyter, and M. Stein. In *Journal of Speech and Hearing Research, 39*(5), October 1996, pp. 527–536. © ASHA, 1996. Reprinted by permission.

Determining if the Patient Is a Candidate for Therapy

If a patient has complicating medical conditions that interfere with rehabilitation, he or she should not be a candidate for therapy until the medical conditions are resolved or stabilized. Other problems such as severe confusion or dementia also make the patient a poor candidate for rehabilitation.

Degree of Aphasia

The degree and type of aphasia are related to the severity of the event and the extent of the brain damage incurred. The patient's status may change daily in the first few weeks as swelling reduces and injured brain cells begin to function. Therefore, it is not clinically smart to make a formal diagnosis in the first two weeks after onset. Once the patient's condition is medically stable, more extensive testing can be done to determine the patient's abilities and weaknesses and then to design an appropriate treatment plan.

Selection of Treatment Goals and Procedures

As mentioned previously, a thorough assessment of the patient's strengths and weaknesses needs to be done prior to initiating therapy. Another consideration in the selection of treatment goals is the ability of family to follow through with treatment. If the patient's spouse is in ill health and their children are not living nearby, there is little likelihood that the treatment goals will be followed through at home. Thus, the clinician needs to determine which goals are the most functional and easily attainable in therapy and also to determine whether or not there are other individuals who may be assisting the patient when he or she returns home.

Spontaneous Recovery

The clinician needs to make a decision as to whether to use therapy techniques that focus on the substitution or the restitution of function. Many studies are being done that focus on treatment efficacy in the area of aphasia treatment and recovery. With limits placed on clinicians with regard to length and frequency of therapy sessions, the clinician must utilize therapy time to the best of his or her ability to restore communicative function to the patient.

The most rapid recovery occurs during the first two months after onset, although spontaneous recovery can take up to six months or longer. During this process, one type of aphasia can evolve into another type. For example, global aphasia may evolve into any of the other types of cortical aphasias. The clinician needs to keep this in mind when selecting treatment procedures.

Spontaneous recovery refers to the natural resolution of impairments. It can last up to several months or only a few weeks. Aphasia is at its worst in the early weeks after onset, and the patient may get some natural return of his or her functions as the swelling recedes and his or her condition becomes more stable medically. Auditory comprehension typically shows the quickest and most dramatic improvement. When allowing spontaneous recovery to run its course, the clinician is ascribing to the "theory of restitution of function," which states that recovery is a physiological process. However, ascribing to the theory of restitution of function also dictates that recovery is time-constrained.

Assisted Recovery

The biggest question that faces a clinician working with patients with aphasia is when to begin treatment. Some clinicians prefer to intervene as soon as the patient's condition is medically stable; others wait until they believe that all spontaneous recovery has run its course although this may be difficult to determine. Still others believe that it is best to treat the patient when he or she is showing improvement.

The second decision that faces the clinician is the issue of what treatment to use. All clinicians agree that the best approaches are those that are implemented using a team approach. The team members were of critical importance in the diagnostic phase, but interaction between the disciplines is even more crucial in the treatment phase. It must be remembered that the most important members of the team are the patient and his or her caregivers. Many times, family members are forced into new roles as the result of a spouse or parent having aphasia. Thus, treatment may need to include helping the family members adapt to their new responsibilities as well as helping the patient to recover language and communication functions.

When the clinician provides assisted recovery, he or she ascribes to the "theory of substitution of function," which assumes that improvement results from system reorganization or compensation. This approach permits treatment as long as learning potential is present (Gonzalez-Rothi, 1990).

Roth and Worthington (2001) write that clients make the greatest improvement when therapy is provided frequently over five to six months with receptive skills improving the greatest, speech production being the next area of most improvement, followed by expressive language skills. The clinician has several options of approaches that can help to reorganize the cortical system. The approach that will be used depends on the evaluation outcome, the patient's medical needs, and the patient's motivation and lifestyle. His or her availability for treatment and the amount of family involvement also affect what approaches, procedures, and goals are selected for therapy. It is also important to include the family in any treatment that is provided. Graham-Keegan and Caspari (1997) make the following suggestions as to how to address a patient with aphasia:

The following are factors to consider when assessing the aphasic person:

1. Are adequate clues available in the first attempted message to give information on content?

2. Are yes/no questions accurate?

3. Can the client indicate when his partner is "on the right track" in pursuit of a message?

4. Does the client expand beyond yes/no in response to questions?

5. Will the client voluntarily switch modalities when one is unsuccessful?

6. Does the client spontaneously use his best expressive modality?

The following are factors when considering the partner:

1. Does the partner make best use of the information given when seeking clarification?

2. When asking yes/no questions to clarify, is there a logical procession from general to specific?

3. Is the frequency of redundant questions appropriate for the client?

4. If the client does not spontaneously use an effective modality, does the partner request it?

5. Is the strategy of encouraging the aphasic person to continue or of asking for a repeat or elaboration likely to result in the aphasic person's giving relevant and intelligible information? (p. 58)

By adjusting conversational expectations and using the above techniques, the patient with aphasia and his or her communication partners should experience more success in exchanging information.

Generally speaking, treatment of aphasia should be designed to "(1) stimulate disrupted processes to promote functional reorganization, (2) teach the use of compensatory strategies to communicate in the face of residual deficits, (3) provide education and counseling to promote adjustment of the patient and family, (4) eliminate 'bad habits' that interfere with successful communication, and (5) promote a suitable communication environment (Simmons-Mackie, 1997, p. 75). Therapy should consist of offering stimulation treatment to enhance language processes, and also training of compensation methods as alternative means of communicating.

The approach that will be used depends on the evaluation outcome, the patient's medical needs, and the patient's motivation and lifestyle. His or her availability for treatment and the amount of family involvement also will affect what approaches, procedures, and goals are selected for therapy.

Addressing Underlying Processes

Luria believed that effective therapy for aphasia relied on leading the cortex into reorganizing itself using cross-modal stimulation. By developing new pathways for receiving and acting on stimuli, improvement in memory and language would be expected. Schuell believed that it was necessary to retrain the ability to reauditorize, or rehear, what has been heard. The belief was that reauditorization would lead to better internal sound organization, and that would, in turn, lead to improved auditory comprehension.

The approach by Luria that addresses the underlying basic cognitive processes is deblocking. Deblocking refers to a system of reorganizing the cortex by using the most intact modalities to trigger the use of other modalities. Hemispheric specialization, in which the right hemisphere is taught to assume some of the responsibilities previously held by the left hemisphere, is an example of deblocking.

Melodic intonation therapy (MIT) and the use of visual imagery are both examples of techniques relying on hemispheric specialization. In the basic research of Backus (1945) on which MIT is based, words and phrases were presented to the patient in a rhythmical, unison manner. In 1973, Albert, Sparks, and Helm explored the use of a singing technique by assigning simple pitch patterns to phrases and sentences to facilitate speech in nonfluent patients. The hypothesis for what became known as MIT was that "functions associated with the intact right hemisphere may be exploited for purposes of rehabilitating speech in left-brain-damaged individuals" (Helm-Estabrooks & Albert, 1991, p. 207).

The most suitable group of candidates for MIT are as follows:

1. Unilateral stroke in left frontal lobe (Broca's area), often extending to the parietal region.

2. Severely limited verbal output with poor speech articulation.

3. Nonfluent or significantly restricted verbal output.

4. Extremely poor speech repetition skills.

5. Moderate to good auditory comprehension.

6. Emotionally stable with good attention span. (Helm-Estabrooks & Albert, 1991; Roth & Worthington, 2001)

There is little proof that this method works.

Reorganization of the representational system is another example of reorganization by teaching a new representational system, which then generalizes to other linguistic behaviors as evidenced by improved auditory comprehension. Visual action therapy (VAT) is an example of such an approach. VAT was developed by Helm and Benson in 1978 after experiencing some success in treating patients with global aphasia using a visual communication system. Known as the VIC system, it used real objects and index cards containing simple drawings. These objects and cards became a representational system for the patients with global aphasia, indicating that these patients retain the basis for a conceptual system of communication. The VAT approach used hand and arm gestures as a communication system. Further modifications included therapy objectives to address buccal or facial apraxia (gestures based on mouth and face movements), proximal limb visual action therapy (gestures based on movements of shoulders, arms, and fingers), and distal limb visual action therapy (finer movements of the hands and fingers than seen in proximal limb visual action therapy) (Roth & Worthington, 2001). All of the modifications use "real objects, line drawings of these objects, and pictures of a simple figure using the objects" (Helm-Estabrooks & Albert, 1991). Each program has seven items. No verbalizations are required. Rather, the patient learns to communicate using gestures. Suitable candidates for limb VAT include those who have unilateral damage to the left hemisphere (particularly in the areas of primary language) or global aphasia with moderate to severe limb apraxia. The best candidates for bucco-facial VAT also include those with left hemisphere damage, particularly in the anterior language areas of the brain, who have severely impaired verbal output but intact verbal comprehension. For both groups, the patient needs to be alert and cooperative, and have a good attention span (Roth & Worthington, 2001).

Treatment efficacy. The determination of the most efficient and effective means by which the clinician provides therapeutic intervention.

Relearning what is lost through application of basic learning principles is the focus of some research being done in studying **treatment efficacy**. This involves reteaching and relearning basic cognitive functions, such as questioning. In these approaches, it is typical to train one behavior in a highly controlled setting and watch for generalization. LaPointe (1990) suggests using a Base 10 behavior management to record ongoing progress in all areas of language (auditory, verbal, visual, graphic).

Compensation Methods

Compensation methods of intervention are basically an attempt to teach interaction of the damaged and intact portions of the brain. In using compensation methods, the clinician accepts the deficits and teaches the patient to compensate using other systems. Examples of compensation methods are the use of sign language or communication boards to facilitate communication when verbal expression is compromised. When using compensation methods, it is also important to teach assertiveness in communication by training the patient to ask others to slow down, repeat, and to use gestures with their speech. The PACE program (Promoting Aphasic Communication Effectiveness) (Davis, 1993; Davis & Wilcox, 1985) is a functional approach to a compensation system. In the PACE program the clinician teaches the patient how to have a communicative exchange in a controlled environment. Verbal, written, and gestural forms of communication are addressed, and success is determined by whether the message was exchanged and understood, no matter which modality was used. PACE addressed the pragmatic aspects of language and clients have been shown to generalize skills learned in treatment. Peach (2001) writes that "PACE is well suited as a means to incorporate compensatory strategies into communication treatment. An additional strength of the approach, however, lies in its us a framework for incorporating traditional language stimulation techniques into a communicatively dynamic context" (p. 506).

Counseling

Regardless of when treatment is begun, the rehabilitation team must provide counseling for the family and patient. Patients who suffer a devastating loss of communication often are afraid, frustrated, angry, and depressed. They may, at various times, feel crazy, stupid, useless, and anxious. This is certainly understandable because when the ability to communicate is lost, the person loses the ability to control his or her own environment. In short, the patient becomes powerless. This may compromise the patient's self-concept and the perception of others regarding the patient.

It is beneficial for patients who have aphasis, and for their family members to participate in group counseling sessions such as the one in Figure 13–11. Families need to understand that a family member with aphasia typically will

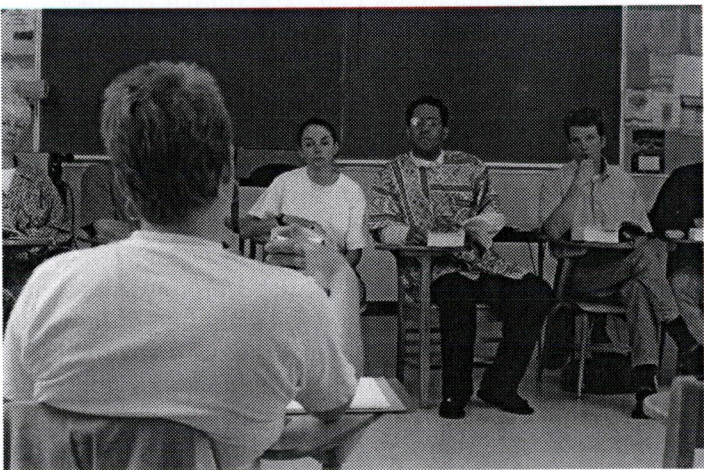

FIGURE 13–11. Support groups can be beneficial to the families of patients who have a neurological deficit such as aphasia or dementia.

think more concretely and may miss subtle humor. He or she may persever-ate, which is the commission of unintentional, repetitive behaviors. Some family members may find this annoying and frustrating. The patient with aphasia also may become overly emotional at times.

Patients may not demonstrate their previous initiative, even if they were highly ambitious and motivated prior to the onset of aphasia. This may re-quire restructuring of family roles, with the nonaphasic family members as-suming some of the responsibilities previously held by the spouse or parent who now has aphasia. In some instances, this may lead to fear and frustration on the part of the family member who assumes new roles, which may be re-pressed as guilt or expressed as anger at the family member for no longer being able to "do his (or her) share" of the household responsibilities.

■ TREATMENT EFFICACY AND FUNCTIONAL OUTCOMES

Treatment efficacy is a topic of great concern for those providing aphasia therapy owing to the inherent multidisciplinary approach and constraints imposed by insurance companies and health maintenance organizations (HMOs). Speech-language pathologists must be able to demonstrate that the therapy techniques utilized in aphasia therapy do, in fact, work effectively to improve the communication status of individuals with aphasia. Olswang (1990) defines treatment efficacy as encompassing several questions includ-ing, "Does treatment work?" "Is one method of treatment more effective than another?" "How does aphasia treatment change the behaviors of the patient?" Holland and colleagues (1996) defined efficacious treatment as "improvements in communication that exceed what can be expected from spontaneous recovery following brain insult" (p. S27).

Several problems are inherent in documenting the effectiveness of treatment for aphasia. One of these problems is that it is difficult to assess how much improvement is due to treatment and how much is the result of spontaneous recovery. A second problem is related to sample size issues. Although this chapter outlined the different types of aphasia as if distinct dividing lines ex-isted among them all, patients frequently display a "graying" of the lines. Individual patients may not have all of the symptoms described as being associated with a particular aphasia, and the symptoms differ from person to person. Even if two patients had identical causative factors, their ages and physical statuses prior to the onset of the aphasia may affect the recovery process differently. It is likewise difficult to match adequate sized samples based on socioeconomic status, gender, and education. The environment after onset and the treatment environments may similarly affect how some patients respond to therapy, so these factors need to be considered as well. In addition, the ethical issue of withholding treatment from some patients in order to have a control population for comparison needs to be addressed. Thus, although individual and group aphasia treatment is effective, it is a challenge to prove.

■ SUMMARY

The assessment and treatment of language disorders, and particularly aphasia, in the adult population present unique challenges for speech-language pathologists. Although a team approach is ideal in all settings with all ages of patients, it is probably most readily available in rehabilitation settings that cater to adults who are recovering from strokes and head injuries that have resulted in aphasia and other deficits. These patients are typically seen in the acute-care hospital until their conditions are medically stable, then they may move to a step-down facility within the hospital where rehabilitation can begin as the patient regains some physical stamina. The next stop in the rehabilitation chain is frequently an inpatient-outpatient rehabilitation facility dedicated to assisting patients in restoring functions and abilities that have been lost due to stroke, head trauma, and other incidents that result in aphasia and physical deficits.

The speech-language pathologist's active participation in the team care of these patients is critical. Speech-language pathologists also must participate in treatment efficacy research to be able to document the benefits of providing therapy to individuals in this patient population.

CASE STUDY

History

Mr. S is a 67-year-old, right-handed native English-speaking male who suffered a stroke on July 23, 2002, resulting in aphasia and a right hemiparesis. He was referred to the University of Florida Speech and Hearing Clinic by a friend. He was evaluated on December 10, 2003.

Mr. S was hospitalized in a local hospital on the day he had the stroke, and after one week of treatment he was transferred to a rehabilitation facility, where he received occupational therapy, physical therapy, and speech therapy.

He has a history of high blood pressure and diabetes of long duration, which are controlled with medication (Diabeta, Procardia, and aspirin). Mrs. S, who was the informant for much of the history, reported that there is a strong family history of strokes. Since the stroke, Mr. S is said to ignore visual stimuli from the right side and has stopped wearing his glasses. He also has a history of hearing loss, and a recommendation of binaural amplification was made at one time.

Mr. S retired from his job of 30 years as a physical plant worker at the University of Florida. He has received a G.E.D., but his formal education was limited to fifth grade. He is not reported to be a big reader, but he does enjoy reading fishing magazines and watching television. He has four children, all of whom live within a 50-mile radius, and several grandchildren.

Current Speech and Language Status

Mrs. S reported that Mr. S's comprehension and speech production have improved greatly in the last few weeks. Since the stroke, he is reported to continue to have difficulty formulating his thoughts, and his speech still contains paraphasic errors. His auditory comprehension is now reported to be quite good. Although he never read much, his reading ability is said to be comparable with his prestroke ability. His handwriting with his nondominant hand is basically illegible. He often has problems with naming. His memory for past events is said to be good; however, his short-term memory may have been affected, as Mrs. S reports he often forgets that he needs to take his medicine. He is sometimes aware of his speech errors and will attempt to self-correct. His speech is not reported to be slurred or slower, but his children say that he does not to speak well on the telephone. No swallowing problems have been reported, although he appears to still have some right-side facial weakness. He has no reported problems with orientation and takes frequent walks in his neighborhood without getting lost. He can take care of his basic needs, including doing some simple cooking, but he needs help with planning and preparing for activities.

Mr. S's main problem is his expressive language. He is said to have problems with word finding, paraphasias, and mistakes on function words such as pronouns (for example, he mistakes "she" for "he").

Assessment and Results

The Western Aphasia Battery (WAB) (Kertesz, 1982) was administered. Results on the WAB yielded an overall aphasia quotient of 69. On the repetition subtest, he scored 56%, having difficulty with repeating the longer sentences. He was 81% accurate in object naming, 100% accurate in sentence completion, and 60% accurate in responsive speech. Word fluency was significantly decreased, as seen when he was able to name only three animals within the time limit.

Mr. S completed the reading subtest with 67% accuracy. He failed to comprehend some of the longer sentences in the sentence reading task, but he was 100% accurate in reading single words. His accuracy dropped in spelling tasks: spelling word recognition was 67% accurate and oral spelling was 17% accurate. Mr. S's writing abilities were significantly decreased. He was able to write his first name recognizably and four of six dictated letters. When asked to write the serial alphabet and the numbers 0 to 20, he produced two letters and two numbers.

Mr. S completed the praxis subtest, achieving 97% accuracy. Within the construction subtests, he received individual scores of 11/30 on the drawing subtests, 3/9 on the block design, and 18/24 on the calculation subtest. His drawings with his nondominant hand were cramped, micrographic, and confined to the extreme right side of the paper. With the exception of the circle and square design, it was not possible to identify the drawings. On the block design, Mr. S was able to place all four blocks together but was unable to reproduce a pattern. On the calculation portion of the test, he was able to complete addition, multiplication, and subtraction problems accurately, but he was not able to complete the division problems.

On the oral speech protocol, Mr. S was able to perform 17 of 20 volitional movements on request, and the other 3 were completed after a model was provided. The sequential oral movements also were performed accurately. The diadochokinetic rate for syllables was slow (about 2 standard deviations below the norm).

An informal probe of Mr. S's ability to formulate "WH-questions" was administered, and he demonstrated great difficulty with the task. In addition, a probe of his narrative conversation was administered by asking him to tell the Cinderella story. He also demonstrated significant difficulty with this task.

Mr. S's abilities can be summed up as follows.

	Strengths	Weaknesses
Communicative	Speech production improving	Conduction aphasia
	Good auditory comprehension	Hearing loss
	Reading intact	Difficulty formulating ideas
	Good long-term memory	Poor naming skills
	Attempts to self-correct	Poor short-term memory
	Good sentence repetition	Mistakes on function words

	Completes oral praxis tests	Unable to write letters
	Answers basic questions	Slow diadochokinesis
Noncommunicative	Family support	Right hemiparesis
	No dysphagia	High blood pressure
	Can do simple chores	Diabetes
	Meets own basic needs	Hemianopsia
	Can do math calculations	Third-grade education
		Illegible writing
		Right-side facial weakness

Conclusions and Recommendations

Mr. S's communication abilities as tested on the WAB and the modified oral motor protocol are consistent with a profile of conduction aphasia with a mild oral-motor involvement.

It is recommended that Mr. S be enrolled in speech-language therapy, and that the family contact an occupational therapist for evaluation of right upper extremity function.

▨   REVIEW QUESTIONS

1. Fluent, well-articulated phonologically correct utterances that make little or no sense to the listener defines
   a. Jargon
   b. Babbling
   c. Semantic paraphasias
   d. Phonemic paraphasias

2. Which of the following statements is most true?
   a. CT scans are superior to MRI scans for the early detection of neurophysiological changes and are typically more sensitive to subtle neuropathologies.
   b. MRI scans are superior to CT scans for the early detection of neurophysiological changes and are typically more sensitive to subtle neuropathologies.

3. The theory of restitution of function states that
   a. Spontaneous recovery is limited by time, usually not extending beyond six months
   b. Recovery is a physiological process

    c. Recovery is a psychological process

    d. a, b, and c

    e. a and b

4. Reading comprehension would be least affected in _____ aphasia.

    a. Wernicke

    b. Transcortical sensory

    c. Conduction

    d. Global

5. Examples of therapy designed to address underlying processes by teaching the right hemisphere to assume some of the responsibility previously held by the left hemisphere are

    a. Melodic intonation therapy and training behaviors in highly controlled settings

    b. Deblocking and base 10 behavior management

    c. PACE and reauditorization

    d. Melodic intonation therapy and visual action therapy

6. A 69-year-old stroke victim exhibits fluent but empty speech, circumlocutions, good articulation, poor reading and auditory comprehension, very poor naming skills, verbal paraphasia, and good repetition skills. What type of aphasia does he have?

    a. Transcortical motor

    b. Wernicke

    c. Broca

    d. Transcortical sensory

7. Transcortical aphasias resemble other types of aphasia except that in transcortical syndromes:

    a. Comprehension is worse

    b. Repetition is remarkably intact

    c. Naming is unimpaired

    d. Paraphasias are less frequent

8. The primary features used to differentially diagnose aphasia are

    a. Naming, presence of physical defects, conversational speech, and repetition skills

    b. Speech fluency, confrontation naming, auditory comprehension, and press of speech

    c. Writing skills, auditory comprehension, reading comprehension, and naming

    d. Naming, conversational speech, auditory comprehension, and repetition skills

9. The fluent aphasias are the result of lesions

    a. Posterior around the auditory association area of the left temporal and/or right parietal lobe

    b. Anterior to the left premotor cortex
    c. Superior to the Sylvian fissure
    d. In the frontal lobe

10. Errors tend to occur closer to the end of a word in the fluent aphasias, but toward the beginning of the word in the nonfluent aphasias.

    a. True
    b. False

■ REFERENCES

Albert, M., Sparks, R.., & Helm, N. (1973). Melodic Intonation Therapy for aphasia. *Archives of Neurology, 29,* 130–131.

Alexander, M. P., & Schmitt, M. A. (1980). The aphasia syndrome of stroke in the left anterior cerebral artery territory. *Archives of Neurology, 37,* 97–100.

American Heart Association (2005). *Heart disease and stroke statistics—2005 update.* Dallas, TX: American Heart Association.

Aronson, A. E. (1991). *Neurology for the medical speech-language pathologist.* Workshop presented in Tampa, FL.

Aten, J., Caliguiri, M., & Holland, A. (1982). The efficacy of functional communication therapy for chronic aphasic patients. *Journal of Speech and Hearing Disorders, 47,* 93–96.

Backus, O. (1945). The rehabilitation of persons with aphasia. In *The rehabilitation of speech.* New York: Harper Bros.

Benson, D. F. (1979). *Aphasia, alexia, and agraphia.* New York: Churchill Livingstone.

Benson, F. (1985). Aphasia. In Heilman, K., & Valenstein, E. (Eds.). *Clinical neuropsychology* (pp. 17–47). New York: Oxford University Press.

Benton, A. L., Hamsher, K., Varney, N. R., & Spreen, O. (1994). *Contributions to neuropsychological assessment.* New York: Oxford University Press.

Beukelman, D., Yorkston, K., & Dowden, P. (1985). *Communication augmentation: A casebook of clinical management.* San Diego: College-Hill.

Bishop, D. V. M. (1983). *Test for reception of grammar.* London: Medical Research Council.

Bogousslavsky, J., & Regli, F. (1990). Anterior cerebral artery territory infarction in the Lausanne Stroke Registry. *Archives of Neurology, 47,* 144–150.

Brookshire, R. H., & Nicholas, L. E. (1980). Sentence verification and language comprehension of aphasic persons. In R. H. Brookshire (Ed.), *Clinical aphasiology: Conference proceedings* (pp. 53–63). Minneapolis, MN: BRK Publishers.

Brookshire, R. H., & Nicholas, L. E. (1982). Comprehension of directly and indirectly pictured verbs by aphasic and nonaphasic listeners. In R. H. Brookshire (Ed.), *Clinical aphasiology: Conference proceedings* (pp. 200–206). Minneapolis, MN: BRK Publishers.

Brookshire, R. H., & Nicholas, L. E. (1985). Consistency of the effects of rate of speech on brain damaged subjects' comprehension of information in narrative discourse. In R. H. Brookshire (Ed.), *Clinical aphasiology: Conference proceedings* (pp. 262–271). Minneapolis, MN: BRK Publishers.

Brookshire, R. H., & Nicholas, L. E. (1997). *The discourse comprehension test* (rev. ed.). Minneapolis, MN: BRK Publishers.

Brown, V. L., Hammill, D. D., & Wiederholt, J. L. (1995). *Test of reading comprehension* (3rd ed.). Austin, TX: Pro-Ed.

Byng, S. (1988). Sentence processing deficits: Theory and therapy. *Cognitive neuropsychology, 5,* 629–676.

Code, C. (1994). Role of the right hemisphere in the treatment of aphasia. In R. Chapey (Ed.), *Language intervention strategies in adult aphasia* (3rd ed.) (pp. 380–386). Baltimore, MD: Williams & Wilkins.

Collins, M. J. (1997). Global aphasia. In L. L. LaPointe (Ed.), *Aphasia and related neurogenic language disorders* (2nd ed.) (pp. 133–150). New York: Thieme.

Davis, G. A. (1993). *A survey of adult aphasia and related language disorders* (2nd ed.). Englewood Cliffs, NJ: Prentice Hall.

Davis, G. A., & Wilcox, M. J. (1985). *Adult aphasia rehabilitation: Applied pragmatics.* San Diego: Singular Publishing Group.

DeMasio, A. R., & Kassel, N. F. (1978). *Transcortical motor aphasia in relation to lesions of the supplementary motor area.* Paper presented at the 30th annual meeting, American Academy of Neurology, Los Angeles, CA.

DeRenzi, E., & Farrari, C. (1978). The reporters test: A sensitive test to detect expressive disturbances in aphasics. *Cortex, 4,* 279–293.

Duffy, R. J., & Duffy, J. R. (1984). *Assessment of nonverbal communication.* Austin, TX: Pro-Ed.

Dunn, L. M., & Dunn, E. S. (1997). *Peabody picture vocabulary test III.* Circle Pines, MN: American Guidance Service.

Emerick, L. L., & Haynes, W. (1986). *Diagnosis and evaluation in speech pathology.* Englewood Cliffs, NJ: Prentice Hall.

Enderby, P., & Crow, E. (1996). Frenchay aphasia screening test: Validity and comparability. *Disability and Rehabilitation, 18,* 238–240.

Enderby, P., Wood, V., Wade, D., & Langton Hewer, R., (1987). The Frenchay aphasia screening test: A short, simple test appropriate for nonspecialists. *International Journal of Rehabilitation Medicine, 8,* 166–170.

Fink, R. B., Martin, N., Schwartz, M. F., Saffran, E. M., & Myers, J. L. (1993). Facilitation of verb retrieval skills in aphasia: A comparison of two approaches. In M. Lemme (Ed.), *Clinical aphasiology, 21* (pp. 263–275). Austin, TX: Pro-Ed.

Frattali, C., Thompson, C. K., Holland, A., Wohl, C. B., & Ferketic, M. (1995). *Functional assessment of communicative skills for adults (ASHA FACS).* Rockville, MD: American Speech-Language-Hearing Association.

Gainotti, G. (1995). The riddle of the right hemisphere's contribution to recovery of language. *European Journal of Communication Disorders, 28*(3), 227–246.

German, D. J. (1990). *The test of adolescent and adult word-finding.* Austin, TX: Pro-Ed.

Geschwind, N. (1965). Disconnexion syndromes in animals and man. *Brain, 88,* 237–294, 585–644.

Gonzalez-Rothi, L. J. (1990). Transcortical aphasias. In L. L. LaPointe (Ed.), *Aphasia and related neurogenic language disorders* (pp. 78–95). New York: Thieme Medical Publishers.

Gonzalez-Rothi, L. (1997). Transcortical motor, sensory, and mixed aphasias. In L. L. LaPointe (Ed.), *Aphasia and related language disorders* (2nd ed.). New York: Thieme.

Goodglass, H. (1993). *Understanding aphasia.* San Diego: Academic Press.

Goodglass, H., & Kaplan, E. (1983a). *The assessment of aphasia and related disorders* (2nd ed.). Philadelphia: Lea & Febiger.

Goodglass, H., & Kaplan, E. (1983b). *The Boston diagnostic aphasia examination.* Philadelphia: Lea & Febiger.

Goodglass, H., Kaplan, E., & Barresi, B. (2001). *Boston diagnostic aphasia examination* (3rd ed.). Philadelphia: Lippincott Williams & Wilkins.

Goodman, R. A., & Caramazza, A. (1986a). *The Johns Hopkins University dysgraphia battery.* Baltimore, MD: The Johns Hopkins University.

Goodman, R. A., & Caramazza, A. (1986b). *The Johns Hopkins University dyslexia battery.* Baltimore, MD: The Johns Hopkins University.

Goss, C. M. (Ed.). (1973). *Gray's anatomy of the human body* (29th American ed.). Philadelphia: Lea & Febiger.

Graham-Keegan, L., & Caspari, I. (1997). Wernicke's aphasia. In L. LaPointe (Ed.), *Aphasia and related neurogenic language disorders* (2nd ed.) (pp. 42–62). New York: Thieme.

Grill, J. J., & Kirwin, M. M. (1989). *Written language assessment.* Novato, CA: Academic Therapy.

Hammill, D. D., & Larson, S. C. (1996). *Test of written language* (3rd ed.). Austin, TX: Pro-Ed.

Hanna, G., Schell, L. M., & Schreiner, R. (1977). *The Nelson reading skills test.* Chicago: Riverside Publishing.

Hegde, M. N. (1994). *A coursebook on aphasia and other neurogenic language disorders.* San Diego: Singular Publishing Group.

Helm-Estabrooks, N. (1991). *Test of oral and limb apraxia.* Austin, TX: Pro-Ed.

Helm-Estabrooks, N., & Albert, M. L. (1991). *Manual of aphasia therapy.* Austin, TX: Pro-Ed.

Helm-Estabrooks, N., Emery, P., & Albert, M. (1987). Treatment of aphasia perseveration (TAP) program. *Archives of Neurology, 44,* 1253–1255.

Helm-Estabrooks, N., Fitzpatrick, P., & Barresi, B. (1982). Visual Action Therapy for global aphasia. *Journal of Speech and Hearing Disorders, 44,* 385–389.

Holland, A. (1970). Case studies in aphasia rehabilitation using programmed instruction. *Journal of Speech and Hearing Disorders, 35,* 377–390.

Holland, A. L. (1980). *Communicative abilities in daily living.* Baltimore, MD: Williams & Wilkins.

Holland, A. L., Fromm, D. S., DeRuyter, F., & Stein, M. (1996, October). Treatment efficacy: Aphasia. *Journal of Speech and Hearing Research, 39,* S27–S36.

Holtzapple, P., Pohlman, K., LaPointe, L. L., & Graham, L. F. (1989). Does SPICA mean PICA? *Clinical Aphasiology, 18,* 131–144.

Howard, D., & Patterson, K. E. (1992). *Pyramids and palm trees.* Bury St. Edmunds, Suffolk, UK: Thames Valley Test Company.

Kaplan, E., Goodglass, H. & Weintraub, S. (1983). *The Boston naming test.* Philadelphia: Lea and Febinger.

Katz, R., & Wertz, R. (1992). Microaphasiology and the computerized clinician. In M. Lemme (Ed.), *Clinical aphasiology conference proceedings* (pp. 7–17). Austin, TX: Pro-Ed.

Kay, J., Lesser, R., & Coltheart, M. (1997). *Psycholinguistic assessments of language processing in aphasia.* Hove, East Sussex, UK: Psychology Press.

Kearns, K. (1985). Response elaboration training for patient-initiated utterances. In R. Brookshire (Ed.), *Clinical aphasiology conference proceedings* (pp. 196–204). Minneapolis, MN: BRK.

Kearns, K. P. (1997). Broca's aphasia. In L. L. LaPointe (Ed.), *Aphasia and related neurogenic language disorders* (pp. 1–41). New York: Thieme Medical Publishers.

Keenan, J. S., & Brassell, E. G. (1975). *Aphasia language performance scales.* Murfreesboro, TN: Pinnacle Press.

Kent, R. D. (1997). *The speech sciences.* San Diego: Singular Publishing Group.

Kertesz, A. (1982). *The western aphasia battery*. New York: Grune and Stratton.

LaPointe, L. L. (1990). *Aphasia and related neurogenic language disorders*. New York: Thieme Medical Publishers.

LaPointe, L. L., Holtzapple, P. A., & Graham, L. F. (1985). The relationship among two measures of auditory comprehension and daily living communication skills. In R. H. Brookshire (Ed.), *Clinical aphasiology: Conference proceedings* (pp. 38–46). Minneapolis, MN: BRK Publishers.

LaPointe, L. L., & Horner, J. (1978, Spring). The functional auditory comprehension test (FACT): Protocol and test format. *FLASHA Journal*, 27–33.

LaPointe, L. L., & Horner, J. (1998). *Reading comprehension battery for aphasia* (2nd ed.). Austin, TX: Pro-Ed.

Lee, L. (1971). *Northwestern syntax screening test*. Evanston: University of Illinois Press.

Lomas, J., Pickard, L., Bester, S., Elbard, H., Finlayson, A., & Zoghaib, C. (1989). The Communicative Effectiveness Index: Development and psychometric evaluation of functional communication measure for adult aphasia. *Journal of Speech and Hearing Disorders, 54*, 113–124.

Luria, A. R. (1958). Brain disorders and language analysis. *Language, Speech, 1*, 14–34.

Luria, A. R. (1970). *Traumatic aphasia: Its syndromes, psychology and treatment*. The Hague: Mouton.

Luria, A. R. (1977). *Neuropsychological studies in aphasia*. Amsterdam: Swets & Zeitlinger BV.

Luria, A. R., & Tsvetkova, L. S. (1968). A modern assessment of the basic forms of aphasia. *Brain and Language, 4*, 129–151.

Markwardt, F. C. (1988). *Peabody individual achievement test-Revised*. Circle Pines, MN: American Guidance Service.

Marshall, R. C. (1994). Management of fluent aphasia patients. In R. Chapey (Ed.), *Language intervention strategies in adult aphasia* (3rd ed.) (pp. 389–406). Baltimore, MD: Williams & Wilkins.

Marshall, R., & Neuburger, S. (1984). Extended comprehension training reconsidered. In R. Brookshire (Ed.), *Clinical aphasiology conference proceedings* (pp. 181–187) Minneapolis, MN: BRK.

McNeil, M. R., & Duffy, J. R. (2001). Primary progressive aphasia. In R. Chapey (Ed.), *Language intervention strategies in aphasia and related neurogenic communication disorders* (4th ed.) (pp. 472–486). Philadelphia; Lippincott, Williams, & Wilkins.

McNeil, M. R., & Prescott, T. E. (1978). *Revised token test*. Baltimore, MD: University Park Press.

Murdoch, B. E. (1988). Computerized tomographic scanning: Its contributions to understanding of the neuroanatomical basis of aphasia. *Aphasiology, 2*, 437–462.

Murray, L. L., & Chapey, R. (2001). Assessment of language disorders in adults. In R. Chapey (Ed.), *Language intervention strategies in aphasia and related neurogenic communication disorders* (4th ed.) (pp. 55–126). Philadelphia: Lippincott Williams & Wilkins.

National Institute of Neurological Disorders and Stroke (2005). www.ninds.nih.gov.

Nelson, H. E. (1984). *New adult reading test (NART)*. Windsor, England: NFER-Nelson.

Newcombe, F., Oldfield, R. C., Ratcliff, G. G., & Wingfield, A. (1971). Recognition and naming of object-drawing by men with focal brain wounds. *Journal of Neurosurgery and Psychiatry, 34*, 329–340.

Newhoff, M., & Apel, K. (1997). Impairments in pragmatics. In L. L. LaPointe (Ed.), *Aphasia and related neurogenic language disorders* (2nd ed.) (pp. 250–264). New York: Thieme.

Obler, L. K., & Albert, M. L. (1979). *The action naming test*. Boston: VA Medical Center.

Olswang, L. B. (1990). Treatment efficacy: The breadth of research. In L. B. Olswang, C. K. Thompson, S. F. Warren, & N. J. Minghetti (Eds.), Treatment efficacy research in communication disorders (pp. 3–17). Rockville, MD: American Speech-Language-Hearing Foundation.

Patronas, N. J., Deveikis, J. P., & Schellinger, D. (1987). The use of computed tomography in studying the brain. In H. G. Mueller & V. C. Geoffrey (Eds.), *Communication disorders in aging: Assessment and management* (pp. 107–134). Washington, DC: Gallaudet University Press.

Payne, J. (1994). *Communication profile: A functional skills survey.* San Antonio, TX: Communication Skill Builders.

Peach, R. K. (2001). Clinical intervention for global aphasia. In R. Chapey (Ed.), *Language intervention strategies in aphasia and related neurogenic communication disorders,* 4th ed., (pp. 487–512). Philadelphia: Lippincott Williams & Wilkins.

Porch, B. E. (1967). *Porch index of communicative ability.* Palo Alto, CA: Consulting Psychologists Press.

Porch, B. (1981). *Porch index of communicative ability,* Vol. 2: *Administration, scoring, and interpretation,* 3rd ed. Palo Alto, CA: Consulting Psychologists Press.

Powell. G. E., Bailey, S., & Clark, E. (1980). A very short form of the Minnesota aphasia test. *British Journal of Social and Clinical Psychology, 19,* 189–194.

Roth, F. P., & Worthington, C. K. (2001). *Treatment resource manual for speech-language pathology* (2nd ed.). Albany, NY: Delmar.

Rubens, A. B. (1976). Transcortical motor aphasia. In H. Whitaker & H. A. Whitaker (Eds.), *Studies in neurolinguistics* (Vol. I). New York: Academic Press.

Sarno, M. (1969). *The functional communication profile.* New York: University Medical Center, Institute of Rehabilitation Medicine.

Sarno, M., & Levita, E. (1971). Natural course of recovery in severe aphasia. *Archives of Physical Medicine and Rehabilitation, 52,* 175–178.

Sarno, M., Silverman, M., & Sands, E. (1970). Speech therapy and language recovery in severe aphasia. *Journal of Speech and Hearing Research, 13,* 606–623.

Schuell, H. (1965). The Minnesota test for differential diagnosis of aphasia. Minneapolis: University of Minnesota Press.

Schuell, H. (1973). *Differential diagnosis of aphasia with the Minnesota test* (2nd ed., rev. by J. W. Sefer). Minneapolis: University of Minnesota Press.

Schuell, H. (1974). *Aphasia theory and therapy.* Baltimore, MD: University Park Press.

Seikel, J. A., King, D. W., & Drumright, D. G. (1997). *Anatomy and physiology for speech, language, and hearing* (exp. ed.). San Diego: Singular Publishing Group.

Shaywitz, S. (2003). *Overcoming dyslexia: A new and complete science-based program for reading problems at any level.* New York: Alfred A. Knopf.

Shewan, C. M. (1979). *Auditory comprehension test for sentences.* Chicago; Biolinguistics Clinical Institutes.

Shewan, C. M. (1988a). Expressive language recovery in aphasia using the Shewan spontaneous language analysis (SSLA) system. *Journal of Communication Disorders, 21,* 155–169.

Shewan, C. M. (1988b). The Shewan spontaneous language analysis (SSLA) system for aphasic adults: Description, reliability, and validity. *Journal of Communication Disorders, 21,* 103–138.

Shewan, C., & Bandur, D. (1986). *Treatment of aphasia: A language-oriented approach.* San Diego: College-Hill.

Shewan, C., & Kertesz, A. (1984). Effects of speech and language treatment on recovery from aphasia. *Brain and Language, 23,* 272–299.

Simmons-Mackie, N. (1997). Conduction aphasia. In L. L. LaPointe (Ed.), *Aphasia and related neurogenic language disorders* (2nd ed.) (pp. 63–90). New York: Thieme.

Sparks, R., Helm, N., & Albert, M. (1974). Aphasia rehabilitation resulting from melodic intonation therapy. *Cortex, 10,* 303–316.

Springer, L. (1991). Facilitating group rehabilitation. *Aphasiology, 5,* 563–566.

Steele, R. D., Weinrich, M., Wertz, R. T., Kleczewska, M. K., & Carlson, G. S. (1989). Computer based visual communication in aphasia. *Neuropsychologia, 27,* 409–426.

Tanner, D. C., & Culberson, W. (1999). *Quick assessment for aphasia.* Oceanside, CA: Academic Communication Associates.

Thompson, C. K., Shapiro, L. P., & Roberts, M. M. (1993). Treatment of sentence production deficits in aphasia: A linguistic-specific approach to wh-interrogative training and generalization. *Aphasiology, 7,* 111–133.

Thurstone, L. L., & Thurstone, T. G. (1962). *Primary mental abilities (Rev.).* Chicago: Science Research Associates.

Tsing, C., & McNeil, M. R. (1997). Nature and management of acquired neurogenic dysgraphias. In L. L. LaPointe (Ed.), *Aphasia and related neurogenic language disorders* (2nd ed.) (pp. 172–200). New York: Thieme.

Wallace, G., & Hammill, D. D. (1997). *Comprehensive receptive and expressive vocabulary test: Adult.* Austin, TX: Pro-Ed.

Waller, M., & Darley, F. L. (1978). The influence of context on the auditory comprehension of paragraphs by aphasic subjects. *Journal of Speech and Hearing Research, 21,* 732–745.

Warden, M. R., & Hutchinson, T. J. (1993). *The writing process test.* Chicago: Riverside.

Watson, R. T., Fleet, S., Gonzalez-Rothi, L. J., & Heilman, K. (1986). Apraxia and the supplementary motor area. *Archives of Neurology, 43,* 787–792.

Webster, D. B. (1997). *Brain dissection and surface anatomy for communication sciences.* San Diego: Singular Publishing Group.

Weiller, C., Isensee, C., Rijntjes, M., Huber, W., Muller, S., Bier, D., Dutschka, K., Woods, R., Noth, J., & Diener, H. D. (1995). Recovery from Wernicke's aphasia: A positron emission tomographic study. *Annals of Neurology, 37*(6), 723–732.

Wertz, R. T. (1986). Language disorders in adults: State of the clinical art. In J. M. Costello & A. L. Holland (Eds.), *Handbook of speech and language disorders* (pp. 759–835). San Diego: College-Hill Press.

Wertz, R. T., LaPointe, L. L., & Rosenbek, J. C. (1994). *Apraxia of speech in adults: The disorder and its management.* New York: Grune and Stratton.

Wertz, R., Collins, M., Weiss, D., Kurtzke, J., Friden, T., Brookshire, R., Pierce, J., Holtzapple, P., Hubbard, D., Porch, B., West, J., Davis, L., Matovitch, G., Morley, G., & Resurreccion, E. (1981). Veterans Administration cooperative study on aphasia: A comparison of individual and group treatment. *Journal of Speech and Hearing Research, 24,* 580–594.

Wertz, R. T., Weiss, D., Aten, J., Brookshire, R., Garcia-Bunuel, L., Holland, A., Kurtzke, J., LaPoiante, L., Milianti, F., Brannegan, R., Greenbaum, H., Marshall, R., Vogel, D., Carter, J., Barnes, N., & Goodman, R. (1986). Comparison of clinic, home, and deferred language treatment for aphasia: A Veteran's Administration cooperative study. *Archives of Neurology, 43,* 653–658.

Westbury, C., & Bub, D. (1997). Primary progressive aphasia: A review of 112 cases. *Brain and Language, 60*(3), 381–406.

Whitney, J. L., & Goldstein, H. (1989). Using self-monitoring to reduce disfluencies in speakers with mild aphasia. *Journal of Speech and Hearing Disorders, 54,* 576–586.

Whurr, R. (1996). *The aphasia screening test* (2nd ed.). San Diego: Singular Publishing Group.

Wiederholt, J. L., & Bryant, B. R. (1992). *Gray oral reading tests* (3rd ed.). Austin, TX: Pro-Ed.

Wilkinson, G. S. (1993). *Wide range achievement test* (3rd ed.). Wilmington, DE: Wide Range.

Wilcox, M. J., Davis, G. A., & Leonard, L. L. (1978). Aphasics' comprehension of contextually conveyed meaning. *Brain and Language, 6,* 362–377.

Williams, M. (1996). *The naming test.* Woodsboro, MD: Cool Spring Software.

Zachman, L., Huisingh, R., Barrett, M., Orman, J., & Blagden, C. (1989). *The WORD test adolescent.* East Moline, IL: LinguiSystems.

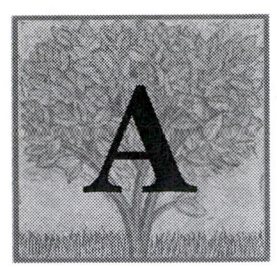

Suggested Reading List on Language Abnormalities in Preschool Children

American Speech-Language-Hearing Association. (1990). The roles of SLPs in service delivery to infants, toddlers, and their families. *Asha, 32*(Suppl. 2), 4.

American Speech-Language-Hearing Association. (1991). Position statement: Augmentative and alternative communication. *Asha, 33*(Suppl. 5), 8.

American Speech-Language-Hearing Association. (1991). Report: Augmentative and alternative communication. *Asha, 33*(Suppl. 5), 9–12.

American Speech-Language-Hearing Association. (1992). Guidelines for meeting the communication needs of persons with severe disabilities. *Asha, 34*(Suppl. 7), 1–8.

American Speech-Language-Hearing Association. (1987). Learning disabilities and the preschool child. *Asha, 29,* 35–38.

American Speech-Language-Hearing Association, Committee on Language Learning Disorders. (1989). Issues in determining eligibility for language intervention. *Asha, 31,* 113–118.

American Speech-Language-Hearing Association, Committee on Augmentative Communication. (1989). Competencies for speech-language pathologists providing services in augmentative communication. *Asha, 31,* 107–110.

American Speech-Language-Hearing Association, Committee on Mental Retardation and Developmental Disabilities. (1989). Mental retardation and developmental disabilities curriculum guide for SLPs and audiologists. *Asha, 31,* 94–96.

Billeaud, F. P. (1998). *Communication disorders in infants and toddlers: Assessment and intervention* (2nd ed.). Boston: Butterworth-Heinemann.

Bloom, L., & Lahey, M. (1978). *Language development and language disorders*. New York: John Wiley & Sons.

Condouris, K., Meyer, E., & Tager-Flusberg, H. (2003, August). The relationship between standardized measures of language and measures of spontaneous speech in children with autism. *American Journal of Speech-Language Pathology, 12*(3), 349–358.

Crystal, D. & Varley, R. (1993). *Introduction to language pathology* (3rd ed.). San Diego: Singular Publishing Group.

Fujiki, M., & Brinton, B. (1995). The performance of younger and older adults with retardation on a series of language tasks. *American Journal of Speech-Language Pathology, 4*, 77–86.

Girolametto, L., Weitzman, E., & Greenberg, J. (2003, August). Training day care staff to facilitate children's language. *American Journal of Speech-Language Pathology, 12*(3), 299–311.

Johnson, B. A. (1995). *Language disorders in children: An introductory clinical perspective*. Albany, NY: Delmar Publishers.

Justice, L. M., Chow, S., Capellini, C., Flanigan, K., & Colton, S. (2003, August). Emergent literacy intervention for vulnerable preschoolers: Relative effects of two approaches. *American Journal of Speech-Language Pathology, 12*(3), 320–332.

Justice, L. M., & Ezell, H. K. (2002, February). Use of storybook reading to increase print awareness in at-risk children. *American Journal of Speech-Language Pathology, 11*(1), 17–29.

La Paro, K. M., Justice, L., Skibbe, L. E., & Pianta, R. C. (2004, November). Relations among maternal, child, and demographic factors and the persistence of preschool language impairment. *American Journal of Speech-Language Pathology, 13*(4), 291–303.

McCauley, R. J. (2001). *Assessment of language disorders in children*. Mahwah, NJ: Lawrence Erlbaum Associates.

Mentis, M., & Lundgren, K. (1995). Effects of prenatal exposure to cocaine and associated risk factors on language development. *Journal of Speech and Hearing Research, 8*(6), 1303–1318.

Nippold, M. A., & Schwarz, I. E. (1996). Children with slow expressive language development: What is the forecast for school achievement? *American Journal of Speech-Language Pathology, 5*, 22–25.

Owens, R. E., Jr. (2004). *Language disorders: A functional approach to assessment and intervention* (4th ed.). Boston: Allyn & Bacon.

Paul, R. (2001). *Language disorders from infancy through adolescence* (2nd ed.). St. Louis, MO: Mosby.

Plante, E., & Vance, R. (1995). Diagnostic accuracy of two tests of preschool language. *American Journal of Speech-Language Pathology, 4*, 70–76.

Roberts, J. E., Mirrett, P., Anderson, K., Burchinal, M., & Neebe, E. (2002, August). Early communication, symbolic behavior, and social profiles of young males with fragile X syndrome. *American Journal of Speech-Language Pathology, 11*(3), 295–304.

Roberts, J. E., Prizant, B., & McWilliam, R. A. (1995, May). Out-of-class versus in-class service delivery in language intervention: Effects on communication interactions with young children. *American Journal of Speech-Language Pathology, 4*, 87–94.

Rossetti, L. M. (1986). *High risk infants: Identification, assessment, and intervention*. San Diego: College-Hill Press.

Rvachew, S., Nowak, M., & Cloutier, G. (2004, August). Effect of phonemic perception training on the speech production and phonological awareness skills of children with expressive phonological delay. *American Journal of Speech-Language Pathology, 13*(3), 250–263.

Rvachew, S., Ohberg, A., Grawburg, M., & Heyding, J. (2003, November). Phonological awareness and phonemic perception in 4-year-old children with delayed expressive phonology skills. *American Journal of Speech-Language Pathology, 12*(4), 463–471.

Snyder, L. E., & Scherer, N. (2004, February). The development of symbolic play and language in toddlers with cleft palate. *American Journal of Speech-Language Pathology, 13*(1), 66–80.

Tiegerman-Farber, E. (1995). *Language and communication intervention in preschool children.* Boston: Allyn and Bacon.

Wolfe, V., Presley, C., & Mesaris, J. (2003, August). The importance of sound identification training in phonological intervention. *American Journal of Speech-Language Pathology, 12*(3), 282–288.

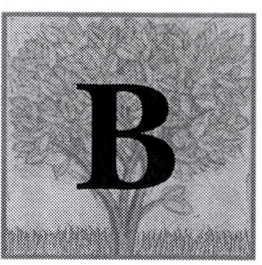

Suggested Reading List on Multicultural Aspects of Language Disorders

American Speech-Language-Hearing Association. (1993). Definitions of communication disorders and variations. *Asha, 35*(Suppl. 10), 33–39.

American Speech-Language-Hearing Association. (1993). Guidelines for gender equity in language use. *Asha, 35*(Suppl. 10), Vol. 35, 42–46.

American Speech-Language-Hearing Association. (1989). ASHA definition: Bilingual speech-language pathologists and audiologists. *Asha, 31,* 93.

American Speech-Language-Hearing Association, Committee on the Status of Racial Minorities. (1983). ASHA position paper on social dialects. *Asha, 25,* 23–24.

Brice, A. E. (2002). *The Hispanic child: Speech, language, culture and education.* Boston: Allyn and Bacon.

Cole, L. (1993, September). Implications of the position on social dialects. *Asha, 25,* 25–27.

Coleman, T. J. (2000). *Clinical management of communication disorders in culturally diverse children.* Boston: Allyn and Bacon.

Craig, H. K., & Washington, J. A. (1995, January). African-American English and linguistic complexity in preschool discourse: A second look. *Language, Speech, and Hearing Services in the Schools, 26,* 87–93.

Craig, H. K., & Washington, J. A. (2002, February). Oral language expectations for African American preschoolers and kindergartners. *American Journal of Speech-Language Pathology, 11*(1), 59–70.

Langdon, H. W., & Cheng, L. L. (1992). *Hispanic children and adults with communication disorders: Assessment and intervention.* Gaithersburg, MD: Aspen Publishers.

Molrine, C. J., & Pierce, R. S. (2002, May). Black and white adults' expressive language performance on three tests of aphasia. *American Journal of Speech-Language Pathology, 11*(2), 139–150.

Rodriguez, B. L., & Olswang, L. B. (2003, November). Mexican-American and Anglo-American Mothers' beliefs and values about child-rearing, education, and language impairment. *American Journal of Speech-Language Pathology, 12*(4), 452–462.

Terrell, B. Y. (1993, November). Multicultural perspectives: Are the issues and questions different? *Asha, 35,* 51–52.

Thomas-Tate, S., Washington, J., & Edwards, J. (2004, May). Standardized assessment of phonological awareness skills in low-income African-American first graders. *American Journal of Speech-Language Pathology, 13*(2), 182–190.

van Keulen, J. E., Weddington, G. T., & DeBose, C. E. (1998). *Speech, language, learning, and the African-American child.* Boston: Allyn and Bacon.

Vaughn-Cooke, F. B. (1993, September). Improving language assessment in minority children. *Asha, 25,* 29–34.

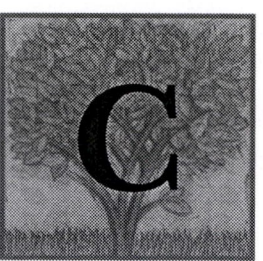

Suggested Reading List on Language Abnormalities in School-Age Children

American Speech-Language-Hearing Association, Committee on Augmentative Communication. (1991, March), Report: Augmentative and alternative communication. *Asha, 33*(Suppl. 5), 9–12.

Barkley, R. A. (2000). Taking charge of ADHD: The complete, authoritative guide for parents (rev. ed.). New York: The Guilford Press.

Bernard-Opitz, V. (1982, February). Pragmatic analysis of the communicative behavior of an autistic child. *Journal of Speech and Hearing Disorders, 47,* 99–110.

Blosser, J. L., & DePompei, R. (2003). Pediatric Traumatic Brain Injury: Proactive intervention (2nd ed.). Clifton Park, NY: Delmar.

Bopp, K. D., Brown, K. E., & Mirenda, P. (2004, February). Speech-language pathologists' roles in the delivery of positive behavior support for individuals with developmental disabilities. *American Journal of Speech-Language Pathology, 13*(1), 5–19.

Brinton, B., & Fujiki, M. (1993, October). Language, social skills, and socio-emotional behavior. *Language, Speech, and Hearing Services in the Schools, 24,* 194–198.

Condouris, K., Meyer, E., & Tager-Flusberg, H. (2003, August). The relationship between standardized measures of language and measures of spontaneous speech in children with autism. *American Journal of Speech-Language Pathology, 12*(3), 349–358.

Ebert, K. A., & Prelock, P. A. (1994, October). Teachers' perceptions of their students with communication disorders. *Language, Speech, and Hearing Services in the Schools, 25,* 211–214.

Ellis, L., Schlaudecker, C., & Regimbal, C., (1995, January). Effectiveness of a collaborative consultation approach to basic concept instruction with kindergarten children. *Language, Speech, and Hearing Services in the Schools, 26,* 69–74.

Fey, M. E., Long, S. H., & Finestack, L. H. (2003, February). Ten principles of grammar facilitation for children with specific language impairments. *American Journal of Speech-Language Pathology, 12*(1), 3–15.

Gallagher, T. (1993, October). Language skill and the development of social competence in school-age children. *Language, Speech, and Hearing Services in the Schools, 24,* 199–205.

Haynes, W. O., Moran, M. J., & Pindzola, R. H. (1999). *Communication disorders in the classroom: An introduction for professionals in school settings.* Dubuque, IA: Kendall/Hunt.

Hummel, L., & Prizant, B. (1993, October). A socioemotional perspective for understanding social difficulties of school-age children with language disorders. *Language, Speech, and Hearing Services in the School, 24,* 216–224.

Kamhi, A. G., & Catts, H. W. (1989). *Reading disabilities: A development language perspective.* Boston: College-Hill Press.

Kaufmann, S. S., Prelock, P. A., Weiler, E. M., Creaghead, N. A., & Donnelly, C. A. (1994, July). Metapragmatic awareness of explanation adequacy: Developing skills for academic success from a collaborative communication skills unit. *Language, Speech, and Hearing Services in the Schools, 25,* 174–180.

Koppenhaver, D. A., Coleman, P. P., Kalman, S. L., & Yoder, D. E. (1991, September). The implications of emergent literacy research for children with developmental disabilities. *American Journal of Speech-Language Pathology, 1,* 38–44.

Kuder, S. J. (2003). *Teaching students with language and communication disabilities* (2nd ed.). Boston: Allyn and Bacon.

Larson, V. L., & McKinley, N. (1995). *Language disorders in older students: Preadolescents and adolescents.* Eau Claire, WI: Thinking Publications.

McCauley, R. J. (2001). *Assessment of language disorders in children.* Mahwah, NJ: Lawrence Erlbaum Associates.

Merritt, D. D., & Culatta, B. (1998). *Language intervention in the classroom.* San Diego: Singular Publishing Group.

Nelson, N. W. (1994, September). Speech-language pathology: Moving toward the 21st century: Traumatic brain injury. *American Journal of Speech-Language Pathology, 3,* 39–41.

Nelson, N. W. (1994, September). School-aged language: Bumpy road or super-expressway to the next millennium? *American Journal of Speech-Language Pathology, 3,* 29–31.

Norris, J. A. (1992, September). Some questions and answers about whole language. *American Journal of Speech-Language Pathology, 1,* 11–14.

Paul, R. (2001). *Language disorders from infancy through adolescence* (2nd ed.). St. Louis, MO: Mosby.

Ratner, V., & Harris, L. (1994). *Understanding language disorders.* Eau Claire, WI: Thinking Publications.

Records, N. L., Tomblin, J. B., & Freese, P. P. (1992, January). The quality of life of young adults with histories of specific language impairment. *American Journal of Speech-Language Pathology, 1,* 44–53.

Reif, S. F. *How to reach and teach ADD/ADHD children.* Eau Claire, WI: Thinking Publications.

Russell, N. K. (1993, April). Educational considerations in traumatic brain injury: The role of the SLP. *Language, Speech, and Hearing Services in the Schools, 24,* 67–75.

Sanger, D. D., Hux, K., & Belau, D. (1997, February). Oral language skills of female juvenile delinquents. *American Journal of Speech-Language Pathology, 6,* 70–76.

Sanger, D., Hux, K., & Griess, K. (1995, January). Educators' opinions about speech-language pathology services in schools. *Language, Speech, and Hearing Services in the Schools, 26,* 75–86.

Semrud-Clikeman, M. (2001). *Traumatic brain injury in children and adolescents: Assessment and intervention.* New York: The Guilford Press.

Sicile-Kira, C. (2004). *Autism spectrum disorders: The complete guide to understanding autism, Asperger's syndrome, pervasive developmental disorder, and other ASDs.* New York: Perigree.

Simon, C. S. (1991). *Communication skills and classroom success.* Eau Claire, WI: Thinking Publications.

Stothard, S. E., Snowling, M. J., Bishop, D. V. M., Chipchase, B. B., & Kaplan, C. A. (1998, April). Language-impaired preschoolers: A follow-up into adolescence. *Journal of Speech, Language, and Hearing Research, 41,* 407–418.

Towne, R. L., & Entwisle, L. M. (1993, April). Metaphoric comprehension in adolescents with traumatic brain injury and in adolescents with language learning disability. *Language, Speech, and Hearing Services in the Schools, 24,* 100–107.

Wagovich, S. A., & Newhoff, M. (2004, November). The single exposure: Partial word knowledge growth through reading. *American Journal of Speech-Language Pathology, 13*(4), 316–328.

Wallach, G. P., & Butler, K. B. (1994). *Language learning disabilities in school-age children and adolescents.* New York: Merrill Publishers.

Wiig, E., & Wilson, C. C. (1994, October). Is a question a question? Passage understanding by preadolescents with learning disabilities. *Language, Speech, and Hearing Services in the Schools, 25,* 241–250.

Wilcox, M. J., Kouri, T. A., & Caswell, S. B. (1991, September). Early language intervention: A comparison of classroom and individual treatment. *American Journal of Speech-Language Pathology, 1,* 49–62.

Suggested Reading List on Language Abnormalities in Adults

Boyle, M. (2004, August). Semantic feature analysis treatment for anomia in two fluent aphasia syndromes. *American Journal of Speech-Language Pathology, 13*(3), 236–249.

Chapey, R. (Ed.). (2001). *Language intervention strategies in aphasia and related neurogenic communication disorders* (4th ed.). Philadelphia: Lippincott Williams & Wilkins.

Davis, G. A. (1993). *A survey of adult aphasia and related language disorders* (2nd ed.). Englewood Cliffs, NJ: Prentice Hall.

Drew, R. L., & Thompson, C. K. (1999, August). Model-based semantic treatment for naming deficits in aphasia. *Journal of Speech, Language, and Hearing Research, 42*(4), 972–989.

Harris, J. L. (1997, August). Reminiscence: A culturally and developmentally appropriate language intervention for older adults. *American Journal of Speech-Language Pathology,* 19–26.

LaPointe, L. L. (1997). *Aphasia and related neurogenic language disorders* (2nd ed.). New York: Thieme.

Marshall, R. C. (1997, February). Aphasia treatment in the early post onset period: Managing our resources effectively. *American Journal of Speech-Language Pathology, 6,* 5–11.

Marshall, R. C., Karow, C. M., Morelli, C. A., Iden, K. K., & Dixon, J. (2003, August). A clinical measure for the assessment of problem solving in brain-injured adults. *American Journal of Speech-Language Pathology, 12*(3), 333–348.

Murdoch, B. E., & Theodoros, D. G. (2001). *Traumatic brain injury: Associated speech, language, and swallowing disorders.* Clifton Park, NY: Delmar.

Parr, S., Byng, S., Gilpin, S., & Ireland, C. (1997). *Talking about aphasia.* Philadelphia: Open University Press.

Payne, J. C. (1997). *Adult neurogenic language disorders: Assessment and treatment.* San Diego: Singular Publishing Group.

Records, N. L., Tomblin, J. B., & Freese, P. R. (1992, January). The quality of life of young adults with histories of specific language impairment. *American Journal of Speech-Language Pathology, 1,* 44–50.

Sacks, O. (1985). *The man who mistook his wife for a hat.* New York: Touchstone.

Shadden, B. B., & Toner, M. A. (1997). *Aging and communication.* Austin, TX: Pro-Ed.

Simmons-Mackie, N. N., & Damico, J. S. (1996, February). The contribution of discourse markers to communicative competence in aphasia. *American Journal of Speech-Language Pathology, 5,* 37–43.

Simmons-Mackie, N., Kingston, D., & Schultz, M. (2004, May). Speaking for another: The management of participant frames in aphasia. *American Journal of Speech-Language Pathology, 13*(2), 114–127.

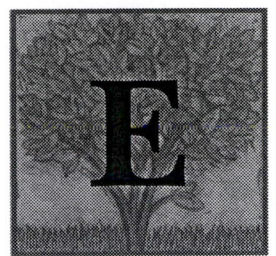

APPENDIX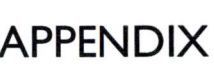

Answers to Review Questions

Chapter 1

1. a
2. d
3. c
4. a
5. b
6. a
7. b
8. b
9. b
10. a

Chapter 2

1. e
2. b
3. d
4. b
5. a
6. b
7. a
8. b
9. b
10. b

Chapter 3

1. b
2. a
3. d
4. d
5. a
6. b
7. b
8. a
9. b
10. b

Chapter 4

1. c
2. b
3. d
4. b
5. a
6. b
7. b
8. a
9. a
10. b

Chapter 5

1. a
2. a
3. b
4. c
5. e
6. a
7. a
8. b
9. b
10. b

Chapter 6

1. b
2. a
3. e
4. d
5. d
6. b
7. a
8. b
9. a
10. a

Chapter 7

1. b
2. c
3. a
4. d
5. b
6. a
7. b
8. a
9. b
10. a

Chapter 8

1. d
2. b
3. b
4. b
5. b
6. d
7. a
8. c
9. b
10. a

Chapter 9

1. b
2. b

3. a
4. b
5. b
6. c
7. b
8. a
9. e
10. a

Chapter 10

1. b
2. b
3. a
4. c
5. b
6. d
7. e
8. h
9. a
10. b

Chapter 11

1. e
2. a
3. e
4. b
5. b
6. a

7. b
8. b
9. b
10. c

Chapter 12

1. d
2. d
3. a
4. a
5. b
6. a
7. c
8. b
9. a
10. a

Chapter 13

1. a
2. b
3. e
4. c
5. d
6. d
7. b
8. d
9. a
10. a

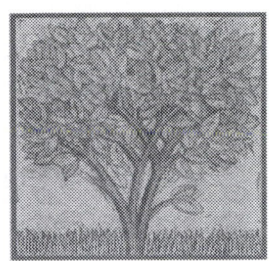

Glossary

Abstract thought processes: Thinking beyond the limits of a fact and developing opinions and expansion on a given piece of information.

Adaptability: The ability to adjust to new or changing circumstances.

Affective control: Inappropriate affect and expression of emotions.

Afferent fibers: Sensory nerve fibers that carry the nerve impulses that arise from sensory stimulation of the sensory end organs to the central nervous system.

Agnosia: The inability to perceive, integrate, and attach meaning to incoming sensory stimuli.

Agrammatism: A symptom frequently associated with Broca's aphasia; the patient is unable to create sentences due to syntactic, morphological, and semantic deficits.

Agraphia: Inability to write.

Acting-out tasks: Tasks in which the clinician offers a set of instructions on what the child must complete; the clinician needs to ascertain that the child is truly responding to the examiner's questions and not performing tasks that he or she knows due to real-world familiarity with the item.

Akinesia: Absence of motor movement.

Alexia: Inability to read, possibly due to neurological impairment.

Alphabetic principle: The dictum governing how specific sounds in a language are represented by specific spelling patterns.

Alternate form reliability: Evaluating the reliability of a test by having the child take two different forms of the same test, then comparing the performance on each form.

Alternating attention: Ability to shift attention between tasks that have different cognitive demands.

Angiography: An x-ray study to study the flow of blood, such as in the arteries.

Anomia: Lack of the ability to recall names of people, common objects, and places.

Aphasia: Impairment of the abilities to comprehend and express language resulting from acquired neurological damage.

Appetite control: The ability to delay gratification, which is typically problematic for children with ADHD.

Apraxia: Inability to coordinate the limb or oral musculature to perform voluntary movements.

Arteriosclerosis: Hardening of the arteries.

Assessment process: The process of interviewing, observing, and testing an individual to determine the nature, extent, and severity of his or her language disorder, delay, or difference.

Associative control: Control that enables a person to maintain a conversation by stating issues that are relevant to the conversation.

Attention deficit disorder: The presence of behavior that typically includes inattention, hyperactivity, and impulsivity that exceeds that expected by children at a given age.

Auditory acuity: The sharpness and clarity with which sound is perceived by the ear.

Auditory agnosia: Inability to make sense of incoming auditory stimuli.

Auditory discrimination: Ability to identify specific sounds by their source or acoustical properties.

Auditory learner: A person who learns primarily by listening.

Auditory memory: Ability to remember sounds, frequently in a specified sequence.

Auditory perception: The identification, interpretation, or organization of sensory data received through the ear.

Auditory processing: A set of skills, including auditory discrimination, auditory analysis, auditory attention, and auditory memory, that integrate what is heard with language.

Auditory processing disorder: Difficulties with functions of language based on input to and feedback from the auditory system, including problems with auditory discrimination, lateralization, recognizing auditory patterns, and localizing sound.

Auditory sequential memory: Ability to remember sounds, words, phrases, and sentences in a specified sequence.

Backward chaining: A series of sequenced behaviors, in which the last steps of the sequence are taught first, working backward to the beginning of the chain; frequently used to teach self-help skills.

Baseline: Preintervention measurement of a patient's skills.

Behavior control: Impulsive behavior due to a poorly organized central nervous system.

Behaviorism: Like empiricism, the belief that a child's language is not innate but develops when verbalisms are positively enforced.

Behavior modification: The implementation of an intervention plan to change, modify, or correct an individual's behavior.

Bradykinesia: Slow motor movements.

Causality: The reactivation of a spectacle or event by bodily movement (e.g., turing the key to have a toy car reactivate).

Central hearing loss: Damage to the eighth nerve in the brain stem or in the cortex.

Cerebral cortex: The outer layer of the brain; the convoluted layer of gray matter that covers each hemisphere of the brain.

Chromosomal disorder: A disorder in the structure and number of chromosomes.

Circumlocution: The use of an indirect manner of expression to describe an object or event when the name cannot be recalled; e.g., saying "That thing you use to unlock the door" instead of "key."

Clinical assumptions: What clinicians judge to be true, although they may not observe or measure attributes related to these events directly.

Clinical facts: Statements made about events that actually took place and were directly observed or measured by the clinician.

Closed-head injury (CHI): A nonpenetrating brain injury in which the skull may be intact or fractured, but the meninges are intact.

Code-switching: The ability of an individual to switch dialects or languages depending on the communicative situation.

Cognition: The process of thinking, using information gained through perception, memory, discrimination, judgment, and other thought processes.

Cognitive determinism: The belief that cognition relies on language for a child to understand his experiences; the child's knowledge of the world is expressed through his language, with meaning preceding form.

Collaboration: Classroom-based or curriculum-based intervention that focuses on learning strategies and using them in materials related to the curriculum.

Collaborative activities: Those activities that involve the joint participation and cooperation of the members of a group.

Collaborative model: Classroom-based or curriculum-based intervention that focuses on learning strategies and using them in materials related to the curriculum.

Conductive hearing loss: A breakdown in the ability of the middle ear to receive the acoustic signals from the environment and then to transmit the acoustical information to the inner ear.

Confrontational naming: The naming of items as the child is confronted with the item by the clinician.

Construct validity: The degree to which a test measures a theoretical construct or trait.

Consultation: A service delivery model in which the speech-language pathologist provides indirect therapy through inservice and input to classroom teachers on appropriate methods for encouraging effective speech and language skills.

Consultative model: A service delivery model in which the speech-language pathologist provides indirect therapy through inservice and input to classroom teachers on appropriate methods for encouraging effective speech and language skills.

Content bias: The effect of a dialectal or cultural difference on the responses of an individual to a test item.

Content validity: A systematic examination of the relevance of the responses given to the test items in order to ascertain how well the test covers a representative sample of the skills to be assessed.

Contrecoup injury: A brain injury occurring opposite from the impact as the brain bounces from the point of impact to the opposite side of the skull.

Correlation coefficient: A number that represents the degree of the relationship between two sets of scores.

Coup injury: Injury at the point of impact, occurring when a blow to the head results in the brain's moving and slamming against the point of impact.

Craniosynostosis: Premature fusion of the bones of the cranium.

Criterion-referenced test: A nonstandardized probe used to study a language construct in more depth than is normally associated with standardized tests.

Criterion-related validity: How effectively a test predicts an individual's behavior or abilities, or both, in specific situations.

CT scans: A computerized reconstruction of the anatomic structures created when narrow x-ray beams focus on a single plane as the scanner rotates around a structure, such as the patient's head.

Culture: The philosophies, ideas, arts, and customs of a group of people that are passed from one generation to the next.

Delayed gratification: The ability to continue providing the correct and expected behaviors even when a delay exists between the response and the provision of reinforcement.

Dementia: A conglomeration of signs and symptoms of central nervous system degeneration that result in progressive and persistent deterioration of intellectual functioning.

Diadochokinetic tasks: Tasks requiring rapid repetitive movements of the articulators; frequently elicited by having the child repeat p^t^k^ as quickly as possible.

Dialect: Systematic, patterned, rule-governed variations in a language.

Diffuse lesion: A lesion in which the damage is spread throughout a large area of the brain or several small areas, resulting in comprehensive deficits.

Discrepancy criterion: The measurable difference between a child's achievement and his expected achievement based on IQ.

Divided attention: Determing how much attention to give to each activity.

Dysarthria: Speech disorder resulting from generalized weakness of the oral musculature.

Dysgraphia: Impaired ability to write, usually due to brain damage.

Dyslexia: Difficulty learning to read, often due to neurological deficit.

Dysnomia: Loss of ability to name people, places, or things; may also be referred to as anomia.

Dysplasia: Abnormal tissue development.

Echolalia: The unmodified involuntary or voluntary repetition of what is said to the child.

EEG: The measurement of electrical activity of the brain taken from electrodes placed on the scalp to detect abnormal neurological signs.

Efferent fibers: Motor nerve fibers that carry impulses from the central nervous system to the muscles and other organs.

Embedded sentences: Compound sentences in which a minimum of two independent clauses are combined to form one sentence.

Embolic stroke: Stroke that results from the traveling of a clot from the location at which it forms.

Emotional regulation: The ability to control one's emotions and express them appropriately based on the myriad components of a setting.

Empiricism: The belief that a child's language is not innate but develops as a result of experiences.

Ethnography: The study of language use for communicative purposes, considering social and cultural factors.

Etiology: Causative factors that lead to any condition, such as a speech or language deficit.

Executive tasks: Activities such as setting goals, initiating tasks, self-monitoring, self-evaluating, keeping schedules, and managing time well.

Exorbitism: Bulging of the eyes beyond the socket of the orbit.

Expressive language: The ability to convey a message through conventional means using words and symbols; the content of what is expressed.

Extrinsic causes: Factors in the environment of the child that interfere with development.

Face validity: How well test items represent what they claim to test.

Fading: The gradual withdrawal of prompts used to facilitate a response.

Fissure: A deep furrow in the brain; also known as a sulcus.

Fluent aphasia: Aphasia in which the initiation and production of speech are intact, but deficits occur in semantics and comprehension.

Focal control: The ability to select what is important and attend to that over all other distractions and information.

Focal lesion: A lesion in which the impact is concentrated in one small area, as of the brain.

Focused attention: The requirement that a child complete an activity, usually under a time constraint.

Forward chaining: A series of sequenced behaviors in which the first steps of the sequence are taught first; the typical chaining approach to teach academic skills.

Functional magnetic resonance imaging (fMRI): An MRI of the brain done while the patient performs specific tasks so the radiologist can visualize mechanisms of the brain activated with specific tasks.

Functional outcome: Terminology coined to define environmentally based results of therapy that can be generalized to the patient's natural settings; expected results of therapy that can readily be integrated into the patient's natural environment.

Generalization: The addition of new stimuli or environmental factors to elicit the same response obtained in a controlled setting.

Genetic: Specific characteristics or traits passed from one generation to the next in the genes.

Glossoptosis: Displacement of the tongue into a downward position.

Graduated prompting: In diagnostic therapy, the co-occurrence of assessment and treatment, with the child being tested for stimulability on a language construct.

Grammatic closure: The ability to determine the missing elements in a sentence.

Gyrus: A rounded elevation in the cerebral hemispheres.

Hematoma: The accumulation of blood below the skin or within the brain.

Hemianesthesia: Lack of sensation on either the right or the left side of the body.

Hemianopsia: Loss of vision in one half of the visual field.

Hemiparesis: Weakness or incomplete paralysis of either the right or the left side of the body.

Hemiplegia: Paralysis of either the right or the left side of the body.

Hemorrhagic stroke: The bursting of the arterial walls in the brain due to aging (loss of elasticity) or high blood pressure; results in intense inflammation and swelling of the surrounding brain tissue.

Homonymous hemianopsia: Loss of the same visual half field (right or left) in both eyes; typically results from a single lesion.

Hydrocephalus: Abnormal accumulation of fluid within the cranium, placing undue pressure on the brain tissues.

Hyperkinetic: Persistent and exaggerated motor movements.

Hyperkinetic dysarthria: A type of dysarthria characterized by involuntary movements, abnormal muscle tone, inappropriate disruption of phonation, and disorders of rate and loudness.

Hyperlexia: Recognizing and reading words exceeding one's cognitive and language levels, yet having no comprehension of what is said or read.

Hypertelorism: Wide placement of the entire bony orbit surrounding the eye.

Hypertension: High blood pressure.

Hyporeflexia: Abnormally low responses when the reflexes are stimulated.

Hypotonia: Abnormally low muscle tone; sometimes referred to as athetosis.

Hypoxia: A decrease in the amount of oxygen delivered to or utilized by a body organ, or both.

Identification tasks: Tasks in which the child is asked to identify a picture or object that is named by the clinician.

Illocutionary force: The intention of a speech act.

Illocutionary stage of development: The social stage of communication development in which the child is interactive and communication efforts are intentional although some of the communication may still be nonverbal.

Impulsitivity: Acting without premeditation, thought, or concern about consequences.

Incidental learning: Learning that results from normal, routine interactions with the environment.

Individualized education plan: Required by IDEA, the academic plan required for all students who are in special education or related services in public schools.

Infarct: Necrotic, or dead, tissue that occurs as a sequela to an ischemic attack.

Intrinsic causes: Factors within the child such as neurological damage.

Ischemic: A deficiency of blood caused by blockage or constriction, and usually from within an artery.

Jargon: Utterances that are fluent and correctly articulated, but make little or no sense to the listener.

Joint attention: The sharing of visual and auditory attention to the same stimulus.

Judgment tasks: Tasks that require the child to make a determination of the accuracy or reasonableness of a statement made by the clinician.

Language acquisition device (LAD): The LAD is not a specific structure, but rather a conglomeration of innate capacity of language that governs the input and output of language form.

Language-based learning disability: A single disorder that manifests itself in different ways at various points in development as communicative contexts and learning tasks change.

Language delay: Acquisition of normal language competencies at a slower rate than would be expected given a child's chronological age and level of functioning.

Language difference: Language behaviors and skills that are not in concert with those of the person's primary speech community or native language.

Language disorder: Any disruption in the learning of language in the absence of primary intellectual, sensory, or emotional deficits.

Language parameters: Aspects of language that form the basis of linguistic functioning.

Learned helplessness: A state of nonaction that a child learns because his or her needs are constantly anticipated by his or her caregivers so that there is little or no need for the child to communicate or initiate communication.

Learning disability: Any one of a heterogeneous set of learning problems that affect the acquisition and use of listening, speaking, writing, reading, mathematical, and reasoning skills.

Lexicon: A composite list of the words and signs that comprise an individual's vocabulary.

Linguistic competence: The language user's underlying knowledge about the system of rules of the language he or she is using.

Linguistic performance: The utilization of the person's linguistic knowledge in daily communication.

Linguistic universals: The shared principles that underlie the variety of languages and form the foundation for a relatively universal structure of language.

Locutionary stage of development: The social stage of communication development during which the child develops intentional, linguistic communication; speech consists primarily of nouns and labels.

Magnetic resonance imaging (MRI): Use of large electromagnets that manipulate the spin of hydrogen molecules to differentiate between different tissues, such as white matter and gray matter.

Maintenance: The independent use of therapy skills in a person's natural settings.

Mean length of utterance (MLU): Average length of a sample of utterances spoken by an individual.

Means-end: A language parameter in which the child has the ability to use foresight in simple problem-solving.

Meningitis: An inflammation of the meninges lining the brain, spinal column, or both.

Mental effort control: Work at concentrating, resulting in mental fatigue when energy is expended on focal control.

Mentalism: Often associated with nativism, the mentalism philosophy posits that one's knowledge is derived from innate mental processes.

Metacognition: The ability to develop alternative ways to solve a problem or resolve a situation, the ability to form hypotheses and task analyze them in a constructive manner, and the capacity to make personal decisions.

Metacognitive skills: Those skills that enable a child to solve problems, form hypotheses, analyze his or her thoughts, and make a decision.

Metalinguistic devices: The ability to think about and analyze language, including the ability to understand humor, multiple meanings, inferences, and figurative language.

Metalinguistics: Skills that allow an individual to think about language in a critical manner and to make judgments with regard to the accuracy and appropriate use of language skills and functions.

Metalinguistic skills: Skills that allow an individual to think about language in a critical manner and to make judgments with regard to the accuracy and appropriate use of language skills and functions.

Metanarrative skills: Ability to analyze stories, extract appropriate details from a story, and comprehend a story.

Metaphor: A figure of speech containing an implied comparison between two things by applying the word or phrase commonly associated with one of the things to another.

Metapragmatics: Conscious and intentional awareness of ways in which to use language effectively in different contexts.

Metapragmatic skills: Conscious and intentional awareness of ways in which to use language effectively in different contexts.

Metathesis: The reversal of the position of two sounds in a word.

Micrognathia: A very small lower jaw that is frequently paired with a recessed chin.

Modality: According to Fillmore, one of two components of sentences that looks at the influence of semantics on grammar, particularly as applied to verb tense, the question form, and negation.

Modeling: The demonstration of a desired behavior to prompt an imitative response.

Morphology: Units of meaning that make up the grammar of language; rules that modify meaning at the word level.

Multi-infarction diseases: Diseases that result in many focal necrotic lesions, causing widespread damage in cortical functioning.

Multimodality approach: An approach to therapy that incorporates information from all sensory systems to teach a conceptual element.

Mutism: Not speaking; may be selective, meaning a child does not talk in certain settings, or elective, meaning there is no organic or physical disability that prevents the child from talking.

Nativism: The capacity to develop language is innate, with language knowledge coming to fruition as the child matures biologically.

Neologism: Unintended substitution of an invented or nonsense word that contains no similarities to the target (intended) word.

Neuritic plaques: Minute areas of degeneration of cortical and subcortical tissues in the brain, also known as senile plaques.

Neurofibrillary tangles: The twisted and tangled neurofibrils in the body of the nerve cells.

Nonfluent aphasia: Slow labored speech, word retrieval deficits, and motor planning deficits due to a lesion or lesions in the anterior language area and left premotor cortex (Broca's area); includes Broca aphasia, transcortical motor aphasia, and global aphasia.

Nonliteral language: Language that is abstract and symbolic.

Orthography: Rule-based spelling.

Otitis media: Inflammation of the middle ear.

Otitis media with effusion: Inflammation of the middle ear accompanied by the accumulation of infected fluid.

Paragrammatism: Use of semantically and morphologically intact sentences which, however, are semantically empty; use of inappropriate words and inflections; associated with fluent aphasias.

Paraphasia: The unintentional substitution of an incorrect word for an intended word.

Parenchymal lesions: Those which extend to matter within the brain tissue such as those that occur as a result of a hemorrhagic stroke.

Penetrating head injury: An open head injury resulting in a fracturing or perforation of the skull with the meninges becoming torn or lacerated.

Percentile score: Percentage of individuals in the standardization sample for an age level who scored below a predetermined raw score.

Perceptual-cognitive skills: The integration of thinking and organizing sensory input.

Peripheral hearing loss: Conductive hearing losses and losses related to malfunction of the inner ear.

Perlocutionary stage of development: The social stage of communication development, during which the child is interactive but uses nonverbal and unintentional communication.

Perpetuating factors: Factors that result in the persistence of a language or communication deficit.

Perseveration: "Getting stuck," usually involuntarily, on a motor, verbal, or nonverbal activity.

PET scan: The observation of patterns of radioactivity in the brain through positive emission tomography.

Phoneme-grapheme correspondence: The association of a printed letter with the sound it masks.

Phoneme synthesis: The act of combining sounds presented in isolation into a single word.

Phonemic awareness: Recognition of the fact that words are made up of sounds and understanding the differences between phonemes.

Phonemic paraphasia: Unintended substitution of a phonemically similar word for the intended word.

Phonemic segmentation: The act of breaking down a word into sounds.

Phonological awareness: An understanding of the distribution and sequencing of phonemes and their relationship to the printed letters.

Phonological processing: Understanding of the sound system of a language.

Phonology: Distribution and sequencing or organization of phonemes within a language.

Physiatrist: A physician who specializes in rehabilitation medicine.

Placebo effect: An inactive treatment that has a suggestive effect on the individual's symptomology.

Polydrug exposed: The use of multiple drugs, including alcohol, by a pregnant mother.

Pragmatics: The social use and functions of language for communication.

Precipitating factors: Factors that result in the onset of the language or communication problem.

Predisposing factors: Factors that dispose or incline an individual toward an impairment related to language and communication skills.

Prelingual hearing loss: A hearing loss acquired prior to the development of speech and language.

Preoperational skills: Skills needed to emerge into conceptual thinking leading to prelogical thought.

Postlingual hearing loss: A hearing loss after the development of speech and language.

Press of speech: Use of excessive content of speech, as if the speaker has to press on.

Presymbolic language: The stage of communication that precedes the use of gestures, words, and actions to denote specific language concepts or words.

Principles: Summary statements of experimental evidence that provide the rules from which treatment procedures are developed.

Procedures: Concrete, measurable, and objective clinical activities based on the experimental evidence, which form the foundation for therapy outlined in principles.

Processing: How the child handles information that is presented to him visually and/or aurally.

Prognathism: Abnormal facial construction in which the upper and/or lower jaws project forward.

Prompt: A supplementary antecedent that is added to the original stimulus to increase the probability of a correct response.

Proposition: According to Fillmore, the second component of a sentence that regulates the relationship between nouns and verbs.

Propositional force: The literal meaning of a sentence.

Prosody: The use of tone and accent to embellish spoken language.

Psycholinguistics: The study of language structures and processes that undergird the ability to speak and understand language.

Psychostimulants: Medications that have antidepressant effects and stimulate the production of dopamine that acts on the frontal lobe to improve executive functions.

Quality control: A person's ability to provide an explanation for his or her own actions.

Rapport: A harmonious connection between two individuals based on mutual respect and a level of trust.

Reliability: The consistency of a test in measuring what it claims to measure in the same individual on reexamination.

Retrograde amnesia: A common sequela of traumatic brain injury that creates difficulty in remembering the events that led up to the accident.

Scaffolding system: A "stair-step" approach to problem solving in a group consisting of students at varying levels of ability in which a high-functioning child provides a model for a lower functioning child.

Screening: The administration of short tests to determine if a child's language is within normal limits or if he or she needs to be referred for a complete diagnostic procedure.

Scripts: Scenarios designed to facilitate language development and the application of language skills to reading.

Segmentation: The breaking down of sentences into words, words into syllables, and syllables into phonemes.

Selective attention: The attention needed to focus on what is important in myriad stimuli.

Semantic paraphasia: Unintended substitution of a semantically similar word for the intended word.

Semantics: The knowledge and ideas a person has about the objects and events in his or her world; the content of language.

Sensorimotor: Skills involving the integration of sensory feedback and motor behaviors.

Sensorimotor stages: Stages of development that precede early symbolic communication, characterized by the development and integration of the sensory and motor systems of the child.

Sensorineural hearing loss: Hearing loss due to malfunctioning of the inner ear or damage to the acoustic nerve.

Sensory integration: The organization and interpretation of input from various sensory systems of the body.

Shaping: The differential reinforcement of successive approximations to a specified target to create a new behavior.

Skill: A sequence of responses that are learned through the coordination of various motor and sensory systems and are eventually organized into complex chains.

Sociolinguistics: The study of social and cultural influences on language structures.

Soft signs: Possible early indicators that, taken as a group, could be warning signs for a possible language-based learning disability.

Speech acts: In a communicative exchange, expressions verbalized by the speaker such as receiving information, giving information, acknowledging an individual (greeting and departing words).

Speech community: A group of people who routinely and frequently use a shared language to interact with each other.

Spontaneous recovery: The unassisted resolution of deficits created by a disease or injury such as a stroke.

Standard deviation: A statistical measurement used to document the disparity between an individual's test score and the mean.

Standardized test: A test that has been evaluated using a sample of individuals that represents a broad cross section of cultural groups. Standardized tests offer norms that allow a comparison of a child's performance on a test with those in the standardization sample.

Standard score: A score obtained by converting the raw score to a weighted raw score which takes into account the average score and the variability of scores of children of that age.

Stereotypes: The unintentional use (can be appropriately or inappropriately) of real or invented or nonsense words or phrases that have little meaning; used frequently by global aphasics.

Stereotypical phrases: Fixed, nonvarying utterances that are often heard produced by others and used in excess by children with social interaction deficits.

Stimulability: The degree to which a child can imitate a language construct presented by the clinician; the less intervention is needed, the more the child is stimulable.

Stroke: A condition caused by blockage or bursting of an artery leading to disruption of blood flow to the brain and resulting in neurologic damage to the area of the brain that is supplied by that artery.

Subcortical pathways: Interconnections in the brain that lie below the cerebral cortex.

Survival language: Knowing the "lingo" associated with peer language, and knowing how to be part of a peer group through appropriate actions and communication styles.

Sustained attention: The ability to remain on task, but without the time constraints of focused attention

Symbolic communication: Communication in which the individual understands the relationships between words and objects and events (i.e., that the words represent the objects and events).

Syndrome: A cluster of characteristics that occur concurrently and form a specific pattern of signs and symptoms.

Syntax: Appropriate rule-based ordering of words in connected discourse.

Tactile defensiveness: A pronounced dislike of being touched, usually accompanied by a negative emotional reaction.

Task analysis: The breaking down of a task into small steps that must be accomplished individually before the whole task can be completed.

Test-retest reliability: Evaluating the reliability of a test by having the child take two different forms of the same test, then comparing the child's performance on each form.

Therapy: The process of establishing and habituating new skills, then generalizing the skills to the client's natural environment.

Thromboembolic stroke: General term for stroke in which the clinician cannot differentiate between a thrombotic or embolic stroke.

Thrombotic stroke: A stroke occurring after the build-up of plaque on the inner walls of a vessel, which blocks the flow of blood; a thrombosis is a clot.

Topic-associated narrative: A series of narratives linked to a topic, with no particular theme or point to the narrative.

Topic-centered narrative: A tightly structured discourse on a single topic or a series of closely related topics and events.

Total-task presentation: A series of sequenced behaviors, all of which must be done completely and in sequence in order to master the skills and be reinforced.

Transformational generative grammar (TGG): A grammar system in which there is a deep structure and a surface structure and a set of rules that govern the combining of words.

Treatment efficacy: The determination of the most efficient and effective means by which the clinician provides therapeutic intervention.

Unilateral neglect: A problem frequently associated with right hemisphere damage that results in difficulty or inability to attend to stimuli received on the side of the body opposite the brain damage.

Validity: The degree to which a test measures what it is designed to measure, and how well it does so.

Vigilance: The attention skills needed to develop and use a memory bank.

Visual learner: A person who learns primarily and most effectively through the visual modality.

Wada Test: The administration of automatic speech tasks following the injection of sodium amytal into the left or right carotid artery to temporarily paralyze one hemisphere.

Whole language: A discovery-based, informal method of integrating cognitive skills, language skills, and curricular goals.

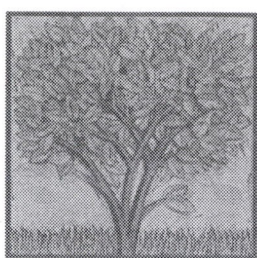

Index

Impulsivity (*continued*)
  definition of, 199, 525
  triggers for, 56–57
Incidental learning, 214, 525
Incidental teaching, 399
Individualized education plans (IEPs), 396–397, 525
Individuals with Disabilities Education Act (IDEA), 143, 220
  assessment mandate of, 380
  focus on transition from school to work, 360, 396–397
  traumatic brain injury definition, 326
Inductive teaching, 400
Infants
  assessment form, sample, 113–118
  assessment of language deficits in, 77–139, 363
  Early Communication Checklist, 96, 133–135
  "failure to thrive" babies, 51–52
  language and communication development in, 6–7
  language disorder causes in, 30–76
  language sampling in, 363
  premature/high-risk, 51–52
  prenatal exposure to alcohol and drugs, 52–57, 167–168, 188–189
  swaddling of, 167
  TBI causes in, 325
Infarcts
  definition of, 452, 525
  due to strokes, 452
  multi-focal, in Alzheimer's disease, 433
  multi-infarction diseases, 422, 435, 528
Intelligence Quotient (IQ), 93
  cognitive impairment classification by, 62
  diadochokinetic tasks and, 177–178
  discrepancy criteria based on, 258, 367–368
  in language-based learning disabilities, 223
  performance, 177, 223
  in preschoolers with cognitive disabilities, 191
  verbal, 177, 223
Intensity of reaction, 156, 157
Interactionism, 7–8
Interactionistic theory of language development, 402
Interaction of language components, 19–21
Interactive environmental frameworks, 147–148
Intervention, models of, 393–396. *See also* Therapy; Treatment
Interviews. *See also* Checklists; Tests
  preassessment, for aphasia/neurological deficits, 454–455

questions for assessment/diagnosis, 83–84, 85
  student, 361–362
Intrinsic causes, 254–255, 525
IQ. *See* Intelligence Quotient
Ischemic, definition of, 452, 525
Ischemic lesions, 452

J

Jargon, 18, 473, 525
Johnson, Lyndon Baines, 161
Joint action routines, 399–400
Joint attention, 145, 525
Judgment tasks, 90, 525

L

Labeling, 31–32
LAD. *See* Language acquisition device
Landau-Kleffner syndrome, 330
Language
  and cognition, relationship of, 32, 331
  curricular demands based on, 214–215
  education, 404–405
  teaching methods, 399–400
  testing, in adults, 460–470
  testing, in school-age children, 357–388
Language acquisition device (LAD), 526
Language age (LA), 212
Language-based learning disabilities, 211–244
  "almost but not quite" children, 213, 215
  assessment and diagnosis of, 258–262
  at risk children, identification of, 215–220
  auditory processing evaluation and, 368
  case study, 236–240
  categories of, 213
  clinical findings, 222–227
  comorbidity with ADD/ADHD, 294
  definition of, 213, 526
  identification of, 213–214
  phonological deficits in, 222–223
  risk factors/red flags for, 213
  semantic deficits in, 224–226
  soft signs of, 217–219
  speech-language pathologist and, 212–213, 217
  stories, in therapy for, 272
  survival language and, 227
  syntactic deficits in, 226
  writing skills in, 223–224
  written language problems, therapy for, 401